THE APPLICANT'S MANUAL OF PHYSICIAN ASSISTANT PROGRAMS 2020

MARK VOLPE, PA-C

BRITTANY HOGAN, PA-C

The Applicant's Manual of Physician Assistant Programs

5th Edition

ISBN-13: 978-1697868661

ISBN-10: 1697868665

Published by Createspace in Charleston, SC

Notice: Physician Assistant program admissions is an ever-changing process. Every effort has been made to ensure that the information in this book is up to date and accurate. However, given the possibility of human error and ongoing changes in admissions processes, neither the authors nor the publisher nor any other party who has been involved in the preparation or publication of this work warrants that the information contained herein is in every respect accurate or complete. They disclaim all responsibility for any errors or omissions or for the results obtained from use of the information contained in this work. Readers are encouraged to confirm the information contained herein with other sources.

About the Authors:

Mark Volpe, MPH, MMSc, PA-C is a Physician Assistant practicing in outpatient internal medicine and urgent care in Connecticut. He graduated from the Yale University PA Program in 2015, where he played a role in several aspects of the admissions process throughout three admissions cycles. He completed his MPH from Southern Connecticut State University and his BS from the University of Connecticut. He has a particular interest in PA program admissions, education, and physician assistant research. During and after Yale, Mark has been published in several peer reviewed journals, served as a special advisor to the BHSc program at Southern Connecticut State University, served on the admissions committee of the University of Saint Joseph PA Program in West Hartford, CT, and is a guest lecturer in their public health and clinical medicine courses. Additionally, Mark precepts students from the Yale University PA Program and the University of Saint Joseph.

Brittany Hogan, MMSc, PA-C is a Physician Assistant practicing in plastic surgery and cosmetic medicine in Massachusetts as well as neurosurgery in Rhode Island. She graduated from the Yale University PA Program in 2016. Brittany earned her BS from Fordham University in 2010, where she played for the division 1 women's soccer team. She worked in New York City as an EEG technician and then in Boston as a health and wellness coach prior to attending PA school. Brittany has numerous publications and has won awards for her scholarly achievements. She has a passion for teaching and mentoring, and precepts students from Johnson & Wales and Bryant University PA programs.

Preface:

We are very excited to bring you the 5th edition of The Applicant's Manual of Physician Assistant Programs. The 2020 edition has been designed not only to include all relevant information regarding each PA program, new and old, in the United States, but also to incorporate feedback from our valued customers to make this book as helpful as possible for future PA applicants. We hope that you enjoy the updates to the current edition of the book, which include:

- The addition of many new PA programs that have established themselves within the past year

- Updated information on the over 240 programs included in the 4th edition

- Inclusion of CASPer and PA-CAT testing requirements for programs that now require these exams

- Insights from interviews with PA Program Directors

- Reformatting for enhanced readability

We wish you the best of luck in your journey towards becoming a Physician Assistant, and hope that this book serves as a useful tool in your search for your perfect PA program.

Best Wishes,

Mark Volpe, MPH, MMSc, PA-C

Brittany Hogan, MMSc, PA-C

Foreword:

How much time do you think you'll spend trying to figure out which PA programs to apply to? As you are probably aware, applying to physician assistant school is a daunting task. By the time CASPA opens you want to be ready to submit your transcripts, letters of recommendations, personal statement, etc. so that your application is one of the first for review by the admissions committee. The more time you spend scouring the internet for those programs that might be the "perfect" fit, the further your application will be delayed.

I can still remember how stressed I was when I was going through the application process; I swear I visited every PA program's web page at least a dozen times a week to figure out which programs I met the minimum requirements for, which ones had mission statements that matched my values and future goals, and so on. Now, there are over 250 established and developing programs! At this point it seems nearly impossible to efficiently research every program in order to determine which school is the best fit for you.

As the founder of myPAresource and mentor to many future PAs in need of shadowing hours, I repeatedly get asked about the application process and how to decide which schools to apply to. Generally my response includes the following mantra: apply early and apply abundantly. I HIGHLY recommend that you NOT limit yourself to a single school, as that can be a terrible mistake. Limiting your options is the reason it takes some applicants 2, 3, or even 4 years to get accepted into PA school. Many programs receive over 1,000 applications for an average of 40 seats. Those are pretty intimidating odds! By applying to a variety of programs, you INSTANTLY increase the likelihood of an interview, which as you know is the first step on the path towards PA school acceptance.

Since graduating from PA school myself and in the time spent mentoring prospective PA students, I have seen how complicated, involved and expensive CASPA has become over the years. With all of the new programs popping up, it can be difficult to narrow down which schools to devote your application budget to. I HIGHLY recommend finding an efficient way to research the programs you're interested in applying to before making haphazard or blind choices within the CASPA system. When I was in your shoes, I sent my application to roughly 13 programs, about half of which I felt qualified for. For 3 of the programs, I didn't even meet the minimum requirements, and for 3 others, I didn't fill out the required supplemental applications. I essentially wasted hundreds of dollars and many hours of my life (neither of which I'll ever get back) because at the time, there wasn't a comprehensive resource to assist in streamlining this expensive and time-consuming process. Now there is.

Because they are so involved in the pre-PA community, Mark and Brittany recognize how much time future PA students spend during the application process simply on research. After all, it's one of the most important parts of the process. PA programs are looking for hard-working students with meticulous attention to detail! As former PA applicants themselves, Mark and Brittany are intimately familiar with how laborious and overwhelming the process can be. As such, they spend many months each year researching every PA program in the country and detailing the requirements and intricacies of each school, which saves you copious amounts of time early on. Chances are you will save money too because you'll know which programs not to apply to based on your applicant statistics and you'll know which programs require supplemental applications. Trust me, I know how hard it is to apply to PA school with all of those fees on a minimum wage salary. The small cost of this resource is well worth the return on investment.

Mark and Brittany have worked hard for five years now with the goal of preventing you from wasting time and energy in search of all of the answers. The Applicant's Manual of Physician Assistant Programs truly is an efficient tool for every future PA student to use during the application process. I urge you to utilize this book to its full potential and let it guide you to those programs that are a good fit for you. Wishing you all the best of luck in the process!

Best,

Brian Palm, PA-C

Emergency Medicine

Founder of myPAresource

Atlanta, GA

TABLE OF CONTENTS

INTRODUCTION

Purpose

Welcome to The Applicant's Manual of Physician Assistant Programs. This guide was formulated for prospective students applying to physician assistant (PA) programs and provides specific, pertinent, detailed information about each accredited PA program in the United States as of January 2020. Applicants should use this guide as a primary resource to investigate each program and to evaluate their own credentials relative to those typically desired by each program. This guide is the first and only of its kind to incorporate all relevant information about each PA program into a single reference, saving the applicant the substantial amount of time it typically takes to explore multiple programs. This guide also provides the applicant with a quick and easy resource that can be referenced throughout the application process.

In the coming pages, we will provide an overview of the PA profession, describe the types of information included in this manual, define key terms used throughout the manual, and provide tips for applicants as they navigate the application process. Additionally, we have included reference links where you can find more information about the topics explored throughout the manual. We hope that you find this to be a useful tool throughout the application process.

Overview of the PA Profession

According to the American Academy of Physician Assistants (AAPA), a PA is a nationally certified and state-licensed medical professional. PAs practice medicine on healthcare teams with physicians and other providers. They practice in all medical specialties and prescribe medication in all 50 states, the District of Columbia, the majority of the U.S. territories and the uniformed services. PAs work in collaboration with physicians and other providers as part of the healthcare team to provide high-quality medical care to patients.

Though the duties of a PA can vary based on their practice setting, experience, and chosen specialty, PAs are trained to perform many of the same tasks as their physician counterparts, including: (1) taking a medical history; (2) performing a physical exam; (3) ordering and interpreting laboratory and imaging tests; (4) diagnosing and treating acute and chronic diseases; (5) counseling patients; (6) assisting in simple and complex surgery; (7) writing prescriptions; and (8) rounding on patients in hospitals, nursing homes, and other settings.

Additionally, some duties of PAs vary based upon state-specific practice laws. In each state, PAs designate a physician with whom they collaborate either remotely or in the workplace and can utilize as a resource in patient care.

PAs are educated in PA programs sponsored by colleges and universities throughout the United States that are accredited by the Accreditation Review Commission on Education for the Physician Assistant (ARC-PA). The ARC-PA sets standards (referred to as "the Standards") that PA programs must meet to remain accredited. The ARC-PA thoroughly evaluates each program to ensure a quality educational experience for all PA students that will adequately prepare them to become certified. Each PA program varies from 24-36 months in duration, and programs award graduates a Master's degree. In the didactic (classroom) phase, programs provide students with education in basic science, behavioral science, clinical medicine, pathophysiology, pharmacology, anatomy, physiology, history taking, physical diagnosis and much more. In the clinical phase, students typically complete over 2,000 hours of rotations in a variety of settings and specialties, which include primary care, internal medicine, obstetrics and gynecology, pediatrics, surgery, emergency medicine, and psychiatry. Some PA programs offer additional core, or required, rotations in other specialties. Most programs offer elective rotations, which allow students to further their knowledge in a particular area of medicine. Examples of elective rotations include dermatology, orthopedics, endocrinology, cardiology, among many others. Upon graduation, PAs are well-trained "generalists", with foundational knowledge in several areas of medicine that they can use to practice general internal medicine or enter into another specialty of their choosing.

After completing a PA program, graduates are eligible to sit for the Physician Assistant National Certification Exam (PANCE), which is created by the National Commission on the Certification of Physician Assistants (NCCPA). Once the PANCE is successfully completed, the credential of physician assistant – certified (PA-C) is given to PAs to denote their certification by the NCCPA. Before practicing, PAs must then complete licensing requirements in the state in which they wish to practice.

PAs are responsible for obtaining continuing medical education credits throughout their career. They must also pass a recertification exam (PANRE) every 10 years to maintain their certification and eligibility to practice. This also ensures that the PA maintains the requisite general medical knowledge to be able to transition into different medical specialties, if desired. Alternative pathways for recertifying are also currently being explored and piloted.

Currently, the PA profession is in a stage of unprecedented growth. There are more than 250 currently accredited PA programs in the United States, over 80 of which were created in the

IMPORTANT ADMISSIONS INFORMATION

ew

ion will review the information provided about each accredited PA program in nt pages. The goal of this section is to help you understand the information given h school, provide you with general information about PA admissions, and also u with tips on navigating the admissions process to put yourself in the best position d. We also provide links and resources for further information.

Information

hool, we provide detailed contact information. This includes the mailing address, one contact, and primary email contact. This information should be used as your ans of communicating with programs when you have program specific questions, bout the application process or your specific application, and for submitting any upplemental information that programs may require. Such information may ial transcripts, updated course grades and GPAs if courses were in progress at application, or updates to other sections of your application such as healthcare awards, research, certifications, or others. Please note that turnover of program orrelate with a change in certain contact information. Be sure to check each bsite for any updates to the listed contact information. Also, be sure to use on responsibly; programs expect you to thoroughly read through their website ting them with general questions, as they routinely receive many inquiries.

ghlights

, we provide information about the program's accreditation status, degree m start date, program length, class capacity, and tuition cost.

last 10 years. An additional 50 programs are in development throug
growth in the United States from 2014-2024 for PAs is predicted a
faster than the national average. Additionally, the median annual
the United States in 2018 was $108,610. The PA profession is also
to countries such as England, Canada, and Australia, where new e
different accrediting bodies and standards are beginning to tra
countries. This may result in expanded opportunities for U.S. tra
in the future.

Links for Further Information

American Academy of Physician Assistants: www.aapa.org

Accreditation Review Commission on Education for the
www.arc-pa.org

International Academy of Physician Associate Educato

National Commission on the Certification of Physician

United States Department of Labor:
www.bls.gov/ooh/healthcare/physician-assistants.htm

Overvi

This sec
subseque
about ea
provide y
to succee

Contact

For each s
primary ph
primary me
questions a
additional s
include offi
the time of
experience,
staff might
program's w
this informat
before conta

Program Hi

In this section
offered, progra

last 10 years. An additional 50 programs are in development throughout the country. The job growth in the United States from 2014-2024 for PAs is predicted at over 30%, which is much faster than the national average. Additionally, the median annual compensation for a PA in the United States in 2018 was $108,610. The PA profession is also expanding internationally to countries such as England, Canada, and Australia, where new educational programs under different accrediting bodies and standards are beginning to train PAs to practice in those countries. This may result in expanded opportunities for U.S. trained PAs to practice abroad in the future.

Links for Further Information

American Academy of Physician Assistants: www.aapa.org

Accreditation Review Commission on Education for the Physician Assistant: www.arc-pa.org

International Academy of Physician Associate Educators: www.iapae.com

National Commission on the Certification of Physician Assistants: www.nccpa.net

United States Department of Labor: www.bls.gov/ooh/healthcare/physician-assistants.htm

IMPORTANT ADMISSIONS INFORMATION

Overview

This section will review the information provided about each accredited PA program in subsequent pages. The goal of this section is to help you understand the information given about each school, provide you with general information about PA admissions, and also provide you with tips on navigating the admissions process to put yourself in the best position to succeed. We also provide links and resources for further information.

Contact Information

For each school, we provide detailed contact information. This includes the mailing address, primary phone contact, and primary email contact. This information should be used as your primary means of communicating with programs when you have program specific questions, questions about the application process or your specific application, and for submitting any additional supplemental information that programs may require. Such information may include official transcripts, updated course grades and GPAs if courses were in progress at the time of application, or updates to other sections of your application such as healthcare experience, awards, research, certifications, or others. Please note that turnover of program staff might correlate with a change in certain contact information. Be sure to check each program's website for any updates to the listed contact information. Also, be sure to use this information responsibly; programs expect you to thoroughly read through their website before contacting them with general questions, as they routinely receive many inquiries.

Program Highlights

In this section, we provide information about the program's accreditation status, degree offered, program start date, program length, class capacity, and tuition cost.

Accreditation

PA programs are accredited by the ARC-PA and given one of several different accreditation statuses listed below:

- **Accreditation** – Provisional is an accreditation status granted when the plans and resource allocation, if fully implemented as planned, of a proposed program that has not yet enrolled students appear to demonstrate the program's ability to meet the ARC-PA Standards, or when a program holding Accreditation – Provisional status appears to demonstrate continued progress in complying with the Standards as it prepares for the graduation of the first class (cohort) of students. Accreditation – Provisional does not guarantee any subsequent accreditation status. Accreditation – Provisional is limited to no more than five years from matriculation of the first cohort. PA students attending programs that are provisionally accredited on admission are eligible to sit for the PANCE upon graduation.

- **Accreditation** – Continued is granted (1) when a currently accredited program is in compliance with the Standards, (2) in the case of a program holding Accreditation – Probation when the program has demonstrated that it is once again in compliance with the Standards, or (3) when a program holding Accreditation – Provisional demonstrates compliance with the Standards after completion of the provisional review process. Accreditation – Continued status remains in effect until the program closes or withdraws from the accreditation process, or until accreditation is withdrawn for failure to comply with the Standards.

- **Accreditation** – Probation is a temporary status of accreditation, limited to two years, that is granted when a program holding an accreditation status of Accreditation – Provisional or Accreditation – Continued does not meet the Standards, and when the capability of the program to provide an acceptable educational experience for its students is threatened. Once placed on probation, a program that fails to comply with accreditation requirements in a timely manner, as specified by the ARC-PA, may be scheduled for a focused site visit and/or risk having its accreditation withdrawn. Programs that are placed on probation are required to teach out current students enrolled in the program, even if accreditation is lost, or find other programs willing to accept their students so that they can graduate and sit for the PANCE.

- **Accreditation** – Administrative Probation is a temporary status granted when a program has not complied with an administrative requirement, such as failure to pay fees or submit required reports. Once placed on Administrative Probation, a program that fails to comply with administrative requirements in a timely manner, as specified by the ARC-PA, may be scheduled for a focused site visit and/or risk having its accreditation withdrawn.

- **Accreditation** – Withheld is a status granted when an entry-level program, seeking Accreditation – Provisional status, is not in compliance with the Standards. The program receiving this accreditation status may voluntarily withdraw from the accreditation process within the 30-day appeal timeframe.

- **Accreditation** – Withdrawn is a status granted when an established program is determined no longer to be in compliance with the Standards and is no longer capable of providing an acceptable educational experience for its students, or when the program has failed to comply with ARC-PA accreditation requirements, actions or procedures. The program may voluntarily withdraw from the accreditation process within the 30-day appeal timeframe.

- **Voluntary Inactive Status** may be granted to programs that temporarily suspend instruction and cease to matriculate students. The conditions of this status are determined program circumstances necessitating this status.

Programs carrying the status "Accreditation – Withdrawn" or that plan to close in the coming year are omitted from this manual, as they are no longer accepting new applicants.

Degree Offered

The degree status is a consideration for students applying to PA programs. This section describes the degree that students will receive upon graduation from an accredited program. All PA programs are required to offer a Master's degree as the degree conferred upon graduation. You will notice in your research that there are many different Master's degrees offered by PA programs including Master of Medical Sciences (MMSc), Master of Physician Assistant Studies (MPAS), and Master of Health Sciences (MHS), among others. These degrees are essentially equivalent, and the degree name should not weigh heavily in your decision on where to apply. Most importantly, any student graduating from an accredited PA program, regardless of degree offered, is eligible to sit for the PANCE to achieve certification.

Program Start Date

Additionally, the start date of the program is important to consider when selecting PA programs. The majority of programs start in August, January, or May each year. However, there are others that start in other months. This becomes important for several reasons. If you are a student who is applying during fall of your senior year in 2020 for admission the following year, you may be eligible for programs that start in May 2021, August 2021, and January 2022. Some students prefer a break after undergraduate studies, and so may not wish to apply to programs that start in May, immediately after their undergraduate education would end. Others may not want to wait seven months to start a program in January, and so instead should apply to programs with earlier start dates. Furthermore, regardless of whether you are a current undergraduate or have been out of school for several years, you may be accepted to programs with varying start dates. Thus, you will need to consider the timing of the program start date, the program length, your current employment position and finances, as well as potential future lost PA wages if you opt for a program that has a longer duration or a later start date in making your final decision about where to attend.

Program Length

The program length is another essential consideration when evaluating PA programs. Most PA programs are 24-36 months in duration. There are pros and cons for both shorter and longer programs. In general, longer programs tend to have more built-in breaks and may offer a slightly lighter per-semester course load compared to shorter, more condensed programs. Though longer programs may offer a seemingly better school-life balance, you may also find them attached to a steeper price tag. Many programs justify a longer period of training with higher tuition. Attending a longer program will also put you into the workforce later than you might otherwise enter if you attended a shorter program. This may be significant for some, especially if you consider the months to a year of lost wages that you would have been earning sooner had you attended a shorter program. Shorter programs of course provide the advantage of decreased time in school, potentially lower tuition, and earlier entry into the workforce. However, they also provide a shorter time for mastering the material and a denser schedule while in school. Choosing program length is largely a personalized decision based on the above-mentioned and other individual factors.

Class Capacity

Another important component of choosing a PA program is its class capacity. The class capacity is the maximum amount of students that a PA program is accredited to enroll per class. Most programs tend to fill their class capacity, but not all do. As an example, Yale is accredited to have a class size of up to 45 students per year, however routinely selects 36-40 students. Programs have class capacities that range from 20-100+ students. Some students are more comfortable in a smaller, more intimate program, while other students may prefer a larger, more robust learning environment. If you are unsure whether you prefer a larger or smaller program, you should apply to both smaller and larger programs and then evaluate each when you visit campus for interviews, information sessions, or other prospective student events.

Tuition

Lastly, in the program highlights we provide you with the tuition of each program. Tuition can vary based on several factors, such as whether the institution is public or private, the institution location, and program resources. We provide you solely with the tuition in this manual, unless there are mandatory fees automatically built into the tuition. For several reasons, we typically do not include other PA school expenses such as books, university fees, and living expenses. Students can mitigate projected expenses in a variety of ways, such as living at home or budgeting finances, using savings, getting financial help from family/friends, and applying for scholarships. Thus, projected expenses provided by each school may not be an accurate depiction of the overall cost of attendance. Additionally, many students choose not to buy some or all of the books recommended by the program. Some programs offer all their rotations locally, while others require significant travel to rotations at an added expense. Thus, the only factor that is universally comparable for all students is the base tuition. Applicants should utilize the tuition information provided to compare tuitions at different programs, but should also research projected cost of living, university fees, books, scholarships and other financial aid opportunities available at different institutions to get a better sense of projected overall program cost.

Links for Further Information

Accreditation Review Commission on Education for the Physician Assistant:
www.arc-pa.org

Physician Assistant Education Association Program Directory:
www.directory.paeaonline.org

Student Statistics

This section provides the most recent available statistics for students accepted into each PA program. Some programs report only some or none of these statistics, and so they are not always available for each program each year. However, for those programs that do report statistics, applicants can compare their statistics to those of the average accepted student to get a sense of how likely or unlikely they might be to receive an interview and ultimately, an offer of acceptance at a given program.

For each program with available statistics, we report the percentage of male and female students as well as the percentage of minority students in each class. We also report the average overall GPA, science GPA and prerequisite GPA for accepted students. These numbers are largely determined by the Central Application Service for Physician Assistants (CASPA), the common application that most students use for the PA application process, and may vary slightly from the GPAs that are reported on your undergraduate or graduate transcripts for several reasons. Firstly, CASPA may use a different formula from your undergraduate or graduate institution to determine GPA. Secondly, CASPA does not accept grade replacement, while some undergraduate and graduate institutions do. This means that if you repeat a course you performed poorly in and attain a better grade the second time, both the initial grade and the grade on the second attempt will be included in your GPA calculations.

In addition, the average Graduate Record Examination (GRE) scores for the quantitative, verbal, and writing sections are reported. Importantly, not all schools require this examination as a part of their admissions requirement. However, it is a good idea to consider taking the GRE, as it will make you eligible to apply to many more programs. Additionally, many programs have cutoff values for the GRE, meaning that students who fail to attain a given score automatically will not be interviewed. Typically this score is around 300 total, or the 50th percentile overall. The degree to which programs emphasize GRE scores in their admissions decisions varies, but it is in your best interest to prepare well so that you can maximize this score, especially if your application is weak in other areas.

We have also included average healthcare experience and average age. Finally, when available, we also provide the student to faculty ratio, which may be an indicator of how much individualized attention is provided to students. You may receive more individualized attention in a program with 100 students and an 8:1 ratio compared to a program with 60 students and a 12:1 ratio. As previously stated, some programs include some or all of this information while others include some variation of these categories or no statistics at all.

We have done our best to include whatever class statistic information programs have made available at the time of publication.

Links for Further Information

Central Application Service for Physician Assistants:
https://portal.caspaonline.org/caspaHelpPages/about-caspaoverview/index.html

Graduate Record Examination: www.gre.org

APPLICATION BASICS

Types of Admissions

There are several basic components of the application process that each applicant should be aware of. Schools generally offer one of two types of admissions: rolling or non-rolling. Rolling admissions means that a school reviews each application as it is received, in the order that it is received, and makes decisions about interview invitations in a chronologic fashion. Thus, students who apply early in the application cycle are at an advantage because their application will be reviewed sooner than those who apply closer to the deadline. Regardless of strength of application, students who apply late in the cycle may not receive an interview simply because all of the class spots or interview spots have been filled. Non-rolling admissions refers to schools that review all of the applications equally and without preference to time of submission (as long as they were received prior to the deadline). For these programs, there is no advantage to applying early, as all applications are reviewed following the application deadline, and invitations to interview are then sent out.

The Common Application

Applicants need to consider whether or not a program participates in CASPA, the centralized application service. Through CASPA, you are able to complete one application online and send one set of documents (e.g., transcripts, letters of recommendation) to them. CASPA will verify your coursework for accuracy, calculate your GPA, and submit your application and attached documents to your designated PA programs. You also enter your personal statement through CASPA, where you describe your motivations for entering the PA profession. More than 90% of programs participate in CASPA. For programs that do not participate in CASPA, students typically need to submit a separate application (and fee) for that program, which may have different content than the CASPA application. It is highly recommended that students review all of the "Before Applying" materials on the CASPA website prior to beginning their application. It is also important to note that once your application is submitted to CASPA, it needs to be verified before it is sent off to the programs as a completed application. This process can take 2-4 weeks and should be taken into consideration to ensure that applicants meet the appropriate deadlines for each program. Further detailed discussion about CASPA is beyond the scope of this text. However, the CASPA website has detailed information for all applicants and offers customer service for individual questions.

Secondary Applications

Applicants also need to investigate whether or not a program requires a secondary application (and fee). These are applications created by some PA programs that students must complete in addition to CASPA. Supplemental applications often ask questions that are specific to the program's mission, interests, and goals. They may also ask for a list of prerequisite coursework, a curriculum vita, or for documentation of other program-specific requirements. Since secondary applications often include essay-style questions, these applications can be time consuming. It is important to plan ahead to complete this application prior to the application deadline for each program.

Yellow Ribbon Schools

The Yellow Ribbon Program is a provision of the law that created the Post-9/11 GI Bill. The Yellow Ribbon Program is available for Institutions of Higher Learning (degree granting institutions) in the U.S. or at a branch of such an institution located outside the U.S. The program allows approved institutions of higher learning and the VA to partially or fully fund tuition and fee expenses that exceed the established thresholds under the Post-9/11 GI Bill. Only Veterans (or dependents under Transfer of Entitlement) at the 100% benefit level qualify. Active duty members and spouses thereof are not eligible for this program. The school's agreement with the VA specifies an amount the school will contribute (and VA will match) to make up all or part of the difference between what the Post-9/11 GI Bill will pay and the unmet tuition and fees charges. The school's agreement with the VA may limit the number of participants in the program and is determined on a first-come, first-served basis.

Application Deadlines

Finally, applicants should be aware of the application deadline. We provide the application deadline listed on the program website. However, it is important to realize that there are several different types of application deadlines, which are color coded on the CASPA application website. Some programs have e-submission deadlines. This means that if you submit your application to CASPA by the program deadline, you have met the deadline for your application, even though CASPA typically takes another 2-4 weeks to process and verify your application. Other programs have complete date deadlines. This means that in order for applicants to meet the deadline, they must have all transcripts, letters of recommendation and other supporting documents submitted to and received by CASPA prior to the deadline. However, the application does not need to be verified (GPA calculated) by CASPA by the deadline for programs with complete date deadlines. Finally, there are programs with verified deadlines, meaning that all supporting documentation and GPA calculations must be completed by CASPA prior to the program deadline. This means you should plan to have your application submitted in its entirety at least 2-4 weeks before program deadlines.

Links for Further Information

Central Application Service for Physician Assistants:

https://portal.caspaonline.org/caspaHelpPages/about-caspaoverview/index.html

Veterans Administration:

https://www.benefits.va.gov/GIBILL/docs/factsheets/Yellow%20Ribbon%20Program.pdf

APPLICATION REQUIREMENTS

Grade Point Average

As expected, every PA program has specific requirements that must be met for admission. Most programs require a 3.0 overall GPA and/or 3.0 science GPA or prerequisite GPA. In order to be a competitive applicant, you should look to exceed these values. In many cases, if your GPA values are less than these minimums, PA programs will not consider your application unless it is exceedingly strong in other areas. As previously stated, courses that were taken multiple times will have both the initial and subsequent grades included in GPA calculations. Furthermore, many PA programs also do consider trends in GPAs. A student who steadily improved their GPA from a 2.5 freshman year to a 4.0 senior year is generally viewed more favorably than one who started out with a 4.0 freshman year and then declined to a 2.5 senior year, even though the overall and science GPAs of the two students might be equivalent.

Prerequisite Coursework

PA programs have specific prerequisite course requirements. These are listed for each program, as well as any other specific information about those prerequisites. Common courses that many programs require include college-level biology, chemistry, organic chemistry, biochemistry, microbiology, genetics, human anatomy, human physiology, psychology, English and statistics. These do vary by program. One common example is that most programs require two semesters of human anatomy and physiology. Most programs will allow you to complete this as either one course in human anatomy and a second course in human physiology, or as a two-semester sequence of human anatomy and physiology combined. It is also important to note whether or not schools require a lab component with certain science classes. Unless specifically listed, labs are not required for prerequisites. For example, "Biology with lab" means that the course must include a lab component. In most cases, the lab portion of the course is expected to be completed in conjunction with the course (as a part of the same series and at the same institution). If a prerequisite is just listed as "Biology", it means that the lab component is not a requirement. However, many schools prefer that you have completed a lab even when it is not required and doing so will make you a more competitive applicant.

Some programs also impose time limits on courses, meaning that students must have taken the courses in the last 5 years or 10 years, as an example, in order for them to meet the prerequisite requirement for that given program. If a course was taken in the distant past, students may need to repeat the course again, or apply for a waiver through the school. In some instances, the time limit may be waived if an applicant has been working directly in the healthcare field for a number of years. Additionally, some programs will allow students to apply while prerequisite courses are still in progress, while others require that all courses be completed prior to application. In general, the more prerequisites completed prior to application the better, because programs can more accurately and completely assess your application if more prerequisite grades are available. Finally, programs differ in terms of what types of college credits they will accept. Some programs accept community college credits while others do not. Some programs accept online coursework, Advanced Placement (AP) courses from high school, or course waivers, while others do not. Though we have attempted to include this information throughout the text for each school, it is in the applicant's best interest to review this information on each program's website, as requirements are constantly evolving. This is especially recommended if your prerequisites were completed in a non-traditional manner.

Furthermore, when possible/applicable, we have made an effort to include "recommended" coursework. These are classes that are not required prerequisites, but may contribute to building a more comprehensive and diversified physician assistant student. If you haven't completed "recommended" courses, don't sweat it. If you have, use this to your advantage. They will be looked upon favorably!

Prerequisite Healthcare Experience

In addition to coursework prerequisites, programs have varying levels of required prerequisite experience. Generally, there are two categories of experience that programs evaluate. The first is direct patient care experience. This refers to experience in which applicants were directly responsible for patient care. Oftentimes, these experiences require a certification. Some examples include medical assistant, emergency medical technician, certified nursing assistant, physical therapy aide, physical therapist, registered nurse, emergency department technician, athletic trainer, paramedic, military medic, and many more. PA programs require anywhere from 0-4000+ hours of direct patient care experience, and in general, the more experience you have, the more favorably your application will be viewed. Typically, paid experience is preferred over volunteer experience, as it usually indicates a higher level of responsibility. However, many programs highly value volunteer experiences, both related to and not related to healthcare. Such positions should be sought out, coveted, and confidently reported in the application. By acquiring more experience, you make yourself a competitive applicant for more programs, especially those that have a high number of required healthcare hours.

The second type of experience is healthcare experience. This includes positions in which applicants performed a role related to healthcare, but that did not involve direct patient contact. Examples include medical secretary, office manager, pharmaceutical sales representative, hospital volunteer, pharmacy technician, medical scribe, and others. It is important to note that the definition of what counts as direct patient contact versus healthcare related experience can sometimes vary by program. If you are unsure which category your experience falls under, you should view the program's website or contact the program directly to inquire. For positions where there was a combination of direct patient care responsibility and non-patient care responsibilities, hours can be divided into each of those categories on the CASPA application. For example, if you worked 2,000 hours as a medical assistant, with 50% of your time devoted to patient care and 50% of your time devoted to clerical work, you would count 1,000 of those hours as direct patient care hours and 1,000 of those hours as healthcare related experience on CASPA. Lastly, many PA programs value and encourage PA shadowing in order to learn the role and responsibilities of the profession, and to ensure you are pursuing a career that is well aligned with your goals and expectations.

CASPA Definitions

In the past several years, CASPA has updated their definitions of patient care experience and healthcare experience, with some controversy. CASPA defines patient care experience as "Experiences in which you are directly responsible for a patient's care. For example, prescribing medication, performing procedures, directing a course of treatment, designing a treatment regimen, actively working on patients as a nurse, paramedic, EMT, CNA, phlebotomist, physical therapist, dental hygienist, etc.". CASPA defines healthcare experience as "Both paid and unpaid work in a health or health-related field where you are not directly responsible for a patient's care, but may still have patient interaction; for example, filling prescriptions, performing clerical work, delivering patient food, cleaning patients and/or their rooms, administering food or medication, taking vitals or other record keeping information, working as a scribe, CNA (depending on job description), medical assistant, etc.". The controversy arises from the fact that most medical assistant and CNA jobs, for example, involve direct patient contact experience yet are included in the healthcare experience definition and not the direct patient care definition.

Overall, our advice remains the same as in previous years. If you directly worked with and cared for patients in the majority of your duties, regardless of your clinical title, it counts as direct patient care experience and should be listed as such on CASPA. If the majority of your duties were clerical or technical and did not involve caring for patients, your hours should be listed as healthcare experience. If your job included some patient care and some clerical work, your hours should be split accordingly on your CASPA application between these two sections.

Standardized Testing

Some programs have required standardized testing while others do not. The most common standardized test requirement for PA programs is the GRE. As previously stated, it is worth taking this exam as it will increase the number of programs you can apply to. Additionally, many programs have cutoff values for the GRE, meaning that if students fail to attain a given score they automatically will not be interviewed. Typically this score is around 300 total, or the 50th percentile overall. Some programs will accept the Medical College Admissions Test (MCAT) in lieu of the GRE, while other programs require the GRE but may waive the requirement if the applicant already holds a graduate degree.

Many PA programs are also turning to the Computer-Based Assessment for Sampling Personal Characteristics (CASPer) as an admission requirement. CASPer tests non-academic characteristics of potential students such as collaboration, communication, empathy, ethics, equity, motivation, problem solving, professionalism, resilience, and self-awareness. These characteristics make for a great future PA, but are sometimes difficult to demonstrate on the CASPA application. By completing the CASPer test, applicants provide programs with an insight into their personal skills prior to the holistic review or the interview phase. This allows programs to look at more than just academic ability and helps them make more informed decisions about which candidates to offer interviews to.

Finally, some programs are starting to require the brand new Physician Assistant - College Assessment Test (PA-CAT) for admissions. The PA-CAT is designed to be a broad-based exam reflecting the common educational experiences of most PA applicants. The PA-CAT will provide evidence-based data on what applicants have learned in prerequisite subject areas prior to applying to PA school.

Topics were chosen based on literature reviews, surveys, and consultations with PA educators who were asked to identify which prerequisites subjects, topics, and concepts are most important for mastery of the demanding PA curriculum. Anatomy and Physiology are given the most emphasis in recognition of what PA students must learn early in the curriculum. Along with Anatomy and Physiology, the PA-CAT will test the following subjects: Microbiology, General Biology, Genetics, General Chemistry (including Organic Chemistry), Biochemistry, Behavioral Sciences, and Statistics. The exam covers a variety of learning targets (objectives) with a focus on the higher-order cognitive level to assess application and understanding.

The PA-CAT will be available commercially in May of 2020. In the future, it is highly likely that it will be the standardized test that most programs require for admissions. As of now there are 18 programs that will be utilizing the PA-CAT for the upcoming cycle. The official list of programs will be released in the near future.

Letters of Recommendation

Lastly, letters of recommendation are a crucial component of the PA admissions application. Most schools require 2-3 letters, and some schools have specific requirements as to who must write and submit the letters. Generally, family members, friends, and personal medical providers are not appropriate letter writers. Applicants should request letters from professors, work supervisors, PAs, nurse practitioners, physicians, volunteer supervisors, or research mentors. Regardless of whom you ask, it is of the utmost importance that the writer knows you well enough to compose a strong letter on your behalf. He/she should be able to attest to attributes such as your academic prowess, clinical experience, rapport with patients, interpersonal skills, perseverance, dedication, motivation, intelligence, scientific aptitude, reliability, and ability to work as part of a team. Remember that a weak or mediocre letter of recommendation can be a red flag for admissions committees, so choose people who you are confident will write great letters. Of note, it is also important to choose people who are reliable and timely. You should provide your letter writers with at least one month of advanced notice so that they have ample time to compose your letter and submit it through CASPA or other application avenues by the appropriate deadline.

Links for Further Information

Central Application Service for Physician Assistants:
https://portal.caspaonline.org/caspaHelpPages/about-caspaoverview/index.html

Physician Assistant Education Association Program Directory:
www.directory.paeaonline.org

Computer-Based Assessment for Sampling Personal Characteristics:
www.takecasper.com

Physician Assistant College Admissions Test (PA-CAT)
https://www.pa-cat.com/about-the-pa-cat/

PROGRAM ATTRIBUTES

Overview

Here we provide key information that helps to distinguish programs from one other and to help you narrow down your list of programs. For each program we provide the mission statement, curriculum structure, PANCE scores, and unique program features (if available).

Mission Statement

Each PA program has a mission statement that affirms a desire to produce well-trained PAs and lists other specific attributes that reflect the focus of the program. Students can ascertain whether or not they might be a good fit for that program based on the program's mission, vision, and goals. Let's examine some examples:

The mission of the Yale School of Medicine Physician Associate Program is to educate individuals to become outstanding clinicians and to foster leaders who will serve their communities and advance the physician assistant profession.

The Physician Assistant Studies Program at the University of South Dakota provides a comprehensive primary care education that prepares graduates to deliver high quality healthcare to meet the needs of patients in South Dakota and the region.

The mission of the Child Health Associate/Physician Assistant Program at the University of Colorado is to provide comprehensive physician assistant education in primary care across the lifespan, with expanded training in pediatrics and care of the medically underserved.

Though each of the above statements is short, they emphasize important qualities about the programs and the types of students they aim to recruit. The PA program at Yale, in addition to creating well-trained PAs, wants to foster leaders that will serve the community and advance the profession. Applicants with aspirations to eventually obtain local or national leadership roles, or with significant amounts of leadership experience in their undergraduate training, prior employment, or volunteer work may align best with the mission statement of Yale and may have a better chance of acceptance than those without leadership aspirations or experience. The PA Program at the University of South Dakota emphasizes primary care in their mission statement, as well as creating providers who will care for patients in South Dakota and the surrounding areas. Thus, applicants with ties to South Dakota and the surrounding states, as well as interest in pursuing a career in primary care will likely have increased chances of admission compared to those who plan to practice in other areas of the country or in different specialties. Finally, the program at the University of Colorado focuses on pediatrics and care of the medically underserved. If you have an interest in pursuing a career in pediatrics, or have prior experience caring for medically underserved populations, you might be a good fit for this program. These examples emphasize the importance of understanding the mission of each PA program and choosing programs that align with your goals and experience.

Curriculum Structure

The curricular structure of each program can vary significantly. In general, programs are divided into two or three different phases: the didactic and clinical phases, with or without a graduate project phase.

Didactic Phase

The first phase is the didactic phase, in which students complete the majority of their coursework, learn to take a history and perform a physical exam, and learn basic clinical and interactive skills. The didactic phase generally ranges from 10-24 months, with most programs ranging from 12-16 months. Within the didactic phase, there are several types of teaching methodologies that may be implemented. Some methods that programs utilize include lectures, discussion, case-based learning, team-based learning, inquiry-based learning, small group work, projects, self-guided learning, clinical skills workshops, or some combination thereof. We provide the duration of the didactic phase, but encourage you to learn about the different types of teaching methods that each program employs (and what they mean) by visiting the program website and asking questions during the interview process.

Clinical Phase

The second phase is the clinical phase of the program, which is primarily focused on clinical exposure and skills development. It is meant to solidify and build on the foundations of the didactic phase through interactions with real patients. It generally consists of a series of clinical rotations or clerkships, interspersed with "call-back days," where students return to campus to take rotation specific examinations, listen to lectures, give presentations, and participate in workshops. The clinical phase typically ranges from 12-18 months. Each rotation itself can range from 2-12 weeks, with most rotations ranging from 4-8 weeks depending on the program. Generally, programs with longer rotations or shorter clinical phases have fewer elective rotations (rotations where students get to choose an area of medicine they would like to explore further). We provide the number of required and elective rotations, as well as the duration of each rotation for each program.

Graduate Project Phase

The third phase of some PA programs is the graduate project phase. Since most programs offer a Master's degree, many have some type of Master's requirement. In some programs, this is a Capstone Project that students must complete within the local community. Other programs require students to complete a literature review on a topic of interest or to complete a research thesis project. There are also some programs that do not require a graduate project at all, though this is becoming less common. For each program, we include the type of project required, if any, as part of the curriculum and graduation requirements. Specifics of each graduate project should be sought out on individual program websites if further details are desired.

PANCE Scores

The PANCE passing rates for each program are an important metric for applicants, as PAs must pass the PANCE in order to be certified and ultimately able to practice. A student who graduates from an accredited program but does not pass the PANCE is not eligible for licensure. Furthermore, the first-time pass rates (the percentage of students who pass the PANCE on the first attempt) are especially important because the chances of passing the PANCE decrease with each attempt, and because the PANCE is an expensive test. Of course, the PANCE is also a metric of the knowledge obtained in PA school and thus how well a program has prepared students to become PAs. For each program, we provide the first-time PANCE pass rates for the most recent year, as well as cumulative pass rates over the last 5 years. For programs with fewer than five graduating classes who have sat for the PANCE exam, it is indicated how many years of data the statistic is based on. The average national PANCE pass rate each year generally ranges from 90-96%.

Unique Program Features

This section provides the distinguishing features, unique opportunities, and interesting aspects of each program. Students are encouraged to use these as talking points during the interview process. This information is gathered both from program websites as well as from the perspectives of currently enrolled students to provide applicants with the most up-to-date information about each program. Example program features include things such as availability of international rotations, new facilities, medical mission trips, dual degree options, research opportunities, and community service experiences.

From the Program Directors

We interviewed over 20 PA Program Directors from around the country to give you additional insight about what they are looking for in prospective PA students. Their answers are noted below:

- **What is one key characteristic you look for in an applicant?**

  "Grit, the ability to overcome obstacles and persevere in spite of adversity."

  "We like to start with the end in mind. Is this person someone who I would want taking care of me or my family in the future?"

  "If I were to have to point out one thing it would be perseverance--we have a soft spot for applicants who try more than once. If they have applied and not been accepted then done something to improve their application and reapply we look favorably on that."

  "We are looking for leadership."

  "Our program looks for applicants who are already demonstrating our mission of competency (academic performance), compassion (volunteerism), and confidence (leadership), so we can fan their flame and transform them into quality PAs who provide excellent mental, physical, and spiritual care of patients in a holistic manner."

  "Resilience."

  "We are looking for a well-rounded applicant who brings both academic achievement and broad life experience to the table. We value applicants who are committed to service to mankind."

"Professional demeanor."

"We are looking for specific people who just want to care for people. Our outreach is primarily to the homeless."

"We look for individuals who would be a good fit for our program. We do like to see passion for becoming a PA but we also want to see why they are choosing our program specifically. I always encourage applicants to do considerable research into various programs to find a good fit prior to applying rather than just selecting every program in the state for instance. All programs are not equal in regards to who they attract so this process is worthwhile."

"We are looking for candidates who demonstrate the following: 1. Evidence of a commitment to underserved practice; 2. Evidence of strong interpersonal skills and the ability to effectively communicate with peers, patients, and superiors in a professional environment; 3. Evidence of a willingness to provide competent compassionate care."

"Commitment to caring. PA students are all smart, dedicated, and driven personalities; but it's the commitment to caring that really makes a person shine as they're preparing to embark on a career that involves caring for others every day for the rest of their lives."

"We like to see that someone has grit. That they have overcome challenges and persevered. PA school is hard, there are no two ways about it. An applicant who has a perfect academic record and has led a charmed life is great, but I would rather have an applicant who has faced adversity and tenaciously pushed their way through."

"One key thing that helps PA students be successful is the presence of grit. This is the ability to demonstrate resilience and overcoming challenges. PA School is incredibly challenging - intelligence and work ethic alone are not enough."

"Maturity. PA programs are rigorous and time intensive. We want candidates who are mature enough to handle the curriculum."

"We look for well rounded applicants who are interested in practicing with underserved communities once they go into practice, in some capacity ranging from volunteering some time in Free Clinics to working primarily in rural or underserved communities."

What can students do to optimize their chances before applying?

"Become familiar with the mission statement of the programs they are interested in and verify that they meet all of the prerequisites. Remember that to be competitive, you need to be well above the average in the categories that matter most to the programs."

"Do not be in too big of a rush. Make sure you have a strongly competitive application before applying. This may mean taking a year or two off from academics to gain more experience. It might mean taking a few more science-based classes (Immunology, Genetics, Molecular & Cell biology, Pharmacology, etc.) to show that you have a strong academic foundation. Students with a lower GPA should consider doing a formal post-bac program or even a master's degree program."

"The required prerequisites are meant to be a guide for applicants to have a better understanding of what we believe will make for a successful student in our program. We expect that many applicants will have grades, test scores and healthcare hours that exceed the minimums in one or more area. Applicants who at least meet the minimum requirements listed on our website will be considered for an interview."

"Our admissions committee reads the entire CASPA application and we like to look beyond academics for involvement in campus activities outside the classroom such as sports, music, clubs and volunteer experiences."

"Complete all the requirements for the particular PA school's list of needs--best to have a full, finished application rather than to have things "hanging". Be patient and take a gap year or two to have a maximum impact."

"We utilize rolling admissions, so early application is strongly encouraged. Evidence of sustained service to the community in a non-medical capacity is valued."

"Obtain as much PA shadowing hours as possible in the primary care and specialty areas as well as in various practice settings. This exposure and insight allows our applicants to better understand the role and responsibility of the PA on the healthcare team and how PAs interact with patients/families, attending MDs/PA colleagues/staff, and other ancillary services."

"Try to excel in an area that we look at including GPA, GRE, or healthcare experience. Having 20,000 hours or a very high GPA or GRE score will help you stand out."

"When it comes down to it, prior coursework and grades are the main element of the application. If grades are the issue, the student would work on increasing their GPA. If grades are not the issue, then gaining some healthcare experience would be helpful. On rare occasion, we recommend re-taking the GRE, but in most cases, this does not really make a difference in our admission process overall."

"Obtain as much experience, including PA-C shadowing, as possible. Try to vary your experiences as well, so that you see what PAs do in the ER vs. family practice vs. orthopedics. It's so helpful to have some exposure into health care before diving into PA school, not to mention most schools have a minimum hour requirement."

"Make sure you meet the requirements for the program to which you are applying. Make it clear that you meet those requirements. For example, if you must shadow a PA for a certain number of hours, make it clear that the person you shadowed was a PA."

"Visit our website and review not just the requirements and prerequisites, but also the admission selection factors, the program mission/goals, and other pertinent program information. Then be sure to address all these items in your CASPA application in some way."

"Demonstration on their application of this interest by volunteering in underserved populations is looked upon favorably."

· Is there one part of the application that you weigh most heavily?

"Health care experience and volunteer experience. Health care experience is more valuable with positions that allow more independent decision making. Volunteer experience should be hands on with individuals in need and not organizing fundraisers or participating in beach or park clean up."

"Overall academic preparation. We look beyond just overall GPA and Science GPA to see if students took full academic loads (15-18 units per term). These are the best predictors of student success and show that they can handle the heavy science load and the pace of a PA program."

"There is not one trait or characteristic that is most important, it is really more of the total individual (application + interview) that determines who will be a good fit for our program."

"For admissions, we look for a student who has performed well in a variety of science courses during high school to include our listed prerequisites. Shadowing a PA is a great way for high school students to gain a better understanding of the PA profession and scope of practice."

"We use a holistic admissions process to look at the applicant as a whole so no one part of the application is weighed more heavily."

"No, we are truly looking for a broadly prepared applicant who has branched out in all areas in ways that are meaningful for a future in health care."

"We take a balanced approach to both academic and non-academic factors in our application review process. Our program reviews applications holistically, assessing each applicant on their entire application rather than setting a "cut point" that all applicants must meet to be successful."

"Prior academic performance determined by the applicants GPA."

"Cumulative and science GPA. There is no way around it. The only data point that correlates with how well students will do in PA school is how well they performed in UG studies. We do have a comprehensive approach to our process, but grades are a large factor for getting the CASPA application on our desk."

"We use a holistic admissions approach that includes the student's overall GPA, prerequisite GPA, patient care hours, GRE scores, community service/leadership, and interview. The 3 major components we look at in terms of scoring are GPA/grades/GRE, patient care hours/ shadowing, and interview; and they're weighted similarly. During the interview, applicants will meet with current PA students, PA faculty, PA graduates and preceptors which allows us to get a good understanding of each applicant as a person, and allows the applicants to get to know who we are as a program."

"An applicant with a GPA that is below the requirement or who hasn't met the healthcare requirements won't be given a second look."

"We do not weight one part of the application more heavily than another."

"There is no one part of the application we weight most heavily—students should have strong academic credentials, health work experiences with meaningful patient contact, leadership skills, and a willingness to volunteer their time in underserved communities.

NOTES:

Prerequisites Completed: Grade:

1. ....
2. ....
3. ....
4. ....
5. ....
6. ....
7. ....
8. ....
9. ....
10. ....

Prerequisites to Be Completed: Semester:

1. ....
2. ....
3. ....
4. ....
5. ....
6. ....
7. ....
8. ....
9. ....
10. ....

Healthcare Experience (type and hours):

GRE:
Verbal:

Quantitative:

Analytical:

PA Shadowing:

Volunteer Experience:

Letter Writers:

Notes on Schools:

List of Schools to Apply to: **Page #**

1. ....

2. ....

3. ....

4. ....

5. ....

6. ....

7. ....

8. ....

9. ....

10. ....

11. ....

12. ....

13. ....

14. ....

15. ....

16. ....

17. ....

18. ....

19. ....

20. ....

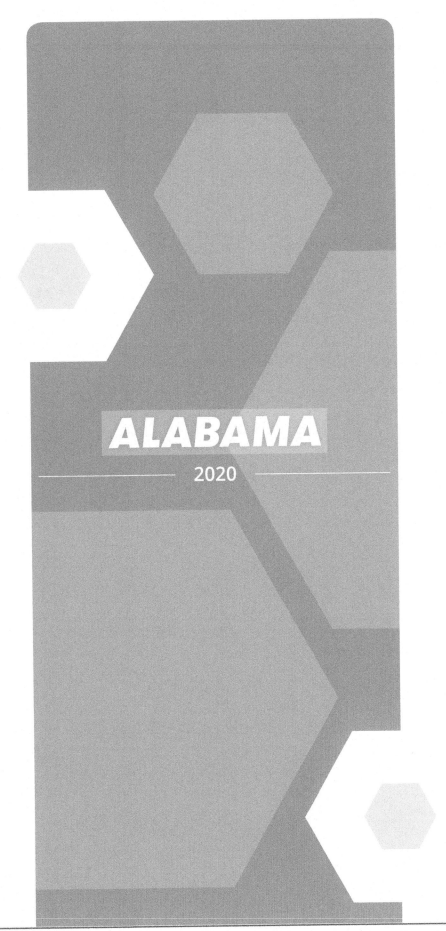

ALABAMA

2020

Samford University

800 Lakeshore Drive
Birmingham, AL 35229
Phone: 205-726-2611
Email: mwcarter@samford.edu

PROGRAM HIGHLIGHTS

Accreditation: Provisional

Degree Offered: Master (MSPAS)

Start Date: August annually

Program Length: 27 months

Class Capacity: Not reported

Tuition: $97,000

CASPA Participant: Yes

Supplemental Application: Yes

Yellow Ribbon: Yes

Admissions: Non-rolling

Application Deadline: August 1

PREREQUISITE COURSEWORK:

General Psychology or Abnormal Psychology or Developmental Psychology (6 credits), Human Anatomy and Physiology with lab (6-8 credits), General Biology I and II with lab (6-8 credits), Microbiology with lab (3-4 credits), General Chemistry I and II with lab (8-9 credits), Statistics (3 credits), Medical Terminology (1 credit). Applicants may have 6 prerequisite credits in progress at the time of application. Prerequisites must be completed with a grade "C" or better.

GPA Requirement: Overall GPA 3.0; Science GPA 3.0; Non-Science GPA 3.0

Healthcare Experience: Preferred, not required

PA Shadowing: Preferred, not required

Required Standardized Testing: GRE or MCAT

Letters of Recommendation: Three required; one each from a professor, supervisor, and PA, MD, DO or CRNP

Seat Deposit: $1,000

SAMFORD UNIVERSITY

MISSION:

The mission of Samford University's Department of Physician Assistant Studies is to nurture and develop students both spiritually and academically to provide empathetic, compassionate medical care and service to the community.

NO CLASS STATISTICS REPORTED

PANCE SCORES

5-year First Time Pass: N/A

Most Recent First Time Pass: N/A (have not graduated a class yet)

CURRICULUM STRUCTURE

Didactic: 15 months

Clinical: 12 months

Rotations: 7 mandatory, 5 elective (each 4 weeks)

UNIQUE PROGRAM FEATURES

Facilities: The program's Experiential Learning and Simulation Center offers discipline specific and interdisciplinary learning opportunities across the simulation continuum. High fidelity simulators respond realistically to care and allow students to practice skills until they are comfortable with assessment and procedures. The center also features adult, pediatric and neonatal simulators and a variety of patient care settings including inpatient hospital rooms, an operating room and even a simulated home unit.

University of Alabama at Birmingham

430 School of Health
Professions Building
1716 9th Avenue South
Birmingham, AL 35294
Phone: 205-975-4237
Email: Askcds@uab.edu

PROGRAM HIGHLIGHTS

Accreditation: Continuing

Degree Offered: Master (MSPAS)

Start Date: August annually

Program Length: 27 months

Class Capacity: 80 students

Tuition: $63,825 (in-state);
$146,280 (out-of-state)

CASPA Participant: Yes

Supplemental Application:
Yes ($75 fee)

Yellow Ribbon: Yes

Admissions: Non-rolling

Application Deadline: August 1

PREREQUISITE COURSEWORK:

Biology (8 credits), Microbiology
with lab preferred (3-4 credits),
Human Anatomy and Physiology
(6-8 credits), General Chemistry
with lab preferred (8-9 credits),
Statistics (3-4 credits), Psychology
(6 credits). All applicants with
9 or fewer semester hours of
prerequisite courses to complete
on Jan 1st of the year of admission
will be considered for admission.

GPA Requirement: Overall GPA 3.0;
Science GPA 3.0; Prerequisite GPA
3.0

Healthcare Experience: Preferred,
not required

PA Shadowing: Preferred, not
required

Required Standardized Testing: GRE
or MCAT

Letters of Recommendation: Three
required; no one specific

Seat Deposit: $300

UNIVERSITY OF ALABAMA AT BIRMINGHAM

MISSION:

The mission of the University of Alabama at Birmingham Physician Assistant Studies Program is to attract and train culturally diverse individuals with the knowledge, skills, and judgment needed to provide competent and compassionate healthcare to all.

CLASS OF 2018

Male: 11%

Female: 89%

Minority: 19%

Overall GPA: 3.66

Science GPA: 3.60

GRE Verbal: 58th percentile

GRE Quantitative: 50th percentile

Average Healthcare Experience: 3,446 hours

Average Age: 24

PANCE SCORES

5-year First Time Pass: 93%

Most Recent First Time Pass: 86%

CURRICULUM STRUCTURE

Didactic: 15 months

Clinical: 12 months

Rotations: 7 mandatory, 5 elective (each 4 weeks)

Master's Research Project Presentation: Required for graduation

UNIQUE PROGRAM FEATURES

Healthcare Screenings for the Homeless: Students can volunteer to provide clinical services at the Firehouse Shelter in Birmingham with faculty from the School of Health Professions.

Admissions Preference: Approximately 50% of students in the Class of 2018 were Alabama residents, while the other 50% came from other states.

Dual Degree: This program offers a dual degree MSPAS-MPH program, where students begin online MPH courses in the spring and summer prior to PA program matriculation in the fall.

PROGRAM HIGHLIGHTS

Accreditation: Continuing

Degree Offered: Master (MHS)

Start Date: May annually

Program Length: 27 months

Class Capacity: 40 students

Tuition: $59,889 (in-state);
$116,154 (out-of-state)

CASPA Participant: Yes

Supplemental Application: Yes ($110 fee)

Yellow Ribbon: Yes

Admissions: Non-rolling

Application Deadline: October 1

PREREQUISITE COURSEWORK

Biology (3 credits), General Chemistry I and II with lab (8 credits), Organic Chemistry or Biochemistry (3 credits), General Microbiology (3 credits), Human Anatomy and Physiology (6 credits), Mathematics (3 credits), Statistics (3 credits), General Psychology (3 credits), Medical Terminology (1 credits). Courses may be in progress at the time of application as long as they are completed 1 semester prior to the start of the program. Students will be given bonus points in the admissions process if they have taken genetics, biochemistry, immunology, physics, pathophysiology or pharmacology coursework.

GPA Requirement: Overall GPA 3.0; Science GPA 3.0; Prerequisite GPA 2.0; Last 60 Credit GPA 3.0

Healthcare Experience: 500 hours

PA Shadowing: Not required

Required Standardized Testing: GRE (minimum of 145 on verbal and quantitative)

Letters of Recommendation: Three required; one from a PA/MD/DO

Seat Deposit: $500

UNIVERSITY OF SOUTH ALABAMA

MISSION:

The mission of the University of South Alabama Physician Assistant Program is to educate compassionate and competent individuals from diverse backgrounds to become highly qualified physician assistants in accordance with the highest professional standards to provide a broad spectrum of preventative and curative healthcare to patients in various communities and clinical settings with physician supervision including underserved populations in Alabama both rural and urban. The emphasis of the program is one of primary care, including a broad foundation in the medical and surgical specialties.

CLASS OF 2021

Male: 23%

Female: 77%

Overall GPA: 3.68

Science GPA: 3.62

Last 60 Credit GPA: 3.80

GRE Verbal: 153

GRE Quantitative: 151

Average Healthcare Experience: 2,353 hours

Average Age: 25

PANCE SCORES

5-year First Time Pass: 95%

Most Recent First Time Pass: 100%

CURRICULUM STRUCTURE

Didactic: 15 months

Clinical: 12 months

Rotations: 7 mandatory, 3 elective (each 4-8 weeks)

Capstone Project: Required for graduation

UNIQUE PROGRAM FEATURES

Primary Care Focus: The program has a focus on primary care and you can read about student experiences on the primary care rotation on their website.

Admissions Preference: There is some preference given to Alabama applicants, but the program will consider applicants from all states. In the class of 2021, approximately 55% are Alabama residents.

Community Service: Students are committed to community service. Recently, the didactic class hosted Craws for a Cause, an annual crawfish boil and silent auction that allowed them to raise money for The Learning Tree.

Rotation Abroad: Students may apply to complete a clinical rotation in Women's Health in Cusco, Peru.

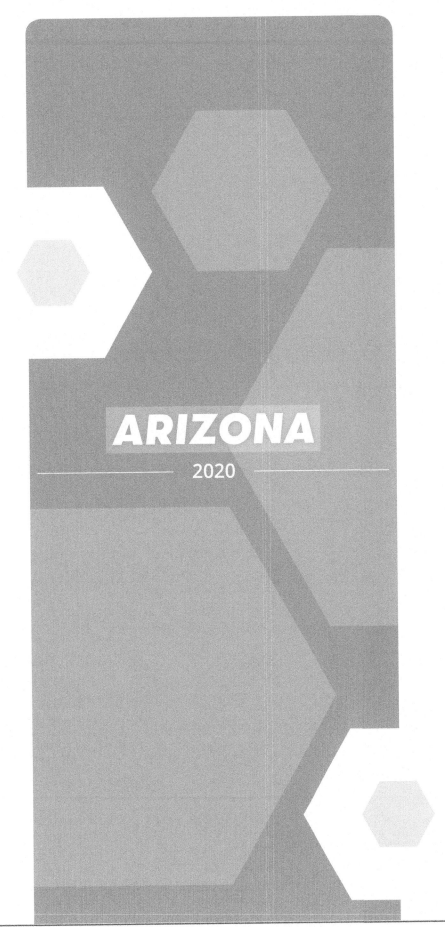

ARIZONA
2020

Arizona School of Health Sciences

5850 E. Still Circle
Mesa, AZ 85206
Phone: 866-626-2878
Email: azadmissions@atsu.edu

PROGRAM HIGHLIGHTS

Accreditation: Continuing
Degree Offered: Master (MSPAS)
Start Date: June annually
Program Length: 26 months
Class Capacity: 70 students
Tuition: $94,796

CASPA Participant: Yes
Supplemental Application:
Yes ($70 fee)
Yellow Ribbon: No
Admissions: Rolling
Application Deadline: September 1

PREREQUISITE COURSEWORK

Human Anatomy with lab (4 credits), Human Physiology with lab (4 credits), Microbiology (3 credits), General Chemistry (4 credits), Organic Chemistry (4 credits), Biochemistry (3 credits), College Statistics (3 credits), Medical Terminology (1 credit), English Composition (3 credits), English Elective (3 credits), Upper Level Sciences (9 credits), Psychology (6 credits). Anatomy, Physiology and Microbiology should be completed within 5 years of the application date. Prerequisites may be in progress at the time of application. It is highly recommended to have at least 12-18 credits of upper division science courses.

GPA Requirement: Overall GPA 3.0; Science GPA 3.0

Healthcare Experience: 1,000 hours

PA Shadowing: Not required

Required Standardized Testing: None

Letters of Recommendation: Three required; one from an employer or supervisor, one from a health care practitioner (MD/DO, PA or NP), and one from a science faculty member

Seat Deposit: $1,500

ARIZONA SCHOOL OF HEALTH SCIENCES

MISSION:

The A.T. Still University Department of Physician Assistant Studies provides a learning-centered education that develops exemplary physician assistants who deliver whole person healthcare with an emphasis on underserved populations.

CLASS OF 2021

Overall GPA: 3.59
Science GPA: 3.54
Average Age: 26

PANCE SCORES

5-year First Time Pass: 96%
Most Recent First Time Pass: 96%

CURRICULUM STRUCTURE

Didactic: 14 months
Clinical: 12 months
Rotations: 7 mandatory, 1 elective (each 6 weeks)

UNIQUE PROGRAM FEATURES

Hometown Scholars Program: This program promotes the provision of high-quality, comprehensive healthcare that is accessible, coordinated, culturally and linguistically competent and community-directed for all underserved populations for applicants interested in pursuing community health. Typically applicants work or volunteer in a community health center and then obtain an endorsement from the community health center leadership, which is used as part of the application process.

Body, Mind, and Spirit Course: This course, which is integrated throughout each didactic term, allows students to explore topics including spirituality in medicine, ethics, inter-professionalism, cross culturalism, and care of diverse patient populations.

Clinical Rotations: Rotations are completed on one of two tracks. The Arizona Track places students throughout the Phoenix, AZ area. The Community Health Centers Track places students into community health centers in Arizona, Texas, California, Louisiana, Georgia, or Oklahoma to complete their rotations.

Midwestern University

19555 N. 59th Avenue
Glendale, AZ 85308
Phone: 623-572-3614
Email: admissaz@midwestern.edu

PROGRAM HIGHLIGHTS

Accreditation: Continuing
Degree Offered: Master (MMS)
Start Date: June annually
Program Length: 27 months
Class Capacity: 86 students
Tuition: $120,779

CASPA Participant: Yes
Supplemental Application: No
Yellow Ribbon: No
Admissions: Rolling
Application Deadline: October 1

PREREQUISITE COURSEWORK

Biology with lab including 4 credits of Anatomy (8 credits), General Chemistry with lab (8 credits), Organic Chemistry with lab (4 credits), Math (3 credits), English Composition (6 credits), Social and Behavioral Sciences (6 credits), Statistics (3 credits). Prerequisites must be completed with a grade "C" or better and can be in progress at the time of application. Recommended courses: Biochemistry.

GPA Requirement: Overall GPA 3.0; Science GPA 3.0; Prerequisite GPA 2.0

Healthcare Experience: Preferred, not required

PA Shadowing: Not required

Required Standardized Testing: GRE (preference for scores >50% in each section), CASPer

Letters of Recommendation: Two required; no one specific

Seat Deposit: $200

MIDWESTERN UNIVERSITY (GLENDALE)

MISSION:

The Midwestern University Physician Assistant Program is committed to educate and mentor students in a setting that cultivates excellence and prepares compassionate, competent physician assistants to serve in a changing healthcare environment.

CLASS OF 2021

Male: 22%

Female: 78%

Overall GPA: 3.66

Science GPA: 3.60

GRE Verbal: 69th percentile

GRE Quantitative: 58th percentile

GRE Analytical: 4.3

Average Age: 25

PANCE SCORES

5-year First Time Pass: 99%

Most Recent First Time Pass: 100%

CURRICULUM STRUCTURE

Didactic: 13.5 months

Clinical: 13.5 months

Rotations: 7 mandatory, 2 elective (each 6 weeks)

Master's Portfolio: Required for graduation

UNIQUE PROGRAM FEATURES

Interprofessional Education: Every first-year PA student participates in a university wide interprofessional course that serves to highlight commonalities between the professions. Program faculty and students also participate in several inter-professional community service opportunities that include providing medical care to the medically underserved communities in the Phoenix area.

Facilities: The program has an onsite cadaver dissection lab and clinical skills/simulation center that students utilize throughout their training.

Northern Arizona University

NAU Graduate College
PO Box 4125
Flagstaff, Arizona 86011
Phone: 602-827-2450
Email: PAProg@nau.edu

PROGRAM HIGHLIGHTS

Accreditation: Continuing

Degree Offered: Master (MPAS)

Start Date: August annually

Program Length: 24 months

Class Capacity: 50 students

Tuition: $75,960 (in-state);
$102,110 (out-of-state, including fees)

CASPA Participant: Yes

Supplemental Application:
Yes ($65 fee)

Yellow Ribbon: Yes

Admissions: Rolling

Application Deadline: September 1

PREREQUISITE COURSEWORK

General Biology I and II (6 credits), Anatomy and Physiology I and II with labs (6 credits), Microbiology with lab (3 credits), General Chemistry I and II with labs (6 credits), Organic Chemistry or Biochemistry (3 credits), Additional Sciences (13 credits). 9 credits of science must be taken in the last 5 years. All prerequisites must be completed at the time of application. AP credits are accepted. Recommended courses: Psychology, Nutrition, Medical Terminology.

GPA Requirement: Overall GPA 3.0; Science GPA 3.0

Healthcare Experience: 500 hours

PA Shadowing: Not required

Required Standardized Testing: GRE (284 or higher is most competitive)

Letters of Recommendation: Three required; preferably from healthcare professionals, employers/supervisors and professors

Seat Deposit: None

NORTHERN ARIZONA UNIVERSITY

MISSION:

The mission of the Northern Arizona University Physician Assistant Studies Program is to recruit individuals of the highest possible quality from diverse backgrounds and life experiences to the profession and to equip them with clinical and professional knowledge, skills and abilities to provide high quality, compassionate medical care for the people of Arizona.

CLASS OF 2020

Male: 20%

Female: 80%

Overall GPA: 3.69

Science GPA: 3.58

Healthcare Experience: 7,502 hours

Average Age: 26

PANCE SCORES

5-year First Time Pass: 97%

Most Recent First Time Pass: 92%

CURRICULUM STRUCTURE

Didactic: 12 months

Clinical: 12 months

Rotations: 7 mandatory, 1 elective (4-8 weeks each)

Capstone Project: Required for graduation

UNIQUE PROGRAM FEATURES

Medical School Partnership: The program is a collaboration between Northern Arizona University and The University of Arizona College of Medicine – Phoenix, which enhances the student experience with access to world-class lecturers, up-to-date technology, simulation centers and inter-professional education.

State Sponsored School: This is the only state school PA program in Arizona and recruits students from Arizona as well as those with ties to the region who plan to practice in Arizona in the future, particularly in rural and underserved areas. Over 90% of graduates take their first job in Arizona. 80% of incoming students come from Arizona.

Homeless Clinic: Students from NAU, Arizona State University, and the University of Arizona work together to run a homeless clinic for the underserved in the Phoenix area.

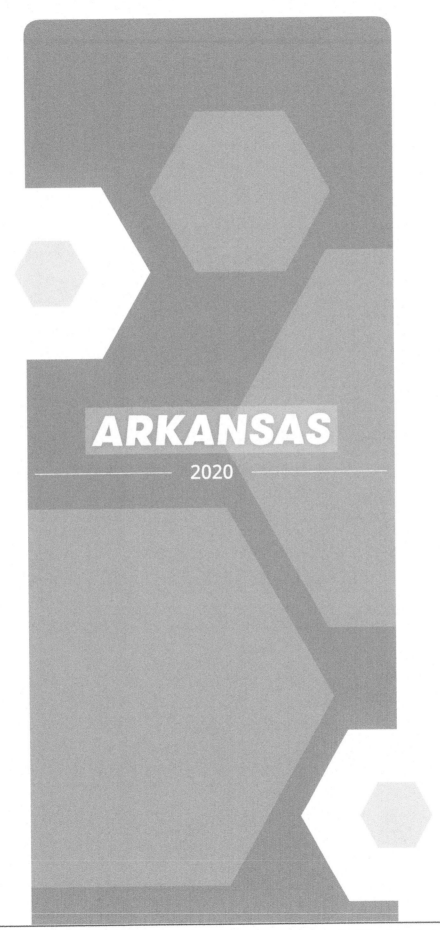

ARKANSAS

2020

Harding University

915 E. Market Ave.
HU Box 12231
Searcy, AR 72149
Phone: 501-279-5642
Email: paprogram@harding.edu

PROGRAM HIGHLIGHTS

Accreditation: Continuing
Degree Offered: Master (MSPAS)
Start Date: August annually
Program Length: 28 months
Class Capacity: 36 students
Tuition: $94,521

CASPA Participant: Yes
Supplemental Application: Yes ($50 fee)
Yellow Ribbon: No
Admissions: Rolling
Application Deadline: November 1

PREREQUISITE COURSEWORK

General Chemistry I and II with labs (8 credits), Organic Chemistry or Biochemistry (3 credits), Microbiology with lab (4 credits), Human Anatomy with lab (4 credits), Human Physiology with lab (4 credits), College Algebra or Precalculus or Calculus or Statistics (3 credits), General or Developmental Psychology (3 credits), Psychology elective (3 credits), Upper Level Biology (3 credits), Medical Terminology (1-3 credits). Only one prerequisite may be left for completion during the spring semester (winter quarter) prior to the program start date the following fall. It is strongly recommended that coursework in Anatomy and Physiology and Microbiology be completed within 7 years prior to applying. The Program may consider applications with a Cumulative Undergraduate GPA below the required 3.0 if it is clear, based on review of the application, that there is strong evidence that the applicant has demonstrated current academic success. This will generally be based on the GPA for the last forty hours of academic work, the academic load being carried, and the level of coursework taken.

GPA Requirement: Overall GPA 3.0; Prerequisite GPA 3.0

Healthcare Experience: 100 hours (strongly recommended)

PA Shadowing: 20 hours (recommended, not required)

Required Standardized Testing: GRE

Letters of Recommendation: Three required; one professional, one academic, one that is not personal recommended

Seat Deposit: $500

HARDING UNIVERSITY

MISSION:

To develop caring physician assistants who practice competent, patient-centered primary care in diverse environments.

CLASS OF 2021

Overall GPA: 3.50

Prerequisite GPA: 3.57

Average Healthcare Experience: 2,172 hours

Average Age: 24

PANCE SCORES

5-year First Time Pass: 95%

Most Recent First Time Pass: 85%

CURRICULUM STRUCTURE

Didactic: 12 months

Clinical: 16 months

Rotations: 6 mandatory, 2 elective, 1 preceptorship (each 6 weeks)

Master's Project: Required for graduation

UNIQUE PROGRAM FEATURES

Christian Faith: The University has strong Christian values and teaches physician assistants who practice within a framework of dependence on God and faith. It also includes a course in Christian Bioethics.

Mission Trip: Each year during spring break, Harding University PA students are invited to participate in a mission trip that is organized through Health Talents International (HTI), a Christian faith-based organization affiliated with the Churches of Christ. During this week-long trip, the students work with licensed health care providers to provide primary health care to the descendants of the Mayan civilization in Guatemala.

University of Arkansas

4301 W. Markham St.
Slot 772
Little Rock, AR 72205
Phone: 501-686-7211
Email: paprogram@uams.edu

PROGRAM HIGHLIGHTS

Accreditation: Continuing

Degree Offered: Master (MPAS)

Start Date: May annually

Program Length: 28 months

Class Capacity: 40 students

Tuition: $44,100 (in-state);
$73,500 (out-of-state)

CASPA Participant: Yes

Supplemental Application: Yes ($40 fee)

Yellow Ribbon: No

Admissions: Rolling

Application Deadline: November 1

PREREQUISITE COURSEWORK

General Biology I and II with lab (8 credits), Human Anatomy with lab (4 credits), Human Physiology with lab (4 credits), Microbiology with lab (4 credits), Medical Genetics (3 credits), General Chemistry I and II with lab (8 credits), Organic Chemistry I with lab (4 credits), General Psychology (3 credits), Biostatistics or Statistics (3 credits). Up to two prerequisites may be outstanding at the time of application. Prerequisites must be completed with a grade "C" or better. Anatomy, Physiology, and Microbiology must have been completed in the last 7 years. AP credits are not accepted. Recommended courses: Medical Terminology, Sociology, Pathophysiology, Embryology, Immunology, Histology, Endocrinology, Bacteriology/Virology, Neuroscience, Cell Biology, Organic Chemistry II, Medical Ethics, Speech.

GPA Requirement: Overall GPA 3.0; Science GPA 3.0

Healthcare Experience: 500 hours

PA Shadowing: Preferred, not required

Required Standardized Testing: GRE

Letters of Recommendation: Three required; one from a physician or PA, one from a university/college professor, and one from a supervisor

Seat Deposit: $300

UNIVERSITY OF ARKANSAS

MISSION:

The mission of the UAMS PA program is to produce PA graduates who will practice transformative patient- and family-centered care with the highest professional standards in any community by: (1) Embracing cultural diversity; (2) Collaborating effectively with all members of the healthcare team; and (3) Contributing to the PA profession through leadership, education, and service.

CLASS OF 2021

Male: 43%

Female: 70%

Minority: 37%

Overall GPA: 3.69

Science GPA: 3.63

GRE Total: 303

Average Healthcare Experience: 4,625 hours

Average Age: 24

PANCE SCORES

5-year First Time Pass: 92%

Most Recent First Time Pass: 89%

CURRICULUM STRUCTURE

Didactic: 13 months

Clinical: 15 months

Rotations: 10 mandatory, 2 elective (each 3-5 weeks)

Capstone Project: Required for graduation

UNIQUE PROGRAM FEATURES

Service Learning: The didactic phase includes a required service-learning component across the lifespan of geriatrics, pediatrics, and adults. This is approximately 10 hours per semester.

Facilities: The program has state-of-the-art facilities including lecture halls, small group spaces, a physical exam laboratory, a clinical skills laboratory, and a simulation center.

Admissions Preference: During admission review, first consideration is given to Arkansas residents.

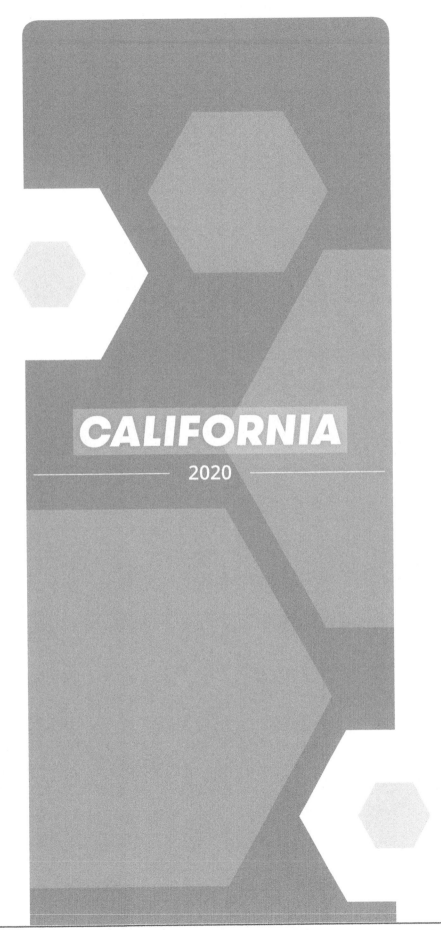

CALIFORNIA
2020

California Baptist University

8432 Magnolia Avenue
Riverside, CA 92504
Phone: 951-552-8515
Email: paprogram@calbaptist.edu

PROGRAM HIGHLIGHTS

Accreditation: Provisional

Degree Offered: Master (MSPAS)

Start Date: September annually

Program Length: 24 months

Class Capacity: 30 students

Tuition: $97,380

CASPA Participant: Yes

Supplemental Application: Yes

Yellow Ribbon: Yes

Admissions: Rolling

Application Deadline: December 1

PREREQUISITE COURSEWORK

Anatomy and Physiology with lab (8 credits), General Chemistry with lab or a combination of Organic, Inorganic and Biochemistry (8-12 credits), Microbiology with lab (3-4 credits), Genetics (2-3 credits), Psychology (3-4 credits), Mathematics (3 credits), English/Writing (6-8 credits), Social Sciences/Humanities (9 credits). Prerequisites must be completed with a grade "C" or better. Science courses taken within the past 5-7 years are recommended. Recommended courses: Biochemistry, Molecular Biology, Statistics, Medical Terminology.

GPA Requirement: Overall GPA 3.2; Science GPA 3.0; Prerequisite GPA 3.0

Healthcare Experience: 1,000 hours

PA Shadowing: Preferred, not required

Required Standardized Testing: None

Letters of Recommendation: Three required; from any of the following: professor, a medical colleague, a supervisor or clergy

Seat Deposit: $500

CALIFORNIA BAPTIST UNIVERSITY

MISSION:

CBU's physician assistant program will prepare graduates who are globally minded and academically prepared to provide quality health care in their communities and to underserved populations.

NO CLASS STATISTICS REPORTED

PANCE SCORES

5-year First Time Pass: 93% (based on one year of data)

Most Recent First Time Pass: 93%

CURRICULUM STRUCTURE

Didactic: 12 months

Clinical: 12 months

Rotations: 8 mandatory, 1 elective (each 5 weeks)

UNIQUE PROGRAM FEATURES

Admissions Preference: The program gives preference to CBU graduates, those with an interest in serving the Inland Empire and shortage areas in California, those with shadowing experience, those with volunteer service, those with global health involvement, and those from underrepresented/underserved populations.

Interviews: Students must pass a basic math and English assessment during the interview process to be considered for admission.

Humanitarian Service: Students engage in humanitarian services through neighborhood outreaches, screening and education at health fairs, required community service hours and serving diverse ethnicities, populations and those with special needs and abilities. Students are given opportunities to see patients alongside the faculty on mobile health units that travel into low socio-economic and underserved areas.

Interprofessional Education: Students from nursing, public health, psychology, athletic training and the PA program take a series of interprofessional seminars together during didactic training.

California State University – Monterey Bay

1450 N. Main Street
Salinas, CA 93906
Phone: 831-772-7070
Email: mspa@csumb.edu

PROGRAM HIGHLIGHTS

Accreditation: Provisional

Degree Offered: Master (MSPA)

Start Date: January annually

Program Length: 28 months

Class Capacity: 33 students

Tuition: $89,498

CASPA Participant: Yes

Supplemental Application: No

Yellow Ribbon: No

Admissions: Rolling

Application Deadline: September 1

PREREQUISITE COURSEWORK

General Biology with lab (8 credits), General Chemistry with lab (8 credits), Microbiology with lab (4 credits), Human Anatomy with lab (4 credits), Human Physiology with lab (4 credits), Statistics (3 credits), English Composition (3 credits), Spanish Language (6 credits or placement exam). All prerequisite coursework is expected to be completed at the time of the application and within 7 years of the application deadline.

GPA Requirement: Overall GPA 3.0; Science GPA 3.0

Healthcare Experience: 1,000 hours

PA Shadowing: 8 hours

Required Standardized Testing: None

Letters of Recommendation: Two required; one should be from PA, NP, MD or DO

Seat Deposit: $100

CALIFORNIA STATE UNIVERSITY - MONTEREY BAY

MISSION:

The mission of the CSUMB Master of Science Physician Assistant program is to train highly-qualified, culturally-resonant, medical providers to serve the health needs of underserved communities.

CLASS OF 2021

Male: 35%

Female: 65%

Overall GPA: 3.43

Science GPA 3.29

Average Healthcare Experience: 5,724 hours

Average Shadowing Experience: 154 hours

Average Volunteer Experience: 1,384 hours

Average Age: 27

PANCE SCORES

5-year First Time Pass: N/A

Most Recent First Time Pass: N/A (have not graduated a class yet)

CURRICULUM STRUCTURE

Didactic: 12 months

Clinical: 16 months

Rotations: 9 mandatory, 1 selective (each 4 weeks)

Graduate Project: Required for graduation

UNIQUE PROGRAM FEATURES

Admissions Preference: Applicants are expected to have 500 hours of community service experience which benefits underserved or disadvantaged populations.

Hybrid Semester: The final hybrid semester includes clinical, didactic, and professional components, and the graduate project. The students will be in clinic on Mondays and Tuesdays and in the classroom Wednesday through Friday.

Medical Spanish: Students take 3 semesters of conversational Spanish during didactic year.

Mission in Practice: This course during didactic year provides students with opportunities to learn about the needs of the local community through service learning and reflection. Potential activities include conducting inter-professional health fairs, mobile rural clinics, and volunteering in homeless communities at a soup kitchen or local shelter.

PROGRAM HIGHLIGHTS

Accreditation: Provisional

Degree Offered: Master (MMS)

Start Date: January annually

Program Length: 24 months

Class Capacity: 50 students

Tuition: $111,200

CASPA Participant: Yes

Supplemental Application: No

Yellow Ribbon: Yes

Admissions: Rolling

Application Deadline: September 1

PREREQUISITE COURSEWORK

Human Anatomy and Physiology I and II with lab (8 credits), General Chemistry I and II with lab (8 credits), General Biology I and II with lab (8 credits), Microbiology with lab (4 credits), Genetics (2 credits), Medical Terminology (1 credit), English Composition (3 credits), General Psychology (3 credits), Intro to Sociology (3 credits), Intro to Statistics (3 credits), Pre-Calculus or Calculus (3 credits). Prerequisites must be completed with a grade "C" or better. AP credits may be accepted for the Pre-calculus or Calculus, Intro to Statistics, General Psychology, English Composition and Intro to Sociology requirements only. Recommended courses: Medical Ethics, Medical Spanish.

GPA Requirement: Overall GPA 3.2; Science GPA 3.2

Healthcare Experience: 1,000 hours

PA Shadowing: Preferred, not required

Required Standardized Testing: GRE

Letters of Recommendation: Three required; one from a PA or MD/DO

Seat Deposit: $1,000

CHAPMAN UNIVERSITY

MISSION:

The mission of the Chapman University MMS PA Studies Program is to provide a personalized, exceptional medical education that inspires compassionate, collaborative, and analytical health care providers who enhance access to high quality care in the community.

CLASS OF 2019

Overall GPA: 3.56

Science GPA: 3.47

GRE Total: 307

Average Healthcare Experience: 2,734 hours

PANCE SCORES

5-year First Time Pass: 92% (based on one year of data)

Most Recent First Time Pass: 92%

CURRICULUM STRUCTURE

Didactic: 12 months

Clinical: 12 months

Rotations: 8 mandatory, 1 elective (each 5 weeks)

Graduate Project: Required for graduation

UNIQUE PROGRAM FEATURES

Bridge Program: Undergraduate Health Science students at Chapman who maintain certain academic criteria are guaranteed an interview and preferential consideration for admission into the program.

Facilities: The PA Program is housed within the state-of-the-art Rinker Health Science Campus, which includes student common areas, exam simulation suites, an anatomy laboratory, two neuromuscular laboratories, and a neurology laboratory.

Scholarships: The program awards a limited number of merit-based scholarships to incoming students who have excelled in the following categories: Academics; Community Service/Volunteerism; Leadership; Diverse Educational and Life Experiences. Scholarships are awarded for one academic year only and are renewable each academic year as long as the scholarship renewal criteria are met.

Charles R. Drew University

1731 E. 120th Street
Los Angeles, CA 90059
Phone: 323-563-4880
Email: admissionsinfo@cdrewu.edu

PROGRAM HIGHLIGHTS

Accreditation: Provisional

Degree Offered: Master (MHS)

Start Date: August annually

Program Length: 27 months

Class Capacity: 26 students

Tuition: $100,324 (including fees)

CASPA Participant: Yes

Supplemental Application: No

Yellow Ribbon: Yes

Admissions: Rolling

Application Deadline: January 15

PREREQUISITE COURSEWORK

General Biology with lab (8 credits), Microbiology with lab (4 credits), Human Anatomy with lab (4 credits), Human Physiology with lab (4 credits), General Chemistry with lab (8 credits), Introduction to Statistics or Biostatistics (3 credits), College Algebra or Higher (3 credits), English Composition (6 credits), Behavioral Sciences (6 credits), Medical Terminology (3 credits). Prerequisites must be completed by May 30th prior to matriculation in August, no more than two can be pending at the time of application, and they should be completed within the last 7 years. Recommended courses: Nutrition, Organic or Biochemistry, Spanish.

GPA Requirement: No minimum (Science and Prerequisite GPAs of 3.0 are preferred)

Healthcare Experience: 2,000 hours (preferred)

PA Shadowing: Preferred, not required

Required Standardized Testing: None

Letters of Recommendation: Three required; no one specific

Seat Deposit: $500

CHARLES R. DREW UNIVERSITY

MISSION:

The mission of the Charles R. Drew University Physician Assistant Program is to support the University Mission and College of Science & Health Mission by preparing a diverse group of uniquely qualified physician assistants who provide excellent medical care with compassion while addressing health disparities, seeking social justice and improving the health of medically underserved communities.

CLASS OF 2020

Science GPA: 3.50

Faculty to Student Ratio: 15:1

Average Healthcare Experience: 5,800 hours

Age Range: 23-33

PANCE SCORES

5-year First Time Pass: 86% (based on one year of data)

Most Recent First Time Pass: 86%

CURRICULUM STRUCTURE

Didactic: 15 months (3 months completed after clinicals)

Clinical: 12 months

Rotations: 7 mandatory, 2 elective (each 4 weeks)

UNIQUE PROGRAM FEATURES

Medical Nutrition: Students complete a medical nutrition therapy course, which provides them with knowledge to manage enteral and parenteral nutrition from pediatrics to geriatrics and allows students to sit for the Certified Nutrition Support Certification Exam and become a Certified Nutrition Support Clinician.

Special Certifications: Students can take seminars to become Certified Diabetes Self-Management Leaders and Certified in Culturally Relevant Urban Trauma.

Social Medicine: The program integrates Social Medicine longitudinally throughout the 27-month master's program, highlighting psychosocial aspects of health and wellbeing. This knowledge is then translated to the community service opportunities at local high schools, in mobile HIV/AIDS testing and outreach, and at farmer's markets, among others.

PROGRAM HIGHLIGHTS

Accreditation: Provisional

Degree Offered: Master (MSPAS)

Start Date: August annually

Program Length: 28 months

Class Capacity: 30 students

Tuition: $107,154 (including fees)

CASPA Participant: Yes

Supplemental Application: No

Yellow Ribbon: Yes

Admissions: Rolling

Application Deadline: November 1

PREREQUISITE COURSEWORK

Biological Sciences with lab (8 credits), Chemistry with lab (8 credits), Human Anatomy with lab (4 credits), Human Physiology with lab (4 credits), Microbiology with lab (4 credits), College Algebra or Higher (3 credits), Statistics (3 credits), General Psychology (3 credits). Anatomy and Physiology must have been taken in the last 10 years. Prerequisites must be completed with a grade "B" or better. Recommended courses: Spanish, Organic Chemistry, Physics, Biochemistry, Medical Terminology, Medical Microbiology, Pharmacology.

GPA Requirement: Overall GPA 3.0; Science GPA 3.0 (last 30 hours)

Healthcare Experience: 500 hours

PA Shadowing: 8 hours

Required Standardized Testing: None

Letters of Recommendation: Three required; one from a PA or NP, MD or DO, or PhD, one from an employer/supervisor, and one from a professor

Seat Deposit: $500

DOMINICAN UNIVERSITY OF CALIFORNIA

MISSION:

The mission of the Dominican University of California Master of Science Physician Assistant Studies (MSPAS) Program is to provide an excellent, interactive learning environment to prepare PAs to provide compassionate, high quality, patient-centered care as members of interdisciplinary healthcare teams. Graduates will be culturally competent, committed to lifelong learning and their professional development. They will be prepared to make significant contributions to the diverse communities that they serve and to the advancement of the PA profession.

NO CLASS STATISTICS REPORTED

PANCE SCORES

5-year First Time Pass: 100% (based on one year of data)

Most Recent First Time Pass: 100%

CURRICULUM STRUCTURE

Didactic: 15 months

Clinical: 13 months

Rotations: 7 mandatory, 2 elective (each 5 weeks)

Capstone Project: Required for graduation

UNIQUE PROGRAM FEATURES

Simulation: The program boasts extensive use of high fidelity medical simulation technology throughout the curriculum.

Continuity Clinic: Students start seeing patients in clinic in the 2nd semester of didactic year.

Admissions Preference: Preference will be given to those who additionally have one or more of the following: Overall and last 30 Science GPA of ≥ 3.50, veteran status, Emergency Medical Tech (EMT) or Paramedic certification, experience as a medical technician in the military, a job in healthcare with direct patient contact or extensive experience with direct patient care, a degree from Dominican University of CA (DUOC), a SES disadvantaged background, residence in a medically-underserved geographic catchment area or residence in a county with geographic proximity to DUOC, foreign language fluency, esp. Spanish, and PA shadowing more hours than required or in multiple settings. In addition, preference is also given to those who have performed volunteer work and completed recommended coursework.

Loma Linda University

24785 Stewart Street
Evans Hall Room 201F
Loma Linda, CA 92350
Phone: 909-558-7295
Email: pa@llu.edu

PROGRAM HIGHLIGHTS

Accreditation: Continuing

Degree Offered: Master (MPA)

Start Date: September annually

Program Length: 24 months

Class Capacity: 36 students

Tuition: $98,476 (including fees)

CASPA Participant: Yes

Supplemental Application: Yes (no fee)

Yellow Ribbon: No

Admissions: Rolling

Application Deadline: October 1

PREREQUISITE COURSEWORK

Human Anatomy and Physiology with lab (8 credits), General Chemistry with lab or a sequence in Inorganic, Organic, and Biochemistry with lab (8 credits), General Microbiology with lab (4 credits), General Psychology, General Sociology or Cultural Anthropology, College-level Algebra or equivalent, English (1 year). A maximum of two total prerequisites may be outstanding at the time of application, with only one science prerequisite outstanding. Prerequisites must be completed with a grade "C" or better. Recommended courses: Statistics, Medical Terminology, Conversational Spanish.

GPA Requirement: Overall GPA 3.0; Science GPA 3.0

Healthcare Experience: 2,000 hours

PA Shadowing: Not required

Required Standardized Testing: None

Letters of Recommendation: Three required; one must be from a currently practicing MD, DO or PA with whom the applicant has worked in a paid patient care position

Seat Deposit: $500

LOMA LINDA UNIVERSITY

MISSION:

The Loma Linda University Department of Physician Assistant Sciences educates primary care physician assistants who will complement the work of physicians by providing health care as active members of a professional healthcare team, excellence and compassion in health care for the whole person, and quality health care for underserved individuals and communities nationally and globally in accordance with the mission of Loma Linda University and the School of Allied Health Professions.

CLASS OF 2020

Male: 53%

Female: 47%

Overall GPA: 3.55

Average Age: 27

PANCE SCORES

5-year First Time Pass: 94%

Most Recent First Time Pass: 97%

CURRICULUM STRUCTURE

Didactic: 12 months

Clinical: 12 months

Rotations: 7 mandatory, 1 elective (each 6 weeks)

Capstone Project: Required for graduation

UNIQUE PROGRAM FEATURES

Primary Care Focus: This program has a primary care focus and specifically, a focus on caring for the underserved.

International Rotations: Currently the program has rotation sites in Honduras, Nepal and Malawi with more sites in development.

Admissions Preference: The program gives preference to Seventh-day Adventists, graduates of Loma Linda, applicants of under-represented populations, applicants with a history of meaningful, continuous involvement in community service, and applicants with current or previous documented military service.

Marshall B. Ketchum University

2575 Yorba Linda Boulevard
Fullerton, CA 92831
Phone: 714-992-7808
Email: PAadmissions@ketchum.edu

PROGRAM HIGHLIGHTS

Accreditation: Continuing

Degree Offered: Master (MMS)

Start Date: August annually

Program Length: 27 months

Class Capacity: 40 students

Tuition: $109,573 (including fees)

CASPA Participant: Yes

Supplemental Application:
Yes ($75 fee)

Yellow Ribbon: No

Admissions: Non-rolling

Application Deadline: November 1

PREREQUISITE COURSEWORK

Biological Sciences, Microbiology with lab, Human Anatomy with lab, Human Physiology with lab, Biochemistry or Organic Chemistry (3 credits), Genetics (3 credits), Statistics (3 credits), General Psychology (3 credits). Two prerequisites may be in progress at the time of application but must be completed by the end of the fall semester of the year prior to matriculation. Prerequisites must be completed with a grade "C" or better. AP credits are accepted for Psychology and Statistics requirements.

GPA Requirement: Overall GPA 3.0; Science GPA 3.0; Last 60 Credit GPA 3.0

Healthcare Experience: 1,000 hours

PA Shadowing: Not required

Required Standardized Testing: None

Letters of Recommendation: Three required; no one specific

Seat Deposit: $1,500

MARSHALL B. KETCHUM UNIVERSITY

MISSION:

Mission: The School of PA Studies' mission is to educate individuals to become compassionate Physician Assistants who provide the highest quality health care in a collaborative environment, are dedicated to their communities, and advance the PA profession.

CLASS OF 2021

Male: 35%

Female: 65%

Overall GPA: 3.55

Science GPA: 3.49

Last 60 Credit GPA: 3.71

Average Healthcare Experience: 9,224 hours

Average age: 27

PANCE SCORES

5-year First Time Pass: 100% (based on four years of data)

Most Recent First Time Pass: 100%

CURRICULUM STRUCTURE

Didactic: 12 months

Clinical: 15 months

Rotations: 7 mandatory, 1 elective (each 6 weeks)

Capstone Project: Required for graduation

UNIQUE PROGRAM FEATURES

Medical Spanish: An elective in medical Spanish is available for interested students.

Interprofessional Education: PA students at Marshall B. Ketchum interact with Optometry and Pharmacy students throughout the curriculum in working on clinical cases and completing coursework in ethics, population health, and public health.

Community Service: The program's students actively engage in community service including health fairs, food banks, professional outreach and elementary school education.

Admissions Preference: Preference is given to military veterans, community service volunteers, and those completing a pre-health professions linkage program from California State University.

Samuel Merritt University

Department of Admissions
3100 Telegraph Avenue
Oakland, CA 94609
Phone: 510-879-0335
Email: deaglin@samuelmerritt.edu

PROGRAM HIGHLIGHTS

Accreditation: Probation

Degree Offered: Master (MPA)

Start Date: September annually

Program Length: 27 months

Class Capacity: 44 students

Tuition: $104,434

CASPA Participant: Yes

Supplemental Application: No

Yellow Ribbon: Yes

Admissions: Non-rolling

Application Deadline: October 1

PREREQUISITE COURSEWORK

Microbiology (4 credits), Human Anatomy (4 credits), Human Physiology (4 credits), Biology elective (4 credits), Statistics (3 credits), Inorganic/General Chemistry (4 credits), Organic Chemistry or General Chemistry II (4 credits). Preference is given to those who have completed courses in the last 5 years. Prerequisites must be completed with a grade "C" or better and completed at the time of application.

GPA Requirement: Overall GPA 3.0; Science GPA 3.0

Healthcare Experience: 1,000 hours

PA Shadowing: 50 hours

Required Standardized Testing: None

Letters of Recommendation: Three required; one from a PA and other references from healthcare providers who have directly supervised the candidate and can comment on how the applicant's work reflects the core values of the program

Seat Deposit: $350

SAMUEL MERRITT UNIVERSITY

MISSION:

The Master Physician Assistant Department at Samuel Merritt University strives to serve the University and the medical community by preparing graduates who are interdependent medical providers, demonstrate commitment to the community and the profession through active leadership, manifest critical and creative thinking, utilize effective communication skills, and who possess the educational foundation for continued growth and development in a changing world of diverse cultures.

CLASS OF 2020

Overall GPA Range:
3.20 - 3.48

Science GPA Range:
3.09 - 3.47

PANCE SCORES

5-year First Time Pass:
90%

Most Recent First Time Pass: 78%

CURRICULUM STRUCTURE

Didactic: 15 months

Clinical: 12 months

Rotations: 7 mandatory, 2 elective (each 4 weeks)

UNIQUE PROGRAM FEATURES

Medical Simulation: The program makes extensive use of high fidelity medical simulation technology and manikins throughout the didactic and clinical curriculum.

International Rotations: International rotations are available to students, as are rotations where students can participate in community health with underserved patients in the San Francisco Bay Area. There are faculty led medical trips to Panama twice yearly.

Community Service: There are many opportunities for community service, one of which is mentoring high school students in the FACES of Future Coalition.

Program Expansion: The program intends to expand to SMU's Fresno campus in the coming years with an additional 25 students.

Southern California University of Health Sciences

16200 Amber Valley Drive
Whittier, CA 90604
Phone: 562-947-8755
Email: mspa@scuhs.edu

PROGRAM HIGHLIGHTS

Accreditation: Provisional

Degree Offered: Master (MSPA)

Start Date: September annually

Program Length: 28 months

Class Capacity: 50 students

Tuition: $104,702 (including fees)

CASPA Participant: Yes

Supplemental Application: No

Yellow Ribbon: No

Admissions: Non-rolling

Application Deadline: January 15

PREREQUISITE COURSEWORK

Chemistry with lab (8 credits), Human Anatomy with lab (4 credits), Human Physiology with lab (4 credits), Microbiology with lab (4 credits), Mathematics (2 credits), Psychology (3 credits), English Composition (3 credits), Sociology or Cultural Anthropology (3 credits), Statistics (3 credits). Prerequisites must be completed by January 15th of the year of matriculation and within the last 7 years. Recommended courses: Medical Terminology, Conversational Spanish.

GPA Requirement: Overall GPA 3.0; Science GPA 3.0

Healthcare Experience: 2,000 hours

PA Shadowing: Not required

Required Standardized Testing: None

Letters of Recommendation: Two required; one academic and one professional letter

Seat Deposit: $1,000

SOUTHERN CALIFORNIA UNIVERSITY OF HEALTH SCIENCES

MISSION:

SCU's Master of Science Physician Assistant program will educate students to become skilled clinical providers for quality integrative healthcare teams. In today's ever-changing healthcare system, our graduates will strive to provide premium healthcare to a diverse population and establish their place as innovative leaders in the delivery of healthcare.

CLASS OF 2020

Male: 39%

Female: 61%

Overall GPA: 3.44

Average Healthcare Experience: 6,961 hours

Average Age: 28

PANCE SCORES

5-year First Time Pass: 84% (based on one year of data)

Most Recent First Time Pass: 84%

CURRICULUM STRUCTURE

Didactic: 16 months

Clinical: 12 months

Rotations: 8 mandatory, 2 elective (each 4-8 weeks)

Capstone: Required for graduation

UNIQUE PROGRAM FEATURES

Integrative Medicine: During core classes, MSPA students study alongside aspiring chiropractors and acupuncturists, creating a rich, vibrant learning environment that emphasizes holistic, interdisciplinary care. Students also complete an integrative medicine rotation.

Technology: IPads are used throughout the curriculum for curriculum delivery and examinations. Students are required to purchase one prior to starting the program.

PROGRAM HIGHLIGHTS

Accreditation: Continuing

Degree Offered: Master (MSPA)

Start Date: August annually

Program Length: 30 months

Class Capacity: 27 students

Tuition: $157,437

CASPA Participant: Yes

Supplemental Application:
Yes (no fee)

Yellow Ribbon: No

Admissions: Rolling

Application Deadline: August 1

PREREQUISITE COURSEWORK

Anatomy (4 credits), Physiology
(4 credits), Chemistry (4 credits),
General Statistics or Biostatistics,
Psychology, 3 upper level science
courses. Courses should be
completed in the last 10 years
and ideally prior to application.
Recommended courses: Human
Biology, Molecular Biology, Cell
Biology, Genetics, Immunology,
Neuroscience, Embryology,
Histology, Microbiology,
Pharmacology, Medical
Terminology.

GPA Requirement: No minimum

Healthcare Experience: 500 hours

PA Shadowing: Not required

Required Standardized Testing: GRE
or MCAT or PA-CAT, Casper

Letters of Recommendation:
Three required; prior employers,
professional colleagues, and
academic advisors are acceptable
references

Seat Deposit: $1,000

STANFORD UNIVERSITY

MISSION:

The Stanford University Master of Science Degree in Physician Assistant Studies Program's mission is to educate and train compassionate and diverse PAs who can provide high-quality patient-centered care, who are dedicated to improving access to healthcare for underserved communities, and who are inspired to become leaders in healthcare, research, and medical education.

CLASS OF 2020 AND 2021

Male: 13%

Female: 87%

Minority: 35%

Overall GPA: 3.66

Science GPA: 3.60

GRE Verbal: 72nd percentile

GRE Quantitative: 80th percentile

GRE Analytical: 76th percentile

Average Healthcare Experience: 3,064 hours

Average Age: 26

PANCE SCORES

5-year First Time Pass: 93%*

Most Recent First Time Pass: 100%*

*Scores from the old 21-month program. The first class of the 30 month program will graduate in 2020.

CURRICULUM STRUCTURE

Didactic: 18 months (including summer break)

Clinical: 12 months

Rotations: 9 mandatory, 3 elective (each 4 weeks)

Capstone Project: Required for graduation

UNIQUE PROGRAM FEATURES

Curriculum: PA students complete some courses with medical students. Students have access to a clinical anatomy lab, academic mentorship, and the Center for Immersive and Simulation-Based Learning.

Admission Factors: The program uses a holistic approach to admissions, selecting students based on academics (40%), health care experience and scholarship (20%), interpersonal and communication skills (10%), community service (10%), supporting materials (10%), and leadership potential (10%).

Capstone Project: Students choose an area of concentration (community health, health services and policy research, clinical research, or medical education) for which they complete extra coursework and their research project.

E4C-PAs: Educators-4-Care-PAs are a special group of clinically practicing PAs within the Stanford health care system who actively serve as teachers and mentors for PA students throughout the program.

PROGRAM HIGHLIGHTS

Accreditation: Continuing

Degree Offered: Master (MSPAS, MPH)

Start Date: August annually

Program Length: 33 months

Class Capacity: 48 students

Tuition: $133,136

CASPA Participant: Yes

Supplemental Application: Yes ($50 fee)

Yellow Ribbon: Yes

Admissions: Rolling

Application Deadline: November 1

PREREQUISITE COURSEWORK

Biological Sciences with lab (8 credits), Chemistry with lab (8 credits), Human Anatomy with lab (4 credits), Human Physiology with lab (4 credits), Microbiology with lab (4 credits), Statistics (3 credits). Anatomy and Physiology must be completed within 5 years of expected matriculation and all courses must be completed at the time of application. Prerequisites must be completed with a grade "C" or better. When reviewing applications, the Committee will focus primarily, though not exclusively, on the most recent 30 units of coursework. AP credits are accepted if listed on your undergraduate transcript.

GPA Requirement: Overall GPA 3.0; Science GPA 3.0

Healthcare Experience: 1,000 hours

PA Shadowing: 20 hours or more (preferred)

Required Standardized Testing: None

Letters of Recommendation: Three required; one from a clinician

Seat Deposit: $1,000

TOURO UNIVERSITY - CALIFORNIA

MISSION:

Through the integration of the Physician Assistant and Public Health disciplines, the mission of the Joint MSPAS/MPH Program is to: 1) Train quality PAs to work with underserved populations, 2) Recruit applicants from these communities or individuals with a demonstrated interest in serving these communities, and 3) Increase access to care for underserved populations.

CLASS OF 2021

Male: 27%

Female: 73%

Minority: 65%

Overall GPA: 3.32

Science GPA: 3.22

Average Age: 26

PANCE SCORES

5-year First Time Pass: 99%

Most Recent First Time Pass: 98%

CURRICULUM STRUCTURE

Didactic: 16.5 months

Clinical: 16.5 months (including MPH fieldwork)

Rotations: 6 mandatory, 2 elective (each 6 weeks)

MPH Capstone: Required for graduation

UNIQUE PROGRAM FEATURES

Dual Degree: All students complete a dual MSPAS/MPH degree program integrating clinical medicine and population health. This is the only program that mandates a dual degree for all PA students.

University of California-Davis

Betty Irene Moor Hall
2570 48th Street
Sacramento, CA 95817
Phone: 916-734-2145
Email:
hs-BettyIreneMooreSON@ucdavis.edu

PROGRAM HIGHLIGHTS

Accreditation: Continuing

Degree Offered: Master (MHS)

Start Date: June annually

Program Length: 27 months

Class Capacity: 65 students

Tuition: $134,990

CASPA Participant: Yes

Supplemental Application: Yes ($105 fee)

Yellow Ribbon: No

Admissions: Non-rolling

Application Deadline: July 15

PREREQUISITE COURSEWORK

Human Anatomy with lab (1 course), Human Physiology with lab (1 course), Chemistry with lab (1 course), Microbiology or Bacteriology with lab (1 course), English Composition (1 course), Social Sciences (2 courses). All must be completed at the time of application and it is desired that Anatomy and Physiology be completed in the last 5 years. Prerequisites must be completed with a grade "C" or better. AP credits are not accepted.

GPA Requirement: Overall GPA 3.0; Science GPA 2.7

Healthcare Experience: 1,000 hours

PA Shadowing: Not required

Required Standardized Testing: None

Letters of Recommendation: Three required; no one specific

Seat Deposit: None

UNIVERSITY OF CALIFORNIA - DAVIS

MISSION:

The mission of the Physician Assistant Program (PA) is to educate health care professionals to deliver care as a member of a healthcare team and to improve the availability of culturally relevant primary health care in underserved populations throughout California.

NO CLASS STATISTICS REPORTED

PANCE SCORES

5-year First Time Pass: 88%

Most Recent First Time Pass: 90%

CURRICULUM STRUCTURE

Didactic: 12 months

Clinical: 15 months (integrated with didactic coursework as well)

Rotations: 9 mandatory, 1 elective (duration not specified)

Master's Thesis: Required for graduation

UNIQUE PROGRAM FEATURES

Interprofessional Education: This is the only program that combines both PA and NP students in the same classroom for the didactic curriculum and includes both the medical school model and nursing model of education blended throughout. Students are exposed to case-based learning and medical simulation.

Primary Care Focus: The program focuses on primary care and encourages graduates to work in primary care, underserved areas, and health professional shortage areas.

Early Clinical Experience: Students begin clinical exposure in the first quarter of studies and work with nursing students and medical students to provide care through the UC Davis Student-Run Clinics.

60

University of California-Davis

University of La Verne

1950 Third Street
La Verne, CA 91750
Phone: 909-448-1475
Email: paprogram@laverne.edu

PROGRAM HIGHLIGHTS

Accreditation: Provisional

Degree Offered: Master (MSPAP)

Start Date: August annually

Program Length: 27 months

Class Capacity: 30 students

Tuition: $100,908

CASPA Participant: Yes

Supplemental Application: No

Yellow Ribbon: Yes

Admissions: Non-rolling

Application Deadline: October 1

PREREQUISITE COURSEWORK

Human Anatomy with lab (4 credits), Human Physiology with lab (4 credits), General Biology with lab (4 credits), General Chemistry I and II with lab (8 credits), Microbiology with lab (3 credits), Psychology (3 credits), Sociology or Anthropology (3 credits), Biostatistics or Statistics (3 credits), Medical Terminology (2 credits), History of Fine Arts (3 credits), Creative and Artistic Expression (3 credits), English/College Writing (6 credits), Speech Communication (2 credits), Philosophy or Religion or Ethics or Critical Thinking (3 credits). All prerequisites must be completed at the time of application and with a grade "C" or better. Human Anatomy and Physiology with lab and Microbiology with lab must have been completed within the last 7 years.

GPA Requirement: Overall GPA 3.0; Science GPA 3.0

Healthcare Experience: Preferred, not required

PA Shadowing: 20 hours

Required Standardized Testing: None

Letters of Recommendation: Three required; one must be from a practicing MD/DO/PA

Seat Deposit: None

UNIVERSITY OF LA VERNE

MISSION:

The mission of the program is to educate diverse, ethical, collaborative and holistic medical providers committed to eliminating health disparities.

NO CLASS STATISTICS REPORTED

PANCE SCORES

5-year First Time Pass: N/A

Most Recent First Time Pass: N/A (have not graduated a class yet)

CURRICULUM STRUCTURE

Didactic: 15 months

Clinical: 12 months

Rotations: 9 mandatory, 1 elective (unspecified duration)

Master's Project: Required for graduation

UNIQUE PROGRAM FEATURES

Admissions Preference: The program will guarantee an interview to veterans, current full-time University of La Verne students, and recent graduates of the university in the last 2 years who meet the admission criteria. The University of La Verne will guarantee an interview to veterans who meet the minimum admission criteria and have applied to the program.

PROGRAM HIGHLIGHTS

Accreditation: Continuing
Degree Offered: Master (MPAP)
Start Date: August annually
Program Length: 33 months
Class Capacity: 60 students
Tuition: $165,960

CASPA Participant: Yes
Supplemental Application: Yes ($50 fee)
Yellow Ribbon: Yes
Admissions: Rolling
Application Deadline: November 1

PREREQUISITE COURSEWORK

General Biology I and II with lab, General Chemistry I and II with lab, Human Anatomy with lab (3 credits), Human Physiology (3 credits), General Microbiology with lab (3 credits), Statistics (3 credits), Introduction to Psychology (3 credits), Spanish (2 semesters), English Composition (2 semesters for international applicants only). All sciences courses must be completed within 10 years of the application deadline and must be completed by the end of the fall semester prior to matriculation. Prerequisites must be completed with a grade "C" or better. AP credits are not accepted. Recommended courses: Medical Terminology.

GPA Requirement: Overall GPA 3.0; Science GPA 2.75

Healthcare Experience: Preferred, not required

PA Shadowing: Preferred, not required

Required Standardized Testing: GRE (295 minimum) or MCAT

Letters of Recommendation: Three required; no one specific

Seat Deposit: $500

UNIVERSITY OF SOUTHERN CALIFORNIA

MISSION:

The Primary Care Physician Assistant Program at USC is dedicated to the advancement of physician assistant education and emphasizes service to the medically underserved. The program is committed to preparing students from diverse backgrounds to practice medicine with physician supervision. Emphasis is placed upon understanding and appreciating diversity. The program aims to prepare its graduates to practice and promote primary health care of the highest quality as part of an interprofessional team.

CLASS OF 2020

Male: 27%

Female: 73%

Minority: 83%

Overall GPA: 3.43

Science GPA: 3.33

GRE Total: 307

MCAT: 504

Average Healthcare Experience: 3,788 hours

Average Community Service: 1,493 hours

PANCE SCORES

5-year First Time Pass: 95%

Most Recent First Time Pass: 86%

CURRICULUM STRUCTURE

Didactic: 12 months preclinical, 4 months post clinical, one summer off

Clinical: 12 months

Rotations: 7 mandatory, 1 elective (duration not specified)

UNIQUE PROGRAM FEATURES

Leadership: The program aims to train PA leaders and has been successful, as graduates have gone on to become members of Congress, President of AAPA and CAPA, as well as various other roles in national and local organizations.

Advocacy Education: Students receive training in advocacy through the Medical Care Organization course and Advanced Topics in Education. Students also volunteer for a program trip to Washington, DC where attendees learn how to advocate for the profession from the AAPA and PAEA staff.

Community Service: Students serve the underserved populations of Los Angeles through student run clinics, food drives, and other initiatives. Evidence of community service is expected of all applicants.

PROGRAM HIGHLIGHTS

Accreditation: Provisional
Degree Offered: Master (MPAS)
Start Date: January annually
Program Length: 27 months
Class Capacity: 45 students
Tuition: $119,252

CASPA Participant: Yes
Supplemental Application: No
Yellow Ribbon: Yes
Admissions: Rolling
Application Deadline: August 1

PREREQUISITE COURSEWORK

General Chemistry with lab (8 credits), Biological Sciences with lab (6 credits), Human Anatomy with lab (4 credits), Human Physiology (4 credits), Microbiology (3 credits), Statistics (3 credits), Psychology (3 credits), English Composition (6 credits). All coursework must be completed prior to submitting your application. AP credits are not accepted.

GPA Requirement: Overall GPA 3.0; Science GPA 3.0

Healthcare Experience: 1,000 hours

PA Shadowing: Preferred, not required

Required Standardized Testing: None

Letters of Recommendation: Two required; no one specific

Seat Deposit: $1,000

UNIVERSITY OF THE PACIFIC

MISSION:

The mission of the Physician Assistant Program at University of the Pacific is to provide students with a superior, learner-centered educational experience that will produce compassionate health care professionals committed to life-long learning and leadership in their careers and communities.

CLASS OF 2021

Male: 25%

Female: 75%

Overall GPA: 3.50

Science GPA: 3.50

Average Healthcare Experience: 4,809 hours

Average Age: 26.1

PANCE SCORES

5-year First Time Pass: 91% (based on one year of data)

Most Recent First Time Pass: 91%

CURRICULUM STRUCTURE

Didactic: 13 months

Clinical: 14 months

Rotations: 9 mandatory, 3 elective (each 4 weeks)

Capstone Project: Required for graduation

UNIQUE PROGRAM FEATURES

Specialty Rotation Pathways: Students can choose from 4 different specialty pathways to complete their 3 elective rotations including emergency medicine, family medicine, surgery, and medicine subspecialties.

Interprofessional Education: The program provides numerous opportunities to interact with students from the school of dentistry, pharmacy and health sciences throughout the curriculum.

Admissions Preference: Some preference is given to veterans, Pacific alumni, and residents of the area.

Photos and Videos: The website has a photo tour of the program and a series of videos aimed to help prospective applicants in applying to the program and preparing for interviews.

**Western University
of Health Sciences**

309 E. Second Street
Pomona, CA 91766
Phone: 909-469-5335
Email: admissions@westernu.edu

PROGRAM HIGHLIGHTS

Accreditation: Continuing

Degree Offered: Master (MSPA)

Start Date: August annually

Program Length: 24 months

Class Capacity: 98 students

Tuition: $88,210

CASPA Participant: Yes

Supplemental Application: Yes ($50 fee)

Yellow Ribbon: No

Admissions: Rolling

Application Deadline: November 1

PREREQUISITE COURSEWORK

College English and English Composition
(6 credits), College Algebra (3 credits),
Human Anatomy and Physiology with
lab (6 credits), Microbiology with lab (3
credits), Genetics (3 credits), Psychology
(3 credits), Sociology (3 credits),
Introductory Statistics (3 credits),
General or Inorganic Chemistry with
lab (6 credits), Humanities (9 credits).
All courses must be completed by the
spring semester prior to matriculation
and no more than one science and non-
science prerequisite may be in progress
after December 31st of the year prior
to matriculation. Science prerequisites
must be completed within 7 years of
the application deadline. Prerequisites
must be completed with a grade "C"
or better. AP credits are not accepted.
Recommended courses: Spanish.

GPA Requirement: Overall GPA 3.0;
Science GPA 3.0; Prerequisite GPA 3.0

Healthcare Experience: Preferred,
not required

PA Shadowing: Preferred, not required

Required Standardized Testing: None

Letters of Recommendation: Two
required; no one specific

Seat Deposit: $1,000

WESTERN UNIVERSITY OF HEALTH SCIENCES

MISSION:

The Department of Physician Assistant Education supports the
University's mission by educating Physician Assistants to deliver
high quality competent and compassionate health care as team
members within the healthcare delivery system.

CLASS OF 2020

Overall GPA: 3.59

Science GPA: 3.55

Prerequisite GPA: 3.72

PANCE SCORES

5-year First Time Pass: 95%

Most Recent First Time Pass: 100%

CURRICULUM STRUCTURE

Didactic: 12 months

Clinical: 12 months

Rotations: 8 mandatory, 3 elective (4 weeks each)

Applied Clinical Project: Required for graduation

UNIQUE PROGRAM FEATURES

Interprofessional Education: PA students complete
case studies with Osteopathic Medicine, PA, Physical
Therapy, Pharmacy, Nursing, Veterinary, Optometry and
Dental students during their didactic curriculum allowing
for collaboration and learning among different healthcare
program students.

Student Experiences: You can read about student
experiences on the program's website under the section
entitled "Testimonials".

Western U Patient Care Center: PA students volunteer
here to provide care working with the pharmacy and
medical students at Western.

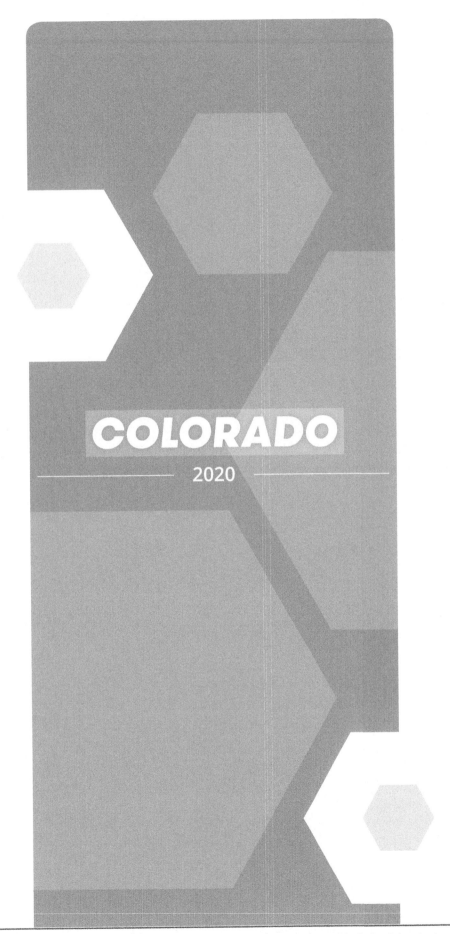

COLORADO

2020

Colorado Mesa University

1100 North Avenue
Grand Junction, CO 81501
Phone: 970-248-1482
Email:
paprogram@coloradomesa.edu

PROGRAM HIGHLIGHTS

Accreditation: Provisional

Degree Offered: Master (MPAS)

Start Date: January annually

Program Length: 27 months

Class Capacity: 16 students

Tuition: $74,000 (in-state);
$123,000 (out-of-state)

CASPA Participant: Yes

Supplemental Application: Yes ($50 fee)

Yellow Ribbon: No

Admissions: Rolling

Application Deadline: September 1

PREREQUISITE COURSEWORK

Human Anatomy with lab (3 credits),
Human Physiology (3 credits), Genetics
(3 credits), Biological Sciences (6 credits),
Chemistry (6 credits), Statistics (3
credits), Psychology (3 credits). Five out
of eight of the prerequisites must be
completed at the time of application.
All prerequisites must be completed no
later than October 1st of the year prior to
matriculation. AP credits are accepted for
Statistics and Psychology requirements
only.

GPA Requirement: Overall GPA 3.0;
Science GPA 3.0; Prerequisite GPA 3.0

Healthcare Experience: 500 hours

PA Shadowing: Preferred, not required

Required Standardized Testing: CASPer

Letters of Recommendation: Three
required; preferred that references be
from a professor, supervisor, and a PA/
NP/MD/DO

Seat Deposit: $500

COLORADO MESA UNIVERSITY

MISSION:

The mission of the CMU Physician Assistant
(PA) Program is to provide a learner-centered
environment that educates competent and
compassionate PAs, committed to leading through
service in their career and communities.

CLASS OF 2021

Prerequisite GPA: 3.61

Average Healthcare Experience: 7,013 hours

Average Community Service Experience: 653 hours

PANCE SCORES

5-year First Time Pass: N/A

Most Recent First Time Pass: N/A (have not graduated
a class yet)

CURRICULUM STRUCTURE

Didactic: 15 months

Clinical: 12 months

Rotations: 8 mandatory, 2 elective (each 4 weeks)

Capstone Project: Required for graduation

UNIQUE PROGRAM FEATURES

Admissions Preference: The school has
a preference for applicants that have a
connection to Western Colorado which
may include living, working, attending
school or other historical connection to
the area.

Red Rocks Community College

5420 Miller Street
Arvada, Colorado 80002
Phone: 303-914-6048
Email: pa.program@rrcc.edu

PROGRAM HIGHLIGHTS

Accreditation: Continuing

Degree Offered: Master (MPAS)

Start Date: August annually

Program Length: 27 months

Class Capacity: 32 students

Tuition: $68,740 (in-state, including fees); $75,466 (out-of-state, including fees)

CASPA Participant: Yes

Supplemental Application: No ($100 fee to apply to program though)

Yellow Ribbon: No

Admissions: Non-rolling

Application Deadline: September 1

PREREQUISITE COURSEWORK

College Algebra or higher (3 credits), Statistics (3 credits), Physics (3 credits), Cell Biology (3 credits), Genetics (3 credits), Human Anatomy and Physiology (6 credits), Organic Chemistry (3 credits). Prerequisites must be completed by September 1st of the year of application and with a grade "C" or better.

GPA Requirement: Prerequisite GPA 3.0

Healthcare Experience: 2,000 hours

PA Shadowing: Not required

Required Standardized Testing: GRE

Letters of Recommendation: Three required; no one specific

Seat Deposit: $750

RED ROCKS COMMUNITY COLLEGE

MISSION:

The mission of the Red Rocks Community College Physician Assistant program is to train clinically competent and compassionate physician assistants to provide primary care to the medically underserved.

CLASS OF 2020

Male: 36%

Female: 64%

Overall GPA: 3.45

Science GPA: 3.38

Average Age: 29.5

PANCE SCORES

5-year First Time Pass: 95%

Most Recent First Time Pass: 100%

CURRICULUM STRUCTURE

Didactic: 13 months

Clinical: 14 months

Rotations: 11 mandatory, 1 elective, 1 preceptorship (each 4 weeks)

Master's Project: Required for graduation

UNIQUE PROGRAM FEATURES

Master's Degree: This is the only community college approved to offer a PA Program Master's Degree.

Community Service: Students in the program are involved in several projects including volunteering at local elementary schools and health career fairs for high school students.

Primary Care Focus: The College has collaborated with Colorado Counties Incorporated, Colorado Municipal League, and the Special Districts Association, which together make up the Colorado Collaboration for Rural Healthcare Access with the goal of increasing the primary care and rural workforce in Colorado.

8401 S. Chambers Road
Parker, CO 80134
Phone: 720-874-2477
Email: admissions@rvu.edu

PROGRAM HIGHLIGHTS

Accreditation: Provisional

Degree Offered: Master (MPAS)

Start Date: September annually

Program Length: 27 months

Class Capacity: 36 students

Tuition: $85,000

CASPA Participant: Yes

Supplemental Application: Yes ($100 fee)

Yellow Ribbon: No

Admissions: Non-rolling

Application Deadline: September 1

PREREQUISITE COURSEWORK

Strongly Recommended: Biology, General Chemistry, Organic Chemistry, Biochemistry, Physics, Statistics, Behavioral Sciences, Social Sciences; Additional coursework such as Genetics, Human Anatomy, Physiology, Microbiology, Cellular Biology, Medical Terminology, Ethics, Humanities, and Communications is recommended. AP credits are not accepted.

GPA Requirement: Overall GPA 2.8

Healthcare Experience: 1,000 hours

PA Shadowing: Not required

Required Standardized Testing: GRE

Letters of Recommendation: Three required; no one specific

Seat Deposit: $500

ROCKY VISTA UNIVERSITY

MISSION:

The mission of the Rocky Vista Physician Assistant Program is to prepare clinically competent, collaborative, and compassionate physician assistants to provide primary care.

CLASS OF 2020

Male: 33%

Female: 67%

Overall GPA: 3.43

Science GPA: 3.29

Average Age: 27

PANCE SCORES

5-year First Time Pass: N/A

Most Recent First Time Pass: N/A (have not graduated a class yet)

CURRICULUM STRUCTURE

Didactic: 8 months

Clinical: 19 months

Rotations: 48 weeks total

Capstone Project: Required for graduation

UNIQUE PROGRAM FEATURES

None reported

PROGRAM HIGHLIGHTS

Accreditation: Continuing

Degree Offered: Master (MPAS)

Start Date: June annually

Program Length: 35 months

Class Capacity: 44 students

Tuition: $54,969 (in-state);
$119,016 (out-of-state)

CASPA Participant: Yes

Supplemental Application:
Yes ($55 fee)

Yellow Ribbon: No

Admissions: Rolling

Application Deadline: September 1

PREREQUISITE COURSEWORK

Chemistry (8 credits), Biology
(14 credits, which must include
3 credits of Anatomy, 3 credits
of Physiology, and 6 credits of
upper division courses), Genetics
(3 credits), Psychology (6 credits),
Statistics (3 credits). The Chemistry
and Biology requirements must
be completed prior to application.
Prerequisites must be completed
with a grade "C" or better. AP credits
are not accepted. Recommended
courses: Biochemistry, Cell Biology,
Immunology, Microbiology.

GPA Requirement: Overall GPA 3.0;
Science GPA 3.0

Healthcare Experience: Preferred,
not required

PA Shadowing: Not required

Required Standardized Testing:
CASPer

Letters of Recommendation: Three
required; no one specific

Seat Deposit: $1,000

UNIVERSITY OF COLORADO

MISSION:

The mission of the Child Health Associate/Physician Assistant Program is to provide comprehensive physician assistant education in primary care across the lifespan, with expanded training in pediatrics and care of the medically underserved.

CLASS OF 2022

Male: 23%

Female: 77%

Minority: 36%

Overall GPA: 3.67

Science GPA: 3.62

Average Healthcare Experience: 1,920 hours

Average Volunteer Experience: 260 hours

Average Age: 26

PANCE SCORES

5-year First Time Pass: 98%

Most Recent First Time Pass: 100%

CURRICULUM STRUCTURE

Didactic: 18 months

Clinical: 18 months

Rotations: Varies based on track

Capstone Project: Required for graduation

UNIQUE PROGRAM FEATURES

Specialized Tracks: The program offers specialized tracks in rural medicine, global health, urban/underserved medicine, LEADS (leadership, education, advocacy, development, and scholarship), and pediatric critical and acute care.

Pediatrics Focus: Though the program prepares PAs to care for patients of all ages, students complete at least three dedicated pediatrics rotations in addition to other rotations such as family medicine, which incorporates the pediatric population.

Colorado Curriculum: The curriculum is based on clinical presentations rather than traditional courses. Students are expected to be self-directed, motivated, and responsible for their own learning using critical thinking and reasoning. Courses emphasize the integration of basic sciences and clinical medicine through the presentation of information in clinical context, employing the use of small group experiences, case-based learning, patient "actors", patient simulators, lectures, and collaborative sessions.

Resident Tuition: Students may petition for residency after their first year living in Colorado. Tuition is $76,318 for the full 3 year program for out-of-state students who are granted residency status after their first year.

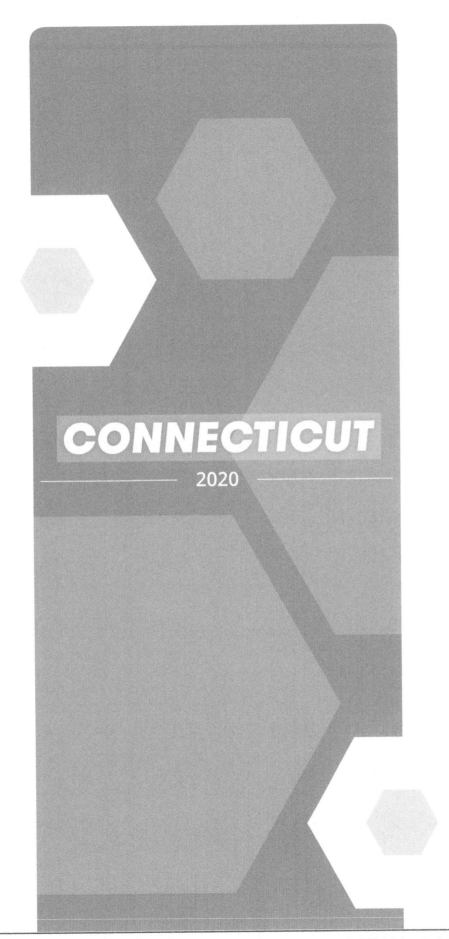

CONNECTICUT
2020

PROGRAM HIGHLIGHTS

Accreditation: Continuing

Degree Offered: Master (MHS)

Start Date: May annually

Program Length: 27 months

Class Capacity: 54 students

Tuition: $101,825

CASPA Participant: Yes

Supplemental Application: No

Yellow Ribbon: Yes

Admissions: Non-rolling

Application Deadline: September 1

PREREQUISITE COURSEWORK

4 semesters of Biology with labs
(to include at least one semester
of Microbiology and 2 semesters
of Anatomy and Physiology), 3
semesters of Chemistry with labs
(to include at least one semester of
Biochemistry or Organic Chemistry),
Pre-calculus or Calculus or
Statistics. There can be a maximum
of two prerequisites in progress at
the time of application and all must
be completed by December 31st of
the year of application.

GPA Requirement: Overall GPA 3.2;
Science GPA 3.2

Healthcare Experience: 2,500 hours

PA Shadowing: Not required

Required Standardized Testing:
None

Letters of Recommendation: Three
required; no one specific

Seat Deposit: $500

QUINNIPIAC UNIVERSITY

MISSION:

The mission of Quinnipiac's PA program is to increase access to quality health care through the education and development of caring, knowledgeable and competent physician assistants who are dedicated to clinical competence, professionalism, leadership, community outreach, and cultural competence.

NO CLASS STATISTICS REPORTED

PANCE SCORES

5-year First Time Pass: 100%

Most Recent First Time Pass: 100%

CURRICULUM STRUCTURE

Didactic: 15 months

Clinical: 12 months

Rotations: 7 mandatory, 2 elective (each 4-6 weeks)

Capstone Project: Required for graduation

UNIQUE PROGRAM FEATURES

Community Service: Students are very active in the local community with mandatory service of 50 hours completed throughout the program.

Facilities: The program is housed within the brand new medical building of the Frank Netter School of Medicine, which features 24 teaching labs, cadaver dissection lab, simulation rooms, 16 standardized patient rooms, multiple team study rooms, an expanded health science library, and a student lounge.

Urban Health Scholars Program: This is a collaboration between the University of Connecticut and the Connecticut Area Health Education Center to provide primary care and health literacy education to urban communities in the state.

Early Clinical Exposure: Students are paired with a physician or PA preceptor one day per week during the didactic curriculum to develop their patient skills prior to rotations.

Sacred Heart University

5151 Park Avenue
Fairfield, CT 06825
Phone: 203-371-7884
Email:
magnusone@sacredheart.edu

PROGRAM HIGHLIGHTS

Accreditation: Provisional

Degree Offered: Master (MPAS)

Start Date: August annually

Program Length: 27 months

Class Capacity: 42 students

Tuition: $102,955

CASPA Participant: Yes

Supplemental Application: No

Yellow Ribbon: Yes

Admissions: Non-rolling

Application Deadline: October 1

PREREQUISITE COURSEWORK

16 units of Biological Sciences to include Microbiology with lab, Human Anatomy with lab, Human Physiology with lab and Upper Level Human Biological Science with lab, Organic Chemistry I and II with lab or Biochemistry with lab, Statistics, General Psychology. Prerequisites must be completed with a grade "C" or better and by the October 1st deadline. AP credits are accepted for the Statistics and Psychology requirements. Recommended courses: Cell Biology, Human Genetics, Immunology, Molecular Biology, Neurobiology, Pathology, Abnormal Psychology, Biochemistry, Biostatistics.

GPA Requirement: Overall GPA 3.0; Prerequisite GPA 3.0

Healthcare Experience: 1,000 hours

PA Shadowing: Not required

Required Standardized Testing: None

Letters of Recommendation: Three required; one from a work supervisor

Seat Deposit: $1,000

SACRED HEART UNIVERSITY

MISSION:

The mission of the SHU program is to provide students with engaging experiences that facilitate lifelong learning, enhance diverse perspectives, emphasize primary care and collaborative practice, and foster a spirit of service with a commitment to continuously improve the health of our communities.

NO CLASS STATISTICS REPORTED

PANCE SCORES

5-year First Time Pass: 85% (based on one year of data)

Most Recent First Time Pass: 85%

CURRICULUM STRUCTURE

Didactic: 12 months

Clinical: 15 months

Rotations: 9 mandatory, 1 elective (each 5 weeks)

Capstone Project: Required for graduation

UNIQUE PROGRAM FEATURES

Holistic Admissions: The SHU Physician Assistant (PA) program uses a holistic admissions process. This is a process by which applicant's cognitive skills, such as GPA, are balanced with non-cognitive variables including but not limited to commitment to service, cultural sensitivity, empathy, capacity for growth, emotional resilience, strength of character, and interpersonal skills.

Facilities: The program is located in Stamford Hospital's newly renovated Tandet Center, which includes brand new lecture halls, a Patient Assessment Suite, and easy access to clinicians at Stamford Hospital.

Capstone Project: Students can choose from several tracks including clinical, global health, community outreach, and PA education.

Interprofessional Education: The program emphasizes education with other health professions including physical therapy, nursing, and occupational therapy students from SHU.

Physician Assistant Institute
126 Park Avenue
Bridgeport, CT 06604
Phone: 203-576-4552
Email: admit@bridgeport.edu

PROGRAM HIGHLIGHTS

Accreditation: Continuing

Degree Offered: Master (MS)

Start Date: January annually

Program Length: 28 months

Class Capacity: 40 students

Tuition: $100,170

CASPA Participant: Yes

Supplemental Application: Yes (no fee)

Yellow Ribbon: Yes

Admissions: Rolling

Application Deadline: August 1

PREREQUISITE COURSEWORK

Anatomy and Physiology with lab (2 semesters), Biology with lab (1 semester), Chemistry with lab (2 semesters), English (1 semester), Psychology (1 semester), Statistics (1 semester), Microbiology (1 semester), Genetics (1 semester), Biochemistry (1 semester). Prerequisites must be completed with a grade "C" or better and within the last 10 years. One course may be in progress at the time of application.

GPA Requirement: Overall GPA 3.0; Science GPA: 3.0

Healthcare Experience: 500 hours

PA Shadowing: Not required

Required Standardized Testing: None

Letters of Recommendation: Three required; preferred sources include a clinical supervisor, a healthcare provider with whom you have had a professional relationship, and an academic professor or employer

Seat Deposit: $1,500

UNIVERSITY OF BRIDGEPORT

MISSION:

The mission of the University of Bridgeport Physician Assistant Institute is to develop clinicians with: dedication to patients; commitment to life-long education; respect for the profession; a global perspective on health care; volunteerism as a professional core value and integrative approach to practice for the benefit of all patients.

NO CLASS STATISTICS REPORTED

PANCE SCORES

5-year First Time Pass: 97%

Most Recent First Time Pass: 97%

CURRICULUM STRUCTURE

Didactic: 15 months

Clinical: 13 months

Rotations: 7 mandatory, 1 elective (each 6 weeks)

Capstone Project: Required for graduation

UNIQUE PROGRAM FEATURES

Integrative Medicine: Students complete coursework in complementary and alternative medicine throughout the didactic curriculum, which includes topics such as chiropractic medicine, acupuncture, and naturopathy to gain perspective into how these professionals might be beneficial to their future patients.

Global Health: The curriculum interweaves global health into many courses, culminating with a Global Health course in the last didactic semester, which offers students the opportunity to investigate the impact of health issues in other countries. There is also a program annual international mission trip.

Community Service: There are a number of annual service opportunities in which students participate including literacy and medical education, food drives, and aid projects for homeless veterans.

University of Saint Joseph

Physician Assistant Studies - Lourdes Hall
1678 Asylum Avenue
West Hartford, CT 06117
Phone: 860-231-5420
Email: pastudiesprogram@usj.edu

PROGRAM HIGHLIGHTS

Accreditation: Provisional

Degree Offered: Master (MSPAS)

Start Date: January annually

Program Length: 28 months

Class Capacity: 45 students

Tuition: $111,457

CASPA Participant: Yes

Supplemental Application: Yes ($50 fee)

Yellow Ribbon: No

Admissions: Rolling

Application Deadline: October 1

PREREQUISITE COURSEWORK

Biology with lab (8 credits), Chemistry with lab (8 credits), Human Anatomy and Physiology with lab (8 credits), Organic Chemistry with lab or Biochemistry (3-4 credits), Microbiology (3 credits), Statistics (3 credits), Psychology (3 credits). Up to two courses may be in progress at the time of application. Courses must have been completed in the last 7 years or require a waiver. Prerequisites must be completed with a grade "C" or better. AP scores of 4 or 5 will be accepted but will not be factored into GPA calculations.

GPA Requirement: Overall GPA 3.0; Prerequisite GPA 3.0

Healthcare Experience: 250 hours

PA Shadowing: Preferred, not required

Required Standardized Testing: None

Letters of Recommendation: Three required; no one specific

Seat Deposit: $1,500

UNIVERSITY OF SAINT JOSEPH

MISSION:

The mission of the University of Saint Joseph Physician Assistant Studies Program is to foster the development of engaged learners into well-qualified Physician Assistants. Intellectual rigor in a spiritually enriched environment will cultivate competent, ethical members of the health care team who demonstrate the highest level of integrity and a commitment to life-long learning. Graduates will exemplify a sense of social responsibility through service to the community and their profession.

NO CLASS STATISTICS REPORTED

PANCE SCORES

5-year First Time Pass: 100% (based on one year of data)

Most Recent First Time Pass: 100%

CURRICULUM STRUCTURE

Didactic: 15 months

Clinical: 13 months

Rotations: 8 mandatory, 1 elective (each 5 weeks)

Capstone Project: Required for graduation

UNIQUE PROGRAM FEATURES

Modular Curriculum: USJ offers the only modular curriculum in the region, where students study one course at a time, mastering the subject materials before moving to the next subject.

Facilities: The program is housed in a brand new state-of-the-art facility including lounge space, lecture halls, group study rooms, an Anatomage table, and physical exam lab.

Admissions Preference: Applicants who have earned a degree at USJ or completed 60 credits at USJ and are currently enrolled will be guaranteed an interview.

Yale School of Medicine

Physician Associate Program
PO Box 208083
New Haven, CT 06520
Phone: 203-785-2860
Email: pa.program@yale.edu

PROGRAM HIGHLIGHTS

Accreditation: Continuing
Degree Offered: Master (MMSc)
Start Date: August annually
Program Length: 28 months
Class Capacity: 40 students
Tuition: $101,080

CASPA Participant: Yes
Supplemental Application: Yes ($50 fee)
Yellow Ribbon: Yes
Admissions: Rolling
Application Deadline: September 1

PREREQUISITE COURSEWORK

Statistics or Calculus (3-5 credits), Human Anatomy (3-5 credits), Human or Animal Physiology (3-5 credits), Organic Chemistry or Biochemistry (3-5 credits), Microbiology (3-5 credits), Genetics (3-5 credits). One course may be in progress at the time of application and must be completed by December 31st with a grade "B" or better.

GPA Requirement: Science GPA 3.0

Healthcare Experience: 1,000 hours (recommended)

PA Shadowing: Preferred, not required

Required Standardized Testing: GRE

Letters of Recommendation: Three required; one from a healthcare professional

Seat Deposit: $1,000

YALE UNIVERSITY SCHOOL OF MEDICINE

MISSION:

The mission of the Yale School of Medicine Physician Associate Program is to educate individuals to become outstanding clinicians and to foster leaders who will serve their communities and advance the physician assistant profession.

CLASS OF 2021

Male: 23%

Female: 77%

Overall GPA: 3.75 (3.44-4.00)

Science GPA: 3.72 (3.35-4.00)

GRE Verbal: 82nd percentile

GRE Quantitative: 69th percentile

GRE Analytical: 84th percentile

Average Healthcare Experience: 2,868 hours

PANCE SCORES

5-year First Time Pass: 98%

Most Recent First Time Pass: 100%

CURRICULUM STRUCTURE

Didactic: 12 months

Clinical: 16 months

Rotations: 10 mandatory, 4 elective (each 4 weeks)

Thesis Project: Required for graduation

UNIQUE PROGRAM FEATURES

International Rotations: Students can utilize an elective rotation to study abroad at pre-approved sites throughout Europe, Asia, Africa, and South America.

Dual Degree Option: Students can apply to both the PA program and School of Public Health at the same time. If accepted to both, students complete a dual MPH/MMSc degree program of 39 months duration.

Early Clinical Exposure: Students learn physical exam skills in groups with medical and nursing students and then visit the hospital in small groups to interview and examine patients throughout year 1.

Surgical Anatomy: Students complete a full-cadaver dissection using surgical cases as a guide to optimize applicability of acquired skills to the operating room setting and clinical practice.

Medication Assisted Treatment: Students earn additional valuable certifications in the practice enhancement course, including the knowledge to be able to prescribe buprenorphine for opiate addiction.

Yale School of Medicine PA Online

7900 Harkins Road
Suite 501
Lanham, MD 20706
Phone: 844-433-9253
Email:
admissions@paonline.yale.edu

PROGRAM HIGHLIGHTS

Accreditation: Provisional

Degree Offered: Master (MMSc)

Start Date: January annually

Program Length: 28 months

Class Capacity: 60 students

Tuition: $101,080

CASPA Participant: No

Supplemental Application:
Yes ($50 fee)

Yellow Ribbon: Yes

Admissions: Rolling

Application Deadline: September 1

PREREQUISITE COURSEWORK

Statistics or Calculus (3-5 credits), Human Anatomy (3-5 credits), Human or Animal Physiology (3-5 credits), Organic Chemistry or Biochemistry (3-5 credits), Microbiology (3-5 credits), Genetics (3-5 credits). Prerequisites must be completed by October 1st and with a grade "B" or better. One prerequisite may be in progress at the time of application.

GPA Requirement: Overall GPA: 2.8; Science GPA 3.0

Healthcare Experience: 1,000 hours (recommended)

PA Shadowing: Preferred, not required

Required Standardized Testing: CASPer (recommended)

Letters of Recommendation: Three required; one academic, one professional, one of the applicant's choice

Seat Deposit: $1,000

YALE UNIVERSITY SCHOOL OF MEDICINE (ONLINE PROGRAM)

MISSION:

The mission of the Yale Physician Assistant (PA) Online Program is to prepare PAs to provide compassionate, high-quality, patient-centered care as members of interdisciplinary teams in a primary care setting.

CLASS OF 2021

Male: 25%

Female: 75%

Overall GPA: 3.35-3.77

Science GPA: 3.26-3.81

Prerequisite GPA: 3.62-4.0

GRE Verbal: 61-93rd percentile

GRE Quantitative: 38-69th percentile

GRE Analytical: 59-92nd percentile

Healthcare Experience: 1,179-11,370 hours

Average Age: 32

PANCE SCORES

5-year First Time Pass: N/A

Most Recent First Time Pass: N/A (have not graduated a class yet)

CURRICULUM STRUCTURE

Didactic: 12 months

Clinical: 16 months

Rotations: 12 mandatory, 3 electives (each 4 weeks)

Master's Capstone: Required for graduation

UNIQUE PROGRAM FEATURES

Unique Curriculum: The didactic portion of the curriculum is completed online, while the clinical portion is completed with in-person experiences in the student's local community. This allows students to learn in their home communities without having to move. There are also several on-campus immersions requiring students to travel to New Haven for one week at a time.

CEED: The Clinical Experience in Early Didactic (CEED) provides first year students in the Yale PA Online program with 120+ hours of direct patient care experience in the didactic year. CEED enables students to apply their didactic learning in a clinical setting and gain experience with responsibilities including physical exams, history taking, presenting to preceptors and reviewing diagnostic tests.

Technology: The program makes innovative use of technology including Focused Lectures in Clinical Knowledge, Online Grand Rounds, Online Standardized Patients, Anatomy Surgical Videos, Anatomy Dissection Videos, EKG Virtual Lab, and Virtual Reality Heart Simulation.

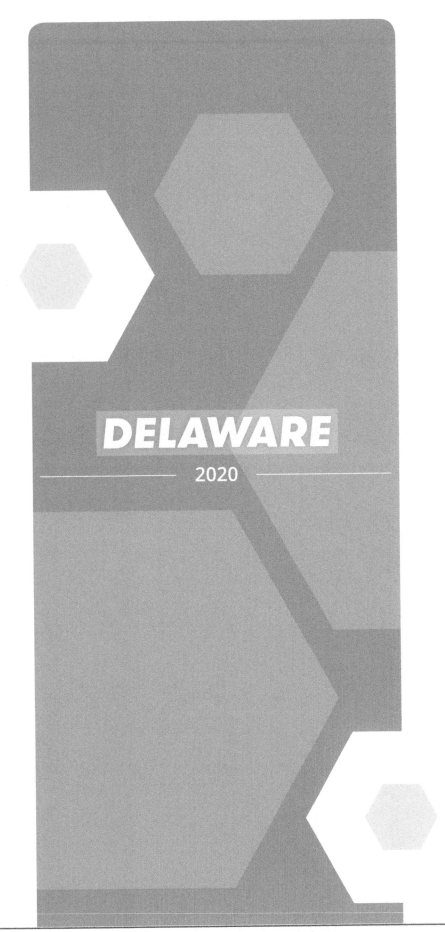

DELAWARE

2020

PROGRAM HIGHLIGHTS

Accreditation: Continuing

Degree Offered: Master (MMS)

Start Date: May annually

Program Length: 24 months

Class Capacity: 49 students

Tuition: $93,042

CASPA Participant: Yes

Supplemental Application: No

Yellow Ribbon: No

Admissions: Rolling

Application Deadline: October 1

PREREQUISITE COURSEWORK

Biological Sciences (5 courses, to include Anatomy, Physiology, and Microbiology; Biochemistry is recommended), Chemistry (3 courses, to include at least one semester of Organic Chemistry), Psychology (1 semester), Statistics (1 semester). Prerequisites must have been completed within the last 10 years. AP credits are accepted if they are listed on your transcript.

GPA Requirement: Overall GPA 3.0 (recommended)

Healthcare Experience: 200 hours

PA Shadowing: Preferred, not required

Required Standardized Testing: GRE or MCAT

Letters of Recommendation: Three required; ideally, one should be from a professor and one from a practicing licensed physician or PA

Seat Deposit: $500

ARCADIA UNIVERSITY

MISSION:

Arcadia University's Physician Assistant Program is dedicated to training highly competent, globally aware physician assistants who are prepared to be life-long learners. The program is committed to fostering excellence in patient care and promoting professionalism, leadership, cultural competency, scholarship, and service.

CLASS OF 2021

Overall GPA	3.65
Science GPA	3.56
GRE Total	312
GRE Analytical	4.30

PANCE SCORES

5-year First Time Pass	100%
Most Recent First Time Pass	99%

CURRICULUM STRUCTURE

Didactic	12 months
Clinical	12 months
Rotations	7 mandatory (each 4-8 weeks), 3 elective (each 4 weeks)

UNIQUE PROGRAM FEATURES

Dual Degree: Students can complete a dual degree MPH with their PA education in 36 months.

Pre-PA Track: There is a 4+2 track available for incoming undergraduates.

Rotations: International rotations are available. To date, Arcadia PA students have studied in over twenty countries around the world, including South Africa, Costa Rica, Guatemala, India, Scotland, England and Belize. More than 65% of students participate in global opportunities.

Community Service: One-week medical mission trips in Appalachia, Panama and Nicaragua are offered to students.

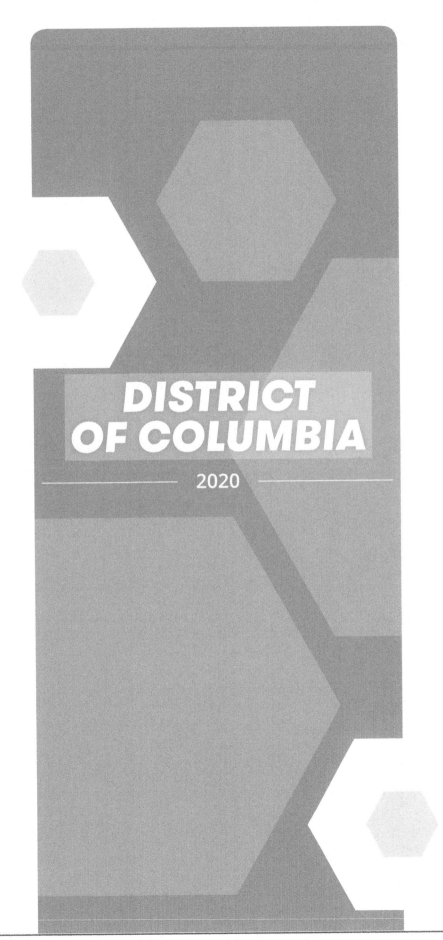

DISTRICT OF COLUMBIA

2020

George Washington University

2100 Pennsylvania Avenue, NW
Suite 300
Washington, DC 20037
Phone: 202-994-7644
Email: paadm@gwu.edu

PROGRAM HIGHLIGHTS

Accreditation: Continuing

Degree Offered: Master (MSHS)

Start Date: June annually

Program Length: 24 months

Class Capacity: 67 students

Tuition: $94,404

CASPA Participant: Yes

Supplemental Application: Yes ($60 fee)

Yellow Ribbon: Yes

Admissions: Rolling

Application Deadline: October 1

PREREQUISITE COURSEWORK

Anatomy (1 semester), Physiology (1 semester), Chemistry (2 semesters, one must be either Organic Chemistry or Biochemistry), Psychology (1 semester), Statistics (1 semester). Prerequisites must be completed with a grade "B-" or better and within the last 10 years. Up to two courses may be in progress at the time of application. AP credits can be used to satisfy the Psychology requirement only. Recommended courses: Developmental Psychology, Abnormal Psychology.

GPA Requirement: Overall GPA 3.0; Science GPA 3.0

Healthcare Experience: 1,000 hours

PA Shadowing: Not required

Required Standardized Testing: GRE

Letters of Recommendation: Two required; preferably from a healthcare professional and an academic instructor

Seat Deposit: $1,000

GEORGE WASHINGTON UNIVERSITY

MISSION:

The George Washington University Physician Assistant Program's mission is to educate physician assistants who demonstrate clinical excellence; embrace diversity, equity and inclusion; advocate for their patients; lead and advance the profession; and serve their communities.

AVERAGE CLASS STATISTICS

Overall GPA: 3.58

Science GPA: 3.57

GRE Verbal: 80th percentile

GRE Quantitative: 60th percentile

GRE Analytical: 4.0

Average Healthcare Experience: 4,000 hours

PANCE SCORES

5-year First Time Pass: 97%

Most Recent First Time Pass: 98%

CURRICULUM STRUCTURE

Didactic: 12 months

Clinical: 12 months

Rotations: 7 mandatory, 1 elective (each 6 weeks)

UNIQUE PROGRAM FEATURES

Dual Degree: Students can complete a 3-year dual MPH/MSHS degree in one of three specialty tracks including Community Oriented Primary Care, Health Policy, and Epidemiology.

Student Society: The Tolton Society is very active in helping students obtain leadership roles, service activities, and establishing a National Medical Challenge Bowl team to compete at the annual PA conference. In addition, students are encouraged to participate in professional advocacy and many descend upon Capitol Hill to discuss issues confronting the PA profession with congressional representatives.

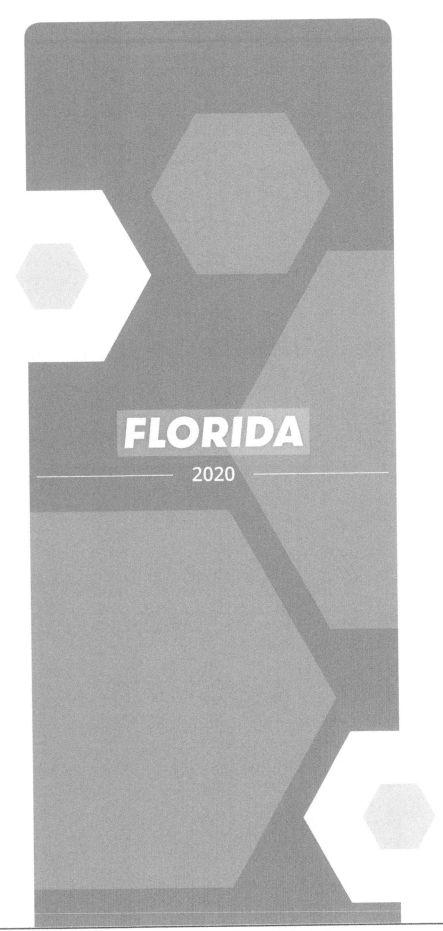

FLORIDA

2020

AdventHealth University

671 Winyah Drive
Orlando, FL 32803
Phone: 407-303-8778
Email: pa.info@ahu.edu

PROGRAM HIGHLIGHTS

Accreditation: Probation
Degree Offered: Master (MSPAS)
Start Date: May annually
Program Length: 27 months
Class Capacity: 30 students
Tuition: $81,130 (including fees)

CASPA Participant: Yes
Supplemental Application: No
Yellow Ribbon: No
Admissions: Non-rolling
Application Deadline: January 15

PREREQUISITE COURSEWORK

Organic Chemistry I and II with lab (8 credits), Anatomy and Physiology I and II with lab (8 credits), General Microbiology with lab (4 credits), Medical Terminology (2 credits), General Psychology (3 credits), Elementary Statistics (3 credits). Science courses should be current within 7 years of program matriculation. Basic Cardiac Life Support certification is required.

GPA Requirement: Overall GPA 3.0; Science GPA 3.0

Healthcare Experience: 2,000 hours (recommended)

PA Shadowing: Preferred, not required

Required Standardized Testing: GRE

Letters of Recommendation: Three required; at least one from a practicing PA or MD/DO and no more than one letter may come from a professor

Seat Deposit: $500

ADVENTHEALTH UNIVERSITY

MISSION:

The Physician Assistant program seeks to educate individuals who desire to become knowledgeable, compassionate and spiritually uplifting healthcare providers. Whether they practice locally, nationally, or globally, it is the intent of this program to graduate individuals who embrace a mission of service to others as they would wish to be done to them.

CLASS OF 2021

Male: 27%

Female: 73%

Overall GPA: 3.60

Science GPA: 3.50

GRE Total: 300

Average Healthcare Experience: 3,883 hours

Average Age: 28

PANCE SCORES

5-year First Time Pass: 92% (based on two years of data)

Most Recent First Time Pass: 100%

CURRICULUM STRUCTURE

Didactic: 15 months

Clinical: 12 months

Rotations: 7 mandatory, 1 elective (each 4-6 weeks)

Capstone Project: Required for graduation

UNIQUE PROGRAM FEATURES

Medical Missions: Students in good standing can participate in a medical mission field project that will be arranged through the University during the clinical year.

Facilities: There is a newly renovated PA lab with 11 fully outfitted patient examination bays where students learn to take histories, perform physical exams, and learn clinical procedures.

Religion: The program curriculum includes courses in practicing faith-based healthcare and includes topics such as human identity, God, spirituality across faith traditions and bioethics.

PROGRAM HIGHLIGHTS

Accreditation: Continuing

Degree Offered: Master (MMSc)

Start Date: August annually

Program Length: 28 months

Class Capacity: 76 students (Miami), 24 students (St. Petersburg)

Tuition: $78,491

CASPA Participant: Yes

Supplemental Application: No

Yellow Ribbon: Yes

Admissions: Rolling

Application Deadline: December 1

PREREQUISITE COURSEWORK

General Chemistry (6 credits), Organic Chemistry or Biochemistry (3 credits), Human Anatomy and Physiology with lab (8 credits), Microbiology with lab (4 credits), Biological Sciences (3 credits), Behavioral/Social Science (6 credits). Courses must be completed within the last 10 years and with a grade "C" or better.

GPA Requirement: Overall GPA 3.0; Science GPA 3.0

Healthcare Experience: Preferred, not required (1,000 hours recommended)

PA Shadowing: Not required
Required Standardized Testing: GRE

Letters of Recommendation: Three required; preferably from clinical work supervisors/coworkers and academic contacts

Seat Deposit: $1,000

BARRY UNIVERSITY

MISSION:

The Barry University Physician Assistant Program educates students in practice of collaborative medicine and encourages life-long learning and professional development. It fosters a technology rich environment and clinical training experiences among diverse patient populations. The program enables students to develop competencies required to meet the health care needs of contemporary society.

NO CLASS STATISTICS REPORTED

PANCE SCORES

5-year First Time Pass: 93%

Most Recent First Time Pass: 95%

CURRICULUM STRUCTURE

Didactic: 16 months (12 pre-clinical and 4 post-clinical)

Clinical: 12 months

Rotations: 7 mandatory, 1 elective (each 6 weeks)

Library Research Paper: Required for graduation

UNIQUE PROGRAM FEATURES

One Program, Two Locations: The program utilizes innovative technology to conduct instructional education via interactive video conferencing. Live lecturers present at one of two locations in Miami or St. Petersburg. Students in the locations without the live lecturer are connected via video conferencing.

Medical Spanish: All students complete a 40-hour total immersion Medical Spanish course.

Florida Gulf Coast University

10501 FGCU BLVD. South
Fort Meyers, FL 33965
Phone: 239-745-4477
Email: paprogram@fgcu.edu

PROGRAM HIGHLIGHTS

Accreditation: Provisional

Degree Offered: Master (MPAS)

Start Date: August annually

Program Length: 27 months

Class Capacity: 20 students

Tuition: $56,000 (in-state, including fees); $139,000 (out-of-state, including fees)

CASPA Participant: Yes

Supplemental Application: Yes (graduate school application $30 fee)

Yellow Ribbon: No

Admissions: Non-rolling

Application Deadline: January 15

PREREQUISITE COURSEWORK

Biology with lab (4 credits), General Chemistry I and II with lab (8 credits), Organic Chemistry or Biochemistry (3 credits), Medical Terminology (3 credits), Human Anatomy and Physiology I and II with lab (8 credits), Microbiology with lab (4-5 credits), Genetics (3 credits). Anatomy, Physiology, Microbiology, and Genetics must be completed within the last 7 years. Prerequisites must be completed with a grade "C" or better and by the end of the fall semester prior to matriculation.

GPA Requirement: Last 60 Upper Division Credits: 3.0; Science BCP GPA: 3.0

Healthcare Experience: 250 hours

PA Shadowing: 20 hours (strongly recommended)

Required Standardized Testing: GRE

Letters of Recommendation: Three required; one from a PA, one from an MD/DO/NP, and one from a professor or any individual who has worked with the applicant in a professional or academic environment for at least 6 months

Seat Deposit: $200

FLORIDA GULF COAST UNIVERSITY

MISSION:

The mission of the MPAS Program at Florida Gulf Coast University is to prepare competent and effective master's level primary-care physician assistant practitioners who will collaboratively practice with physicians and other members of the healthcare team.

NO CLASS STATISTICS REPORTED

PANCE SCORES

5-year First Time Pass: N/A

Most Recent First Time Pass: N/A (have not graduated a class yet)

CURRICULUM STRUCTURE

Didactic: 15 months

Clinical: 12 months

Rotations: 9 mandatory, 3 selective (each 4 weeks)

Capstone Project: Required for graduation

UNIQUE PROGRAM FEATURES

Rotations: Students will complete all of their rotations in the state of Florida and are not allowed to do out-of-state rotations.

Community Service: Students in the program recently completed projects with Anthrex, The Lions Club, and Special Equestrians.

Herbert Wertheim College of Medicine

9250 West Flagler Street
Miami, FL 33174
Phone: 305-348-6567
Email: paschool@fiu.edu

PROGRAM HIGHLIGHTS

Accreditation: Continuing

Degree Offered: Master (MPAS)

Start Date: July annually

Program Length: 27 months

Class Capacity: 45 students

Tuition: $91,142 (in-state, including fees); $93,534 (out-of-state, including fees)

CASPA Participant: Yes

Supplemental Application: Yes ($30 fee)

Yellow Ribbon: No

Admissions: Rolling

Application Deadline: January 15

PREREQUISITE COURSEWORK

Statistics (3 credits), Medical Terminology (1 credit), General Chemistry I and II with lab (8 credits), General Biology I with lab or Zoology with lab (4 credits), General Microbiology (4 credits), Human Anatomy and Physiology with lab (8 credits), Organic Chemistry I with lab (4 credits), Biochemistry with lab (4 credits), Genetics (3 credits). Prerequisites must be completed with a grade "C" or better, within the last 7 years, and must be completed by the fall semester prior to the application deadline.

GPA Requirement: Overall GPA 3.0; Science GPA 3.0; Upper Division GPA 3.0

Healthcare Experience: 1,000 hours (preferred)

PA Shadowing: Preferred, not required

Required Standardized Testing: GRE

Letters of Recommendation: Two required; highly recommended that one be from a PA and the other may be from a MD/DO, PA, NP, or any individual who has worked with the applicant in a professional or educational environment

Seat Deposit: $750

FLORIDA INTERNATIONAL UNIVERSITY HERBERT WERTHEIM COLLEGE OF MEDICINE

MISSION:

The Florida International University Herbert Wertheim College of Medicine Master in Physician Assistant Studies program prepares a diverse, dynamic workforce of competent and compassionate graduate-level health care professionals who are qualified to practice collaboratively on primary care and specialty interprofessional teams, serve their communities, and advance the physician assistant profession.

CLASS OF 2020

Male: 22%

Female: 78%

Minority: 47%

Overall GPA: 3.47

Science GPA: 3.39

GRE Verbal: 151

GRE Quantitative: 151

PANCE SCORES

5-year First Time Pass: 84% (based on two years of data)

Most Recent First Time Pass: 91%

CURRICULUM STRUCTURE

Didactic: 15 months

Clinical: 12 months

Rotations: 7 mandatory, 2 elective (each 4-5 weeks)

Signature Paper: Required for graduation

UNIQUE PROGRAM FEATURES

Admissions Preference: Approximately 80-90% of students each year are selected from Florida.

Student Profiles: Prospective students can also find out more about the MPAS student experience by visiting the MPAS student profiles section of the website.

Florida State University

1115 West Call Street
Tallahassee, FL 32306
Phone: 850-644-1732
Email: painfo@med.fsu.edu

PROGRAM HIGHLIGHTS

Accreditation: Provisional

Degree Offered: Master (MSPAP)

Start Date: August annually

Program Length: 27 months

Class Capacity: 60 students

Tuition: $65,333 (in-state); $88,667 (out-of-state)

CASPA Participant: Yes

Supplemental Application: Yes ($30 fee)

Yellow Ribbon: Yes

Admissions: Rolling

Application Deadline: October 1

PREREQUISITE COURSEWORK

Human Anatomy with lab (4 credits), Human Physiology with lab (4 credits), Biology with lab (8 credits), Microbiology with lab (4 credits), General Chemistry with lab (8 credits), Organic Chemistry with lab (3 credits), Biochemistry (3 credits), Genetics (3 credits), Statistics (3 credits), College Algebra or higher (3 credits), English Composition (6 credits), General Psychology (3 credits), Medical Terminology (1 course). There is no expiration date for prerequisite coursework; however, all prerequisites must be completed at the time of application.

GPA Requirement: Overall GPA 3.0; Science GPA 3.0

Healthcare Experience: 500 hours

PA Shadowing: Preferred, not required

Required Standardized Testing: GRE, CASPer

Letters of Recommendation: Three required; it is suggested that at least one be from a healthcare provider and one from a science faculty member who taught the applicant

Seat Deposit: None

FLORIDA STATE UNIVERSITY

MISSION:

The mission of the Florida State University School of Physician Assistant Practice is to educate and prepare physician assistants to practice patient-centered healthcare in any clinical setting and to be responsive to community needs, especially through service to elder, rural, minority and underserved populations throughout the state of Florida.

CLASS OF 2020

Minority: 32%

Overall GPA: 3.51

Science GPA: 3.47

GRE Verbal: 152

GRE Quantitative: 152

Average Age: 24

PANCE SCORES

5-year First Time Pass: N/A

Most Recent First Time Pass: N/A (have not graduated a class yet)

CURRICULUM STRUCTURE

Didactic: 15 months

Clinical: 12 months

Rotations: 8 mandatory, 1 elective (duration not specified)

Research Project: Required for graduation

UNIQUE PROGRAM FEATURES

Admissions Preference: Preference is given to Florida residents, residents of South Georgia and South Alabama whose county border is contiguous with Florida, and US Military Veterans.

UWF Pipeline Program: Residents of the Florida panhandle who are willing to return to Pensacola for clinical rotations and who meet additional requirements can apply through the pipeline program and are given additional consideration and preference.

Mental Health: The program employs a class psychologist and the school has other special resources available for students to help them work through program stress, general anxiety, crisis intervention, depression, or even family and relationship issues.

PROGRAM HIGHLIGHTS

Accreditation: Provisional

Degree Offered: Master (MPAS)

Start Date: August annually

Program Length: 24 months

Class Capacity: Not specified

Tuition: $105,570

CASPA Participant: Yes

Supplemental Application: No

Yellow Ribbon: No

Admissions: Non-rolling

Application Deadline: December 1

PREREQUISITE COURSEWORK

General Chemistry with lab (8 credits), Human Anatomy with lab (4 credits), Human Physiology with lab (4 credits), Genetics (3 credits), Medical Terminology (1-3 credits), Statistics (3 credits), Microbiology with lab (4 credits), Psychology (3 credits). Courses must be completed within the last 10 years. Recommended courses: Cadaver Anatomy Lab, Biochemistry, Organic Chemistry, Introduction to Pharmacology.

GPA Requirement: Overall GPA 3.0; Science GPA 3.0; Prerequisite GPA 3.0

Healthcare Experience: 30 hours of medical experience or shadowing a PA

PA Shadowing: As above

Required Standardized Testing: CASPer

Letters of Recommendation: Three required; no one specific

Seat Deposit: Not reported

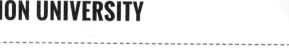

GANNON UNIVERSITY

MISSION:

The Gannon University Ruskin Physician Assistant Program strives to provide a stimulating learning environment, highly qualified and motivated faculty, as well as modern facilities that offer Physician Assistant students the opportunity to become well-prepared primary care providers who are leaders in their field and community.

CLASS OF 2021

Overall GPA: 3.40

Prerequisite GPA: 3.50

PANCE SCORES

5-year First Time Pass: N/A

Most Recent First Time Pass: N/A (have not graduated a class yet)

CURRICULUM STRUCTURE

Didactic: 12 months

Clinical: 12 months

Rotations: 7 mandatory, 1 elective (5 weeks each)

Capstone Project: Required for graduation

UNIQUE PROGRAM FEATURES

Didactic Experience: Didactic courses are taught both in-person and online.

Keiser University

1900 W. Commercial Blvd.
Fort Lauderdale, FL 33309
Phone: 954-776-4456
Email:
paprogram@keiseruniversity.edu

PROGRAM HIGHLIGHTS

Accreditation: Probation

Degree Offered: Master (MSPA)

Start Date: January annually

Program Length: 24 months

Class Capacity: 40 students

Tuition: $92,189 (including fees)

CASPA Participant: Yes

Supplemental Application: Yes ($55 fee)

Yellow Ribbon: Yes

Admissions: Rolling

Application Deadline: November 1

PREREQUISITE COURSEWORK

College Math (3 credits), English (6 credits), Humanities (3 credits), Social Science (3 credits), Behavioral Sciences (6 credits), Medical Terminology (2 credits), General Biology or Zoology with lab (4 credits), General Chemistry I and II with lab (8 credits), Microbiology with lab (4 credits), Biochemistry or Organic Chemistry (3 credits), Anatomy and Physiology I and II with lab (8 credits), Genetics (3 credits). Natural Science courses must be completed within the last 10 years and up to two prerequisites may be in progress at the time of application. Prerequisites must be completed with a grade "C" or better.

GPA Requirement: Overall GPA 2.75; Science GPA 3.0; Prerequisite GPA 3.0

Healthcare Experience: 100 hours

PA Shadowing: 20 hours

Required Standardized Testing: GRE (minimum score of 294)

Letters of Recommendation: Three required; one from a PA, one from a practicing health care provider, and one personal reference

Seat Deposit: $1,145

KEISER UNIVERSITY

MISSION:

The Keiser University physician assistant program provides an environment that fosters quality academic and clinical education. The program, in collaboration with the community, provides physician assistants who excel in integrative patient care, education and service to benefit the public. The program promotes lifelong responsibility for ongoing learning and active participation in a changing healthcare environment.

NO CLASS STATISTICS REPORTED

PANCE SCORES

5-year First Time Pass: 92%

Most Recent First Time Pass: 89%

CURRICULUM STRUCTURE

Didactic: 12 months

Clinical: 12 months

Rotations: 7 mandatory, 2 elective (each 5 weeks)

Graduate Project: Required for graduation

UNIQUE PROGRAM FEATURES

None reported

MDC Medical Campus

950 NW 20th St. Suite 2204
Miami, FL 33127
Phone: 305-237-4103
Email: mdcpaprogram@mdc.edu

PROGRAM HIGHLIGHTS

Accreditation: Continuing

Degree Offered: Bachelor, Masters (MMS)

Start Date: August annually

Program Length: 27 months

Class Capacity: 55 students

Tuition: $31,866 (in-state); $77,347 (out-of-state)

CASPA Participant: No

Supplemental Application: Yes ($25 fee)

Yellow Ribbon: No

Admissions: Not reported

Application Deadline: November 15

PREREQUISITE COURSEWORK

English Composition, Fundamentals of Speech, Humanities, Introduction to Psychology, General Chemistry I and II with lab, Anatomy and Physiology I and II with lab, Microbiology with lab, College Algebra, Statistical Methods, Introduction to Healthcare with lab. All natural science courses taken more than 5 years ago must be repeated. Recommended courses: College Algebra, Medical Terminology, English Communication II.

GPA Requirement: Overall GPA 3.0; Science GPA 3.0

Healthcare Experience: Preferred, not required

PA Shadowing: 50 hours (recommended)

Required Standardized Testing: PA-CAT

Letters of Recommendation: Three required; no one specific

Seat Deposit: $500

MIAMI-DADE COLLEGE

MISSION:

The mission of the PA program is to: (1) Provide high quality education and training opportunities in primary care for students from diverse cultural backgrounds interested in providing health care services to the medically under-served residents in urban and rural communities, especially in Florida; (2) Promote and maintain high academic and professional standards; (3) Participate in professional activities and continuing education to promote life-long learning; (4) Prepare each graduate with a level of didactic and clinical competence that provides successful entry into the profession.

NO CLASS STATISTICS REPORTED

PANCE SCORES

5-year First Time Pass: 92%

Most Recent First Time Pass: 96%

CURRICULUM STRUCTURE

Didactic: 12 months

Clinical: 12 months

Rotations: 8 mandatory (each 4-8 weeks)

UNIQUE PROGRAM FEATURES

Admissions Test: Required of applicants who make the initial cut and consists of 100 multiple choice questions in anatomy, physiology, medical terminology, microbiology and math.

Admissions Preference: This program gives preference to Miami-Dade County residents; however, all applicants are considered.

MMS Degree: The Master of Health Science curriculum consists of 28 credits of required courses through Nova Southeastern's online platform while simultaneously completing the PA program courses at Miami Dade College Medical Campus. It will be required for students matriculating in the year 2020 and thereafter.

Nova Southeastern University

College of Health Care Sciences
3200 S. University Drive
Fort Lauderdale, FL 33328
Phone: 954-262-1251
Email: dickman@nova.edu

PROGRAM HIGHLIGHTS

Accreditation: Continuing

Degree Offered: Master (MMS)

Start Date: May annually

Program Length: 27 months

Class Capacity: 75 students

Tuition: $80,827

CASPA Participant: Yes

Supplemental Application: Yes ($50 fee)

Yellow Ribbon: No

Admissions: Rolling

Application Deadline: December 1

PREREQUISITE COURSEWORK

College Math (3 credits), English (6 credits), Humanities/Arts (3 credits), Social Sciences (9 credits), General Chemistry I and II with lab (8 credits), Microbiology with lab (4 credits), General Biology or Zoology with lab (4 credits), Human Anatomy and Physiology (6 credits), Biochemistry (3 credits), Genetics (3 credits), Medical Terminology (1 credit). Science prerequisites must be completed by the end of the fall semester prior to matriculation. The remaining prerequisites must be completed by the time of matriculation. Prerequisites must be completed with a grade "C" or better. Recommended courses: Biochemistry lab, Anatomy lab, Physiology lab, Statistics.

GPA Requirement: Overall GPA 3.0; Science GPA 3.0

Healthcare Experience: Preferred, not required

PA Shadowing: Not specified

Required Standardized Testing: GRE

Letters of Recommendation: Two required; one from a PA and one from another healthcare professional

Seat Deposit: $1,000

NOVA SOUTHEASTERN UNIVERSITY, FORT LAUDERDALE

MISSION:

To provide a primary care training program designed for, and dedicated to, producing competent physician assistants who will provide quality health care in rural, urban, underserved, and culturally diverse communities; to increase the accessibility of quality health care in the primary care setting; to prepare students for lifelong learning and leadership roles; and to promote the physician assistant profession.

NO CLASS STATISTICS REPORTED

PANCE SCORES

5-year First Time Pass: 98%

Most Recent First Time Pass: 99%

CURRICULUM STRUCTURE

Didactic: 15 months

Clinical: 12 months

Rotations: 7 mandatory, 3 elective (each 3-6 weeks)

Graduate Project: Required for graduation

UNIQUE PROGRAM FEATURES

Dual Degree Program: Students in any of Nova's PA programs can complete a dual degree MMS/MPH program by simultaneously taking online MPH courses during the PA program. Students typically finish the MPH shortly after the MMS.

Instructional Technology: Instruction is provided using the latest, state-of-the-art educational technologies and methods. Computer-based patient simulators and an audience-response system enhance the educational process by providing a safe learning environment for students to demonstrate their knowledge and skills.

Nova Southeastern University

3650 Colonial Court
Fort Myers, FL 33913
Phone: 239-274-1020
Email: rs1152@nova.edu

PROGRAM HIGHLIGHTS

Accreditation: Continuing

Degree Offered: Master (MMS)

Start Date: June annually

Program Length: 27 months

Class Capacity: 54 students

Tuition: $80,827

CASPA Participant: Yes

Supplemental Application: Yes ($50 fee)

Yellow Ribbon: No

Admissions: Rolling

Application Deadline: December 1

PREREQUISITE COURSEWORK

College Math (3 credits), English (6 credits), Humanities/Arts (3 credits), Social Sciences (9 credits), General Chemistry I and II with lab (8 credits), Microbiology with lab (4 credits), General Biology or Zoology with lab (4 credits), Human Anatomy and Physiology (6 credits), Biochemistry (3 credits), Genetics (3 credits), Medical Terminology (1 credit). Prerequisites must be completed with a grade "C" or better. Recommended courses: Biochemistry lab, Anatomy lab, Physiology lab, Statistics.

GPA Requirement: Overall GPA 3.0; Science GPA 3.0

Healthcare Experience: Preferred, not required

PA Shadowing: Not specified

Required Standardized Testing: GRE

Letters of Recommendation: Two required; one from a PA and one from a healthcare professional

Seat Deposit: $1,000

NOVA SOUTHEASTERN UNIVERSITY, FORT MYERS

MISSION:

The NSU Physician Assistant Program - Fort Myers endeavors to provide an exemplary educational experience that emphasizes primary medical care, enables graduates to demonstrate competency and skill in a variety of clinical and cultural settings, provides health care experiences in medically underserved communities, prepares students for lifelong learning, prepares students for leadership roles and cultivates professionalism throughout the program.

NO CLASS STATISTICS REPORTED

PANCE SCORES

5-year First Time Pass: 96%

Most Recent First Time Pass: 92%

CURRICULUM STRUCTURE

Didactic: 14.5 months

Clinical: 12.5 months

Rotations: 6 mandatory, 3 elective (each 4-6 weeks)

Graduate Project: Required for graduation

UNIQUE PROGRAM FEATURES

Dual Degree Program: Students in any of Nova's PA programs can complete a dual degree MMS/MPH program by simultaneously taking online MPH courses during the PA program. Students typically finish the MPH shortly after the MMS.

Rotations: The program requires some clinical rotations in rural or underserved communities.

PROGRAM HIGHLIGHTS

Accreditation: Continuing

Degree Offered: Master (MMS)

Start Date: June annually

Program Length: 27 months

Class Capacity: 60 students

Tuition: $80,827

CASPA Participant: Yes

Supplemental Application: Yes ($50 fee)

Yellow Ribbon: No

Admissions: Rolling

Application Deadline: December 1

PREREQUISITE COURSEWORK

College Math (3 credits), English (6 credits), Humanities/Arts (3 credits), Social Sciences (9 credits), General Chemistry I and II with lab (8 credits), Microbiology with lab (4 credits), General Biology or Zoology with lab (4 credits), Human Anatomy and Physiology (6 credits), Biochemistry (3 credits), Human Genetics (3 credits), Medical Terminology (1 credit). Prerequisites must be completed with a grade "C" or better. Recommended courses: Biochemistry lab, Anatomy lab, Physiology lab, Statistics.

GPA Requirement: Overall GPA 3.0; Science GPA 3.0

Healthcare Experience: Preferred, not required

PA Shadowing: Not specified

Required Standardized Testing: GRE

Letters of Recommendation: Two required; one from a PA and one from a healthcare professional

Seat Deposit: $1,000

NOVA SOUTHEASTERN UNIVERSITY, JACKSONVILLE

MISSION:

To provide an exemplary educational experience, which emphasizes primary medical care, yet will enable graduates to manifest competency and skill in a variety of clinical environments; to develop the necessary skills to pursue lifelong learning; to foster leadership qualities, which will enable graduates to improve access to quality, affordable health care; and to heighten the status of the physician assistant profession.

NO CLASS STATISTICS REPORTED

PANCE SCORES

5-year First Time Pass: 94%

Most Recent First Time Pass: 95%

CURRICULUM STRUCTURE

Didactic: 15 months

Clinical: 12 months

Rotations: 6 mandatory, 3 elective (each 4-6 weeks)

Graduate Project: Required for graduation

UNIQUE PROGRAM FEATURES

Dual Degree Program: Students in any of Nova's PA programs can complete a dual degree MMS/MPH program by simultaneously taking only MPH courses during the PA program. Students typically finish the MPH shortly after the MMS.

Undergraduate Dual Admission Program: Nova Southeastern University's College of Health Care Sciences has established an articulation agreement with Florida State College of Jacksonville for a select number of highly motivated, qualified students interested in pursuing professional studies in the Physician Assistant Program.

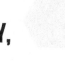

Nova Southeastern University

4850 Millenia Blvd
Orlando, FL 32839
Phone: 407-264-5150
Email: sara.kimble@nova.edu

PROGRAM HIGHLIGHTS

Accreditation: Continuing

Degree Offered: Master (MMS)

Start Date: May annually

Program Length: 27 months

Class Capacity: 64 students

Tuition: $80,827

CASPA Participant: Yes

Supplemental Application: Yes ($50 fee)

Yellow Ribbon: No

Admissions: Rolling

Application Deadline: December 1

PREREQUISITE COURSEWORK

College Algebra (3 credits), English (6 credits), Humanities/Arts (3 credits), Social Sciences (9 credits), General Chemistry I and II with lab (8 credits), Microbiology with lab (4 credits), General Biology or Zoology with lab (4 credits), Human Anatomy and Physiology (6 credits), Biochemistry (3 credits), Human Genetics (3 credits), Medical Terminology (1 credit). Prerequisites must be completed with a grade "C" or better. Recommended courses: Biochemistry lab, Anatomy lab, Physiology lab, Statistics.

GPA Requirement: Overall GPA 3.0; Science GPA 3.0

Healthcare Experience: Preferred, not required

PA Shadowing: Not specified

Required Standardized Testing: GRE

Letters of Recommendation: Two required; one from a PA and one from a healthcare professional

Seat Deposit: $1,000

NOVA SOUTHEASTERN UNIVERSITY, ORLANDO

MISSION:

To provide a high quality training program designed for and dedicated to producing culturally competent physician assistants who will provide quality health care in rural, urban, underserved, and culturally diverse communities; to provide an exemplary educational experience, which emphasizes primary medical care, yet will enable graduates to manifest competency and skill in a variety of clinical environments; to inspire graduates to pursue lifelong learning; to foster leadership qualities that will enable graduates to improve access to quality and affordable healthcare; and to heighten the stature of the physician assistant profession by training quality graduates.

NO CLASS STATISTICS REPORTED

PANCE SCORES

5-year First Time Pass: 99%

Most Recent First Time Pass: 97%

CURRICULUM STRUCTURE

Didactic: 15 months

Clinical: 12 months

Rotations: 7 mandatory, 1 selective, 1 elective (each 4-6 weeks)

Graduate Project: Required for graduation

UNIQUE PROGRAM FEATURES

Dual Degree Program: Students in any of Nova's PA programs can complete a dual degree MMS/MPH program by simultaneously taking only MPH courses during the PA program. Students typically finish the MPH shortly after the MMS.

South University, Tampa

4401 North Himes Avenue
Tampa, FL 33614
Phone: 813-393-3720
Email: paprogramtampa@
southuniversity.edu

PROGRAM HIGHLIGHTS

Accreditation: Continuing

Degree Offered: Master (MSPA)

Start Date: January annually

Program Length: 27 months

Class Capacity: 48 students

Tuition: $84,600

CASPA Participant: Yes

Supplemental Application: No

Yellow Ribbon: Yes

Admissions: Non-rolling

Application Deadline: August 1

PREREQUISITE COURSEWORK

Human Anatomy (1 semester), Human Physiology (1 semester), General Biology (2 semesters), General Chemistry (2 semesters), Biochemistry or Organic Chemistry (1 semester), Microbiology (1 semester). Prerequisites must be completed with a grade "C" or better. AP credits are accepted.

GPA Requirement: Overall GPA 3.0; Science GPA 3.0

Healthcare Experience: Preferred, not required

PA Shadowing: Not required

Required Standardized Testing: GRE (preference for those with scores >50th percentile), CASPer

Letters of Recommendation: Three required; at least one must be from an MD/DO/PA/NP

Seat Deposit: $500

SOUTH UNIVERSITY, TAMPA

MISSION:

The South University Physician Assistant program exists to educate a diverse student population as providers of high quality, cost-efficient health care who will make a positive difference while practicing the art and science of medicine with physician direction.

CLASS OF 2021

Male: 19%

Female: 81%

Minority: 39%

Overall GPA: 3.39

PANCE SCORES

5-year First Time Pass: 95%

Most Recent First Time Pass: 97%

CURRICULUM STRUCTURE

Didactic: 15 months

Clinical: 12 months

Rotations: 7 mandatory, 1 elective (each 6 weeks)

UNIQUE PROGRAM FEATURES

None reported

University of Florida College of Medicine

PO Box 100176
Gainesville, FL 32610
Phone: 352-294-8150
Email: keri.stone@medicine.ufl.edu

PROGRAM HIGHLIGHTS

Accreditation: Continuing

Degree Offered: Master (MPAS)

Start Date: June annually

Program Length: 24 months

Class Capacity: 60 students

Tuition: $55,320 (in-state);
$122,994 (out-of-state)

CASPA Participant: Yes

Supplemental Application: Yes ($30 fee)

Yellow Ribbon: No

Admissions: Rolling

Application Deadline: September 1

PREREQUISITE COURSEWORK

Human Anatomy and Physiology with lab (6-8 credits), Microbiology with lab (3-5 credits), General Chemistry I and II with lab (8-11 credits), Statistics (3 credits), Medical Terminology (1 credit). Prerequisites must be completed with a grade "C" or better and by the end of the fall semester prior to the program's academic year beginning in late June. Preference is given to applicants whose courses are no older than 5 years. AP credits are not accepted. Recommended courses: Biochemistry, Biostatistics, Cell Biology, Cell Physiology, Embryology, Epidemiology, Genetics, Histology, Immunology, Molecular Genetics, Organic Chemistry, Parasitology, Pathogenic Bacteriology, Virology, as well as other non-science courses.

GPA Requirement: None (but successful applicants rarely fall below overall and science GPAs of 3.0)

Healthcare Experience: 2,000 hours (recommended)

PA Shadowing: Preferred, not required

Required Standardized Testing: GRE (preference for those with scores > 300), CASPer

Letters of Recommendation: Three required; at least one should be from a physician who has supervised the applicant in a clinical setting, one from a PA who is familiar with the applicant's clinical work, and one from another health professional who has worked alongside the applicant and/or is familiar with the applicant's clinical skills

Seat Deposit: $200

UNIVERSITY OF FLORIDA

MISSION:

The mission of the School of Physician Assistant Studies is to educate students to become Physician Assistants that will serve the people of Florida and the nation as part of a multidisciplinary healthcare team in a diverse and ever changing healthcare environment.

CLASS OF 2021

Male: 35%

Female: 65%

Minority: 43%

Overall GPA: 3.50

Science GPA: 3.40

GRE Verbal: 155

GRE Quantitative: 154

GRE Analytical: 4.2

Average Healthcare Experience: 2.3 years

Average Age: 25

PANCE SCORES

5-year First Time Pass: 99%

Most Recent First Time Pass: 100%

CURRICULUM STRUCTURE

Didactic: 12 months

Clinical: 12 months

Rotations: 9 mandatory, 1 Internal Medicine selective, 2 elective (each 4 weeks)

Capstone Project: Required for graduation

UNIQUE PROGRAM FEATURES

Community Service: Students have several community service opportunities throughout the curriculum. Most notably, students work in student-run, free healthcare clinics that are sponsored by the College of Medicine during their first and second year. Each student completes one primary care rotation in a rural area.

Facilities: The program boasts state-of-the-art facilities and robust simulation technology, which is provided to the students in the new school of medicine building.

Admissions Preference: This is a state school and each year 60-80% of students are residents of Florida.

Student Blog: The program frequently updates the student blog which provides information about current students, their backgrounds, and the program overall. You can view on the website.

University of South Florida

12901 Bruce B. Downs Boulevard
MDC5
Tampa, FL 33612
Phone: 813-974-8926
Email: paprogram@health.usf.edu

PROGRAM HIGHLIGHTS

Accreditation: Provisional

Degree Offered: Master (MPAS)

Start Date: May annually

Program Length: 24 months

Class Capacity: 50 students

Tuition: $68,166 (in-state);
$129,066 (out-of-state)

CASPA Participant: Yes

Supplemental Application: No

Yellow Ribbon: No

Admissions: Rolling

Application Deadline: November 1

PREREQUISITE COURSEWORK

Statistics (1 semester), Biology
with lab (1 semester), Microbiology
with lab (1 semester), Organic
Chemistry with lab (1 semester),
Biochemistry or Organic Chemistry
II (1 semester), Anatomy and
Physiology with lab (2 semesters),
Medical Terminology (1 course).
Prerequisites must be completed
by the end of December prior to
the year of matriculation. AP credits
are not accepted.

GPA Requirement: Overall GPA 3.0;
Science GPA 3.0

Healthcare Experience: 500 hours

PA Shadowing: Preferred, not
required

Required Standardized Testing: GRE

Letters of Recommendation: Three
required; one from a supervisor in
a clinical setting

Seat Deposit: $200

UNIVERSITY OF SOUTH FLORIDA

MISSION:

To provide a scholarly environment in which students from diverse backgrounds will receive the requisite knowledge and skills to equip them to deliver high-quality, culturally sensitive, and compassionate healthcare in collaboration with physicians in an interdisciplinary healthcare team.

CLASS OF 2021

Male: 14%

Female: 86%

Overall GPA: 3.80

Science GPA: 3.72

GRE Verbal: 69th percentile

GRE Quantitative: 62nd percentile

Average Healthcare Experience: 2,864 hours

PANCE SCORES

5-year First Time Pass: N/A

Most Recent First Time Pass: N/A (have not graduated a class yet)

CURRICULUM STRUCTURE

Didactic: 12 months

Clinical: 12 months

Rotations: 7 mandatory, 2 elective (each 5 weeks)

Capstone Research Project: Required for graduation

UNIQUE PROGRAM FEATURES

Educational Resources: Students have access to world class facilities within the Morsani College of Medicine and 4 libraries including the USF Health Sciences Library as well as the main campus library.

Admissions: Approximately 80-90% of accepted students are from Florida each year.

University of Tampa

401 W. Kennedy Blvd.
Box 11F
Tampa, FL 33606
Phone: 813-257-3071
Email: pam@ut.edu

PROGRAM HIGHLIGHTS

Accreditation: Provisional

Degree Offered: Master (MPAM)

Start Date: August annually

Program Length: 27 months

Class Capacity: 48 students

Tuition: $100,450

CASPA Participant: Yes

Supplemental Application: Yes (no fee)

Yellow Ribbon: Yes

Admissions: Non-rolling

Application Deadline: September 1

PREREQUISITE COURSEWORK

General Biology I and II with lab (2 semesters), Microbiology with lab (1 semester), Anatomy and Physiology I and II with lab (2 semesters), General Chemistry I and II with lab (2 semesters), Statistics (1 semester). Prerequisite courses must be completed with a "C" or better and those greater than 10 years from the date of graduation (degree during which prerequisites were completed) will not be accepted unless the applicant has provided direct patient care for at least 4,000 hours within the last 10 years from Sept. 1 of the year applied. AP credits may be accepted. Recommended Courses: Medical Terminology, Biochemistry, Genetics, Organic Chemistry, Educational Psychology, Biostatistics.

GPA Requirement: Prerequisite GPA 3.0; Last 60 Hour GPA 3.0

Healthcare Experience: 500 hours (recommended)

PA Shadowing: Preferred, not required

Required Standardized Testing: None

Letters of Recommendation: Three required; faculty, coaches, employers, patients or health care providers with whom the applicant has a shadow or work history

Seat Deposit: $1,000

UNIVERSITY OF TAMPA

MISSION:

To provide a scholarly environment in which students from diverse backgrounds will receive the requisite knowledge and skills to equip them to deliver high-quality, culturally sensitive, and compassionate healthcare in collaboration with physicians in an interdisciplinary healthcare team.

CLASS OF 2021

Male: 35%

Female: 65%

Overall GPA: 3.45

Prerequisite GPA: 3.52

Last 60 Credit Hours GPA: 3.59

Average Healthcare Experience: 5,424 hours

PANCE SCORES

5-year First Time Pass: N/A

Most Recent First Time Pass: N/A (have not graduated a class yet)

CURRICULUM STRUCTURE

Didactic: 15 months

Clinical: 12 months

Rotations: 7 mandatory, 2 elective (each 4-6 weeks)

Capstone Research Project: Required for graduation

UNIQUE PROGRAM FEATURES

Admissions Preference: Preference is given to those with community service or mission work > 250 hours, leadership activities > 1 year, a graduate degree earned in any discipline, military service, and to UT alumni.

Additional Certifications: Included in the curriculum are BLS, ACLS, PALS, pre-hospital trauma and life support, and ultrasound-guided procedure certification.

Facilities: UT's PA program is housed in the new Graduate and Health Studies Building, which provides 30,000 square feet of medical training space on two floors. The PA unit includes a simulation center with both high fidelity simulators and standardized patients to allow for competency-based training and assessment. The PA program incorporates cutting-edge technology throughout the curriculum including the Anatomage table, SynDaver and i-Human patients.

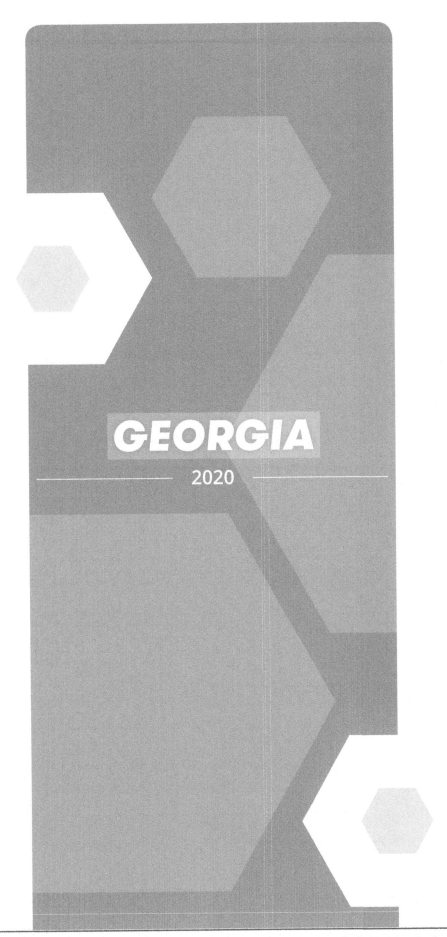

GEORGIA

2020

Augusta University

1120 15th Street
EC-3304
Augusta, GA 30912
Phone: 706-721-3247
Email: paprogram@augusta.edu

PROGRAM HIGHLIGHTS

Accreditation: Continuing

Degree Offered: Master (MPA)

Start Date: May annually

Program Length: 27 months

Class Capacity: 44 students

Tuition: $48,825 (in-state);
$97,650 (out-of-state)

CASPA Participant: No

Supplemental Application: No

Yellow Ribbon: Yes

Admissions: Rolling

Application Deadline: October 15

PREREQUISITE COURSEWORK

General Chemistry I and II with lab (8 credits),
Biology I and II with lab (8 credits), Human Anatomy
and Physiology with lab (4 credits), General
Psychology (3 credits), Organic Chemistry I with lab
(4 credits), Statistics (3 credits), Microbiology with
lab (4 credits). The program also has several other
prerequisites divided into different categories
that are typically completed as general education
requirements in a Bachelor degree program
(please see website). Recommended courses:
Anatomy and Physiology II with Lab, Comparative
Vertebrae Anatomy, Organic Chemistry II,
Histology, Biochemistry, Evolution, Human Growth
and Development, Abnormal Psychology, Cell and
Molecular Biology, Genetics, Embryology, Physics.

GPA Requirement: Overall GPA 3.0;
Science GPA 3.0

Healthcare Experience: 100 hours

PA Shadowing: 100 hours (suggested in two
different clinical settings)

Required Standardized Testing: GRE (290
minimum), CASPer

Letters of Recommendation: Three required; at
least one reference from a PA from each of the
clinical settings observed by the applicant is highly
recommended

Seat Deposit: $500

AUGUSTA UNIVERSITY

MISSION:

To develop physician assistants with the knowledge and skills to practice in all aspects of medicine from a primary care perspective and to meet the needs of society through education, discovery and service.

CLASS OF 2020

Male: 18%

Female: 82%

Overall GPA: 3.65

Science GPA: 3.55

GRE Total: 305

Average Age: 25

PANCE SCORES

5-year First Time Pass: 96%

Most Recent First Time Pass: 98%

CURRICULUM STRUCTURE

Didactic: 15 months

Clinical: 12 months

Rotations: 8 mandatory, 1 elective (each 4 weeks)

Research Project: Required for graduation

UNIQUE PROGRAM FEATURES

Facilities: Students have a full anatomy dissection lab and large simulation laboratory to learn clinical skills as well as a fully equipped surgical suite.

Free Clinic: Students run a free monthly health promotion and disease prevention clinic in conjunction with a soup kitchen to serve the underserved community.

Admissions: Approximately 90% of students are from Georgia in each class.

Emory University

1462 Clifton Rd NE, Suite 276
Atlanta, GA 30322
Phone: 404-727-7825
Email: pa_admissions@emory.edu

PROGRAM HIGHLIGHTS

Accreditation: Continuing

Degree Offered: Master (MMSc)

Start Date: August annually

Program Length: 29 months

Class Capacity: 54 students

Tuition: $102,000

CASPA Participant: Yes

Supplemental Application: Yes ($75 fee)

Yellow Ribbon: Yes

Admissions: Rolling

Application Deadline: September 1

PREREQUISITE COURSEWORK

Biology with lab (4 credits), General Chemistry with lab (8 credits), Human Anatomy and Physiology with lab (8 credits), Organic Chemistry or Biochemistry (3 credits), Statistics or Biostatistics (3 credits). Prerequisites must be completed by December of the application year and with a grade "C" or better. Recommended courses: Microbiology, Genetics.

GPA Requirement: Overall GPA 3.0; Science GPA 3.0

Healthcare Experience: 2,000 hours

PA Shadowing: Preferred, not required

Required Standardized Testing: GRE (preferred Verbal > 153, Quantitative > 144, Analytical > 4)

Letters of Recommendation: Two required; no one specific

Seat Deposit: $1,000

EMORY UNIVERSITY

MISSION:

Our mission is to recruit, educate and mentor a diverse group of students to become highly regarded, sought after physician assistants providing compassionate health care of the highest quality. To that end we create an educational environment that promotes an understanding of human needs and ethical issues as well as the acquisition and application of patient-oriented clinical knowledge and skills.

CLASS OF 2021

Male: 24%

Female: 76%

Overall GPA: 3.60

Science GPA: 3.53

GRE Verbal: 152

GRE Quantitative: 153

GRE Analytical: 4.3

Average Healthcare Experience: 6,781 hours

Average Volunteer Experience: 2,160 hours

Average Age: 27.6

PANCE SCORES

5-year First Time Pass: 92%

Most Recent First Time Pass: 77%

CURRICULUM STRUCTURE

Didactic: 17 months

Clinical: 12 months

Rotations: 7 mandatory, 3 elective (each 5 weeks)

Thesis Project: Required for graduation

UNIQUE PROGRAM FEATURES

Dual Degree: Emory offers a dual MPH/MMSc degree program through the Rollins School of Public Health, which typically takes just over 3 years to complete.

Farmworker Health Project: For the past 22 years, students have cared for over 27,000 farm workers, traveling to farms, fieldside areas, sheds, stores, and churches to set up clinics working with other health professions students. There are several other community service projects students participate in as well with more details on their website, as well as several other clinic opportunities.

Social Medicine Elective: Students may participate in a four-week elective during their clinical year that aims to deepen their understanding of the social determinants of health and patient advocacy while learning strategies to overcome health disparities through service learning and experiential activities in the community.

Mercer University

3001 Mercer University Drive
Davis Building, Suite 213
Atlanta, GA 30341
Phone: 678-547-6305
Email: paprogram@mercer.edu

PROGRAM HIGHLIGHTS

Accreditation: Continuing
Degree Offered: Master (MMSc)
Start Date: January annually
Program Length: 28 months
Class Capacity: 70 students
Tuition: $82,425

CASPA Participant: Yes
Supplemental Application: Yes ($25 fee)
Yellow Ribbon: No
Admissions: Non-rolling
Application Deadline: March 1

PREREQUISITE COURSEWORK

General Chemistry I and II with lab (2 courses), Organic Chemistry (1 course), Biochemistry (1 course), General Biology I and II with lab (2 courses), Human Anatomy and Physiology I and II with lab (2 courses), Microbiology with lab (1 course), English Composition or Intensive writing (2 courses), Statistics or Biostatistics (1 course), General or Introductory Psychology (1 course). Anatomy and Physiology should be completed within the last 10 years. Prerequisites must be completed with a grade "C" or better. AP credits are accepted for scores 3 or better.

GPA Requirement: Overall GPA 3.0; Science GPA 2.9

Healthcare Experience: 1,000 hours

PA Shadowing: Preferred, not required

Required Standardized Testing: GRE (combined score of 300 and analytical score of 3.5 required)

Letters of Recommendation: Three required; one from a practicing PA, MD, or DO, one from a college-level instructor, and one from a non-relative

Seat Deposit: $1,000

MERCER UNIVERSITY

MISSION:

The mission of the Department of Physician Assistant Studies is to educate patient-centered medical providers of the highest quality who are critical thinkers, leaders, and life-long learners.

CLASS OF 2020

Overall GPA: 3.89

Science GPA: 3.47

GRE Total: 310

Average Healthcare Experience: 3,029 hours

PANCE SCORES

5-year First Time Pass: 98%

Most Recent First Time Pass: 100%

CURRICULUM STRUCTURE

Didactic: 13 months

Clinical: 15 months

Rotations: 9 mandatory, 2 elective (each 5 weeks)

Senior Seminar Project: Required for graduation

UNIQUE PROGRAM FEATURES

Godsey-Matthews Student Society: The society is very active and was awarded the Outstanding Silver Student Society Award by SAAAPA in 2014 and the Outstanding Bronze Student Society Award in 2012.

Good Samaritan Health Clinic: Didactic and clinical Mercer PA students partner with faculty and other healthcare providers to extend medical care to the underinsured and uninsured patients in the community.

Medical Mission Trips: Students have recently traveled to Haiti, Nicaragua, Madagascar and Ecuador to deliver healthcare.

Dual Degree: A combined MMSc/MPH program is offered, which adds approximately 1 year to the PA program duration.

Morehouse School of Medicine

720 Westview Drive
Atlanta, GA 30310
Phone: 404-756-1254
Email: pas@msm.edu

PROGRAM HIGHLIGHTS

Accreditation: Provisional

Degree Offered: Master (MSM)

Start Date: June annually

Program Length: 28 months

Class Capacity: 20 students

Tuition: $95,000

CASPA Participant: Yes

Supplemental Application: No

Yellow Ribbon: No

Admissions: Rolling

Application Deadline: October 1

PREREQUISITE COURSEWORK

Biology with lab (8 credits), Microbiology (3 credits), Organic Chemistry I with lab (4 credits), Organic Chemistry II with lab or Biochemistry (4 credits), Human Anatomy and Physiology I and II (6-8 credits), Statistics (3 credits), Psychology (3 credits). A 3.0 GPA for last 60 hours of undergraduate coursework will be considered for candidates with less than a 3.0 cumulative undergraduate GPA. Prerequisites must be completed with a grade of "C" or better and within the last 7 years. AP credits are not accepted.

GPA Requirement: Overall GPA 3.0; Science GPA 3.0

Healthcare Experience: 500 hours

PA Shadowing: Preferred, not required

Required Standardized Testing: GRE or MCAT

Letters of Recommendation: Three required; recommended to be from a PA or physician, academic professor and former employer

Seat Deposit: $500

MOREHOUSE SCHOOL OF MEDICINE

MISSION:

The mission of the Morehouse School of Medicine Physician Assistant Program is to lead the creation and advancement of health equity by empowering and educating the next generation of physician assistants to achieve academic, personal, and professional success and become committed life-long learners who will provide compassionate, high quality, patient-centered care to meet the primary health care needs of the urban and rural underserved populations in Georgia and the nation.

NO CLASS STATISTICS REPORTED

PANCE SCORES

5-year First Time Pass: N/A

Most Recent First Time Pass: N/A (have not graduated a class yet)

CURRICULUM STRUCTURE

Didactic: 13 months

Clinical: 15 months

Rotations: 7 mandatory, 1 elective (each 4-8 weeks)

Capstone Project: Required for graduation

UNIQUE PROGRAM FEATURES

Admissions Preference: The school awards additional admissions points for those who are residents of Georgia or those with Georgia heritage, rural residents, veterans, populations under-represented in medicine, and Atlanta University school of MSM Pipeline Program participants.

South University

709 Mall Boulevard
Savannah, GA 31406
Phone: 912-201-8171
Email:
paprogram@southuniversity.edu

PROGRAM HIGHLIGHTS

Accreditation: Continuing

Degree Offered: Master (MSPA)

Start Date: January annually

Program Length: 27 months

Class Capacity: 70 students

Tuition: $88,610 (including fees)

CASPA Participant: Yes

Supplemental Application: No

Yellow Ribbon: Yes

Admissions: Non-rolling

Application Deadline: August 1

PREREQUISITE COURSEWORK

Human Anatomy with lab (1 course), Human Physiology with lab (1 course), General Biology I and II (2 courses), General Chemistry I and II with lab (2 courses), Biochemistry or Organic Chemistry with lab (1 course), Microbiology with lab (1 course). Prerequisites must be completed with a grade "C" or better. AP credits are accepted.

GPA Requirement: Overall GPA 3.0; Science GPA 3.0

Healthcare Experience: Preferred, not required

PA Shadowing: Preferred, not required

Required Standardized Testing: GRE (preference given to those with scores at or above the 50th percentile), CASPer

Letters of Recommendation: Three required; one from an MD/DO/PA/NP

Seat Deposit: $500

SOUTH UNIVERSITY

MISSION:

The South University, Savannah Physician Assistant Studies program exists to educate a diverse student population as providers of high quality, cost-efficient health care who will make a positive difference while practicing the art and science of medicine with physician direction.

CLASS OF 2021

Male: 19%

Female: 81%

Minority: 10%

Overall GPA: 3.65

Average Healthcare Experience: 2,431 hours

Average Age: 24

PANCE SCORES

5-year First Time Pass: 96%

Most Recent First Time Pass: 97%

CURRICULUM STRUCTURE

Didactic: 15 months

Clinical: 12 months

Rotations: 7 mandatory, 1 elective (each 5 weeks)

UNIQUE PROGRAM FEATURES

Early Clinical Exposure: The program offers early patient contact to students during the didactic year to begin to correlate classroom learning with patient care.

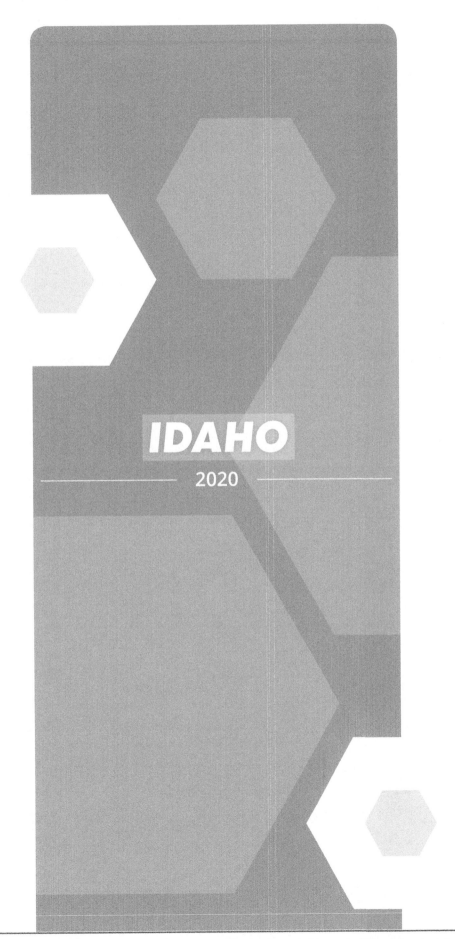

IDAHO

2020

PROGRAM HIGHLIGHTS

Accreditation: Continuing

Degree Offered: Master (MPAS)

Start Date: August annually

Program Length: 24 months

Class Capacity: 72 students

Tuition: $71,658 (in-state); $120,666 (out-of-state)

CASPA Participant: Yes

Supplemental Application: Yes ($60 fee)

Yellow Ribbon: Yes

Admissions: Non-rolling

Application Deadline: November 1

PREREQUISITE COURSEWORK

Microbiology, Biochemistry, Human Anatomy, Human Psychology, Statistics, Abnormal Psychology or Developmental Psychology. First time applicants may have two courses in progress at the time of application, while reapplicants must have completed all coursework prior to reapplying. Prerequisites must be completed with a grade "C" or better. Recommended courses: Advanced Anatomy and Physiology, Immunology, Genetics, Endocrinology, Psychology, Sociology, Anthropology, Health Education, Gender Studies, Spanish.

GPA Requirement: Prerequisite GPA 3.0

Healthcare Experience: Preferred, not required

PA Shadowing: Preferred, not required

Required Standardized Testing: GRE, CASPer

Letters of Recommendation: Three required; no one specific

Seat Deposit: $750

IDAHO STATE UNIVERSITY

MISSION:

The mission of the Idaho State University Physician Assistant program is to train PAs through service-oriented, multimodal, innovative learning. Graduates from ISUs PA Program will be highly competent, compassionate health care providers dedicated to serving individuals and their communities.

CLASS OF 2021

Prerequisite GPA: 3.87

GRE Verbal: 77th percentile

GRE Quantitative: 61st percentile

PANCE SCORES

5-year First Time Pass: 96%

Most Recent First Time Pass: 93%

CURRICULUM STRUCTURE

Didactic: 12 months

Clinical: 12 months

Rotations: 7 mandatory, 1 elective (duration not specified)

Capstone Project: Required for graduation

UNIQUE PROGRAM FEATURES

Medical Spanish: Students can pursue individual Spanish for Healthcare Professions courses or complete a 15-credit sequence to earn a graduate certificate in Spanish for Healthcare Professions.

Opioid Course: Students can complete a course in Medication Assisted Therapy for opioid addiction.

International Activity: Students can participate in medical missions to the Dominican Republic or Peru, and have the opportunity to complete an international rotation in Belize.

One Program, Three Campuses: The program is offered simultaneously on three campuses in Pocatello, Meridian, and Caldwell to encompass the total 72 student class size.

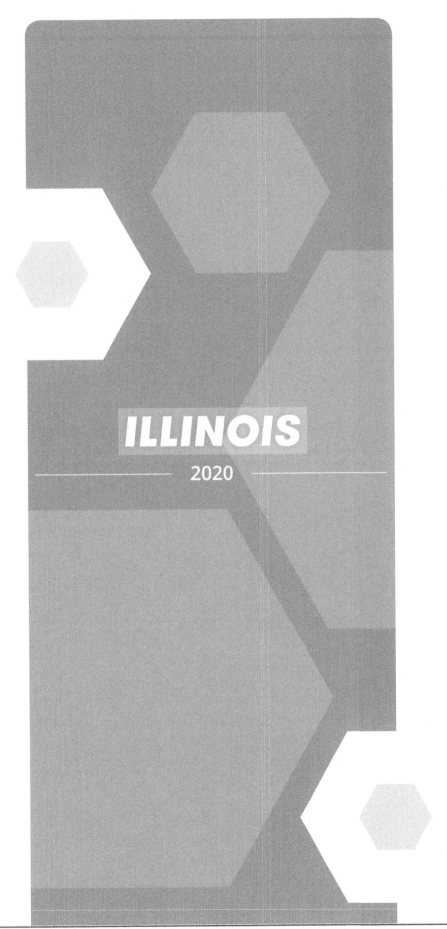

ILLINOIS

2020

PROGRAM HIGHLIGHTS

Accreditation: Provisional

Degree Offered: Master (MPAS)

Start Date: January annually

Program Length: 24 months

Class Capacity: 30 students

Tuition: $99,890 (including fees)

CASPA Participant: Yes

Supplemental Application: No

Yellow Ribbon: Yes

Admissions: Rolling

Application Deadline: August 1

PREREQUISITE COURSEWORK

Human or Vertebrate Anatomy (4 credits), Human or Vertebrate Physiology (3 credits), Biochemistry (3 credits), Microbiology with lab (4 credits), General or Organic Chemistry with lab (4 credits), Additional Biology or Chemistry (3 credits), Statistics (3 credits), Psychology (3 credits), Humanities and Social Sciences (9 credits). The most competitive applicants will have completed courses in the last 7 years and all courses must be completed by September 1st. Prerequisites must be completed with a grade "C" or better. AP credits are not accepted.

GPA Requirement: Overall GPA 3.0; Science GPA 3.0

Healthcare Experience: 1,000 hours

PA Shadowing: 15 hours

Required Standardized Testing: GRE

Letters of Recommendation: Three required; strongly recommended to have one each from a professor, a supervisor and a PA

Seat Deposit: $1,000

DOMINICAN UNIVERSITY OF ILLINOIS

MISSION:

The mission of the Dominican University Physician Assistant Studies program is to produce graduate level physician assistants to provide highly competent patient-centered and compassionate health care in collaboration with physicians. Our physician assistants will serve as an integral member of an inter-professional healthcare team. Our graduates will demonstrate leadership, service and lifelong learning.

CLASS OF 2021

Male: 27%

Female: 73%

Minority: 23%

Overall GPA: 3.56

Science GPA 3.47

GRE Verbal: 51st percentile

GRE Quantitative: 51st percentile

GRE Analytical: 71st percentile

Average Healthcare Experience: 3,696 hours

Average Age: 25

PANCE SCORES

5-year First Time Pass: 77% (based on one year of data plus two additional test takers)

Most Recent First Time Pass: 76%

CURRICULUM STRUCTURE

Didactic: 12 months

Clinical: 12 months

Rotations: 7 mandatory, 1 selective, 2 elective (4 weeks each)

Evidence-Based Research Project: Required for graduation

UNIQUE PROGRAM FEATURES

Medical Spanish: All students complete a basic Spanish course as part of the last didactic semester.

Hybrid Anatomy: The anatomy course will be taught with both traditional cadaveric study and also virtual cadavers using the Anatomage Table.

Community Service: All PA program faculty, staff, and students are required to complete at least one community service project annually.

Midwestern University

555 31st Street
Downers Grove, IL 60515
Phone: 630-515-6034
Email: admissil@midwestern.edu

PROGRAM HIGHLIGHTS

Accreditation: Continuing

Degree Offered: Master (MMS)

Start Date: June annually

Program Length: 27 months

Class Capacity: 86 students

Tuition: $116,186

CASPA Participant: Yes

Supplemental Application: No

Yellow Ribbon: No

Admissions: Rolling

Application Deadline: October 1

PREREQUISITE COURSEWORK

Biology with lab (4 credits), Anatomy
(4 credits), General Chemistry with
lab (8 credits), Organic Chemistry
with lab (4 credits), Math (3 credits),
Statistics (3 credits), English
Composition (6 credits), Social and
Behavioral Sciences (6 credits).
All courses must be completed
by December 31st of the year of
application. Prerequisites must
be completed with a grade "C" or
better. AP credits are accepted.

GPA Requirement: Overall GPA 3.0;
Science GPA 3.0

Healthcare Experience: Preferred,
not required

PA Shadowing: Preferred, not
required

Required Standardized Testing: GRE
(50th percentile expected for each
section), CASPer

Letters of Recommendation: Two
required; no one specific

Seat Deposit: $200

MIDWESTERN UNIVERSITY (DOWNERS GROVE)

MISSION:

The mission of the Midwestern University Physician Assistant (PA)
Program is to develop competent and compassionate physician
assistants who will make meaningful contributions to their patients,
community, and profession.

CLASS OF 2021

Male: 12%

Female: 88%

Overall GPA: 3.79

Science GPA: 3.76

GRE Verbal: 56th percentile

GRE Quantitative: 55th percentile

GRE Writing: 69th percentile

Average Age: 24

PANCE SCORES

5-year First Time Pass: 99%

Most Recent First Time Pass: 100%

CURRICULUM STRUCTURE

Didactic: 12 months

Clinical: 15 months

Rotations: 8 mandatory, 2 elective (each 4-6 weeks)

Capstone Project: Required for graduation

UNIQUE PROGRAM FEATURES

Diverse Rotations: Students will be assigned to rotations
that exemplify the geographic and demographic diversity of
the region including inpatient and outpatient settings as well
as rotations in urban, suburban, and rural communities.

Northwestern University

240 E. Huron Street
McGaw Pavilion Suite 1-200
Chicago, IL 60625
Phone: 312-503-1851
Email:
paprogram@northwestern.edu

PROGRAM HIGHLIGHTS

Accreditation: Continuing

Degree Offered: Master (MMS)

Start Date: June annually

Program Length: 24 months

Class Capacity: 36 students

Tuition: $95,904

CASPA Participant: Yes

Supplemental Application: Yes ($50 fee)

Yellow Ribbon: Yes

Admissions: Rolling

Application Deadline: October 1

PREREQUISITE COURSEWORK

Biochemistry (1 semester), Microbiology (1 semester), Statistics (1 semester), Medical Terminology (1 semester), Anatomy and Physiology (2 semesters). At most two prerequisites may be in progress during the fall prior to admission and one in the spring prior to admission. Prerequisites must be completed with a grade "C" or better in the last 7 years. AP courses will be accepted as long as classes appear on a college transcript with assigned credits.

GPA Requirement: Overall GPA 2.8

Healthcare Experience: 1,000 hours

PA Shadowing: Preferred, not required

Required Standardized Testing: GRE

Letters of Recommendation: Three required; at least one from a healthcare provider

Seat Deposit: $1,000

NORTHWESTERN UNIVERSITY

MISSION:

The mission of the Northwestern University Feinberg School of Medicine Physician Assistant (PA) Program is to prepare PAs to provide compassionate, high quality, patient-centered care as members of interdisciplinary teams. The graduates will be culturally competent, committed to continuous learning and professional development, and make significant contributions to communities and the advancement of the PA profession.

CLASS OF 2021

Male: 22%

Female: 78%

Minority: 14%

Overall GPA: 3.65

Science GPA: 3.61

Prerequisite GPA: 3.77

GRE Verbal: 77th percentile

GRE Quantitative: 69th percentile

GRE Analytical: 4.5

Average Healthcare Experience: 5,033 hours

Average Age: 26

PANCE SCORES

5-year First Time Pass: 100%

Most Recent First Time Pass: 100%

CURRICULUM STRUCTURE

Didactic: 12 months

Clinical: 12 months

Rotations: 7 mandatory, 4 elective (each 4 weeks)

Master's Project: Required for graduation

UNIQUE PROGRAM FEATURES

Problem Based Learning: This program utilizes problem-based learning for much of the didactic curriculum. Students work in small groups of 6-8 students on clinical problems and also collaborate with medical students to solve simulated cases.

Interprofessional Education: Students from the MD, PA, and DPT programs began an interprofessional teamwork learning initiative in 2016 where students learn to work together as teams.

Facilities: Students have 24-hour access to world-class facilities including an anatomy laboratory, simulation technology and immersive learning center, clinical education center, health-sciences library, small group rooms, and several of the area's top hospitals for clinical learning.

Medical Spanish: Students take a medical Spanish course in the final didactic semester.

3333 Green Bay Road
North Chicago, IL 60064
Phone: 847-578-8302
Email:
pa.admissions@rosalindfranklin.edu

PROGRAM HIGHLIGHTS

Accreditation: Continuing

Degree Offered: Master (MS)

Start Date: May annually

Program Length: 24 months

Class Capacity: 67 students

Tuition: $86,174

CASPA Participant: Yes

Supplemental Application: No ($35 extra fee to apply)

Yellow Ribbon: No

Admissions: Rolling

Application Deadline: December 1

PREREQUISITE COURSEWORK

Biochemistry (3 credits), Human Anatomy (3 credits), Human Physiology (3 credits), Introduction to Psychology (3 credits), Microbiology (3 credits). Up to three courses may be outstanding at the time of application. Prerequisites must be completed with a grade "C" or better. Recommended courses: Statistics, Research Design, Technical Writing, Medical Terminology, Medical Ethics, Child, Developmental or Abnormal Psychology.

GPA Requirement: Overall GPA 2.75; Science GPA 2.75

Healthcare Experience: Preferred, not required

PA Shadowing: Preferred, not required

Required Standardized Testing: GRE

Letters of Recommendation: Two required; one should be from an instructor who can attest to the applicant's scholastic aptitude, and one from a healthcare professional with whom the applicant has worked

Seat Deposit: $500

ROSALIND FRANKLIN UNIVERSITY OF MEDICINE

MISSION:

The mission of the Physician Assistant Program is to educate and prepare competent, compassionate, and ethical physician assistant leaders who, as integral members of the inter-professional healthcare team, will provide quality medical care.

CLASS OF 2020

Overall GPA: 3.58

Science GPA: 3.55

GRE Total: 312

Average Age: 25

PANCE SCORES

5-year First Time Pass: 99%

Most Recent First Time Pass: 98%

CURRICULUM STRUCTURE

Didactic: 12 months

Clinical: 12 months

Rotations: 6 mandatory, 2 elective (each 6 weeks)

Master's Project: Required for graduation

UNIQUE PROGRAM FEATURES

Community Service: PA students participate in several activities in the community, such as Kid's First Health Fair, Healthy Families Clinic, Interprofessional Community Clinic, and Community Care Connection.

Research Day: Students deliver poster presentations of their Master's projects as part of the University-wide research day each spring.

Creative Arts Collection: Students, faculty, and alumni maintain a creative arts collection and are encouraged to submit pieces in the form of short story, photography, drawing or painting to the peer-reviewed collection.

Admissions Preference: Students are given additional admissions consideration who are Black or African American, American Indian, Spanish/ Hispanic/Latino/Latina, males, any person who has served honorably in the armed forces of the United States, any person who is socially-disadvantaged or first generation college, a student in the DePaul Pathways Honors Program or the Early Opportunity Program, and an RFUMS student (i.e. biomedical sciences program).

PROGRAM HIGHLIGHTS

Accreditation: Continuing

Degree Offered: Master (MSPAS)

Start Date: June annually

Program Length: 30 months

Class Capacity: 30 students

Tuition: $100,848

CASPA Participant: Yes

Supplemental Application: Yes ($40 fee)

Yellow Ribbon: Yes

Admissions: Rolling

Application Deadline: October 1

PREREQUISITE COURSEWORK

Biochemistry, Human Anatomy, Human Physiology, Microbiology, Psychology, Statistics. Science courses should be taken within the last 7 years. Candidates must have completed at least four prerequisites before applying. Prerequisites must be completed with a grade "C" or better. AP credits are not accepted.

GPA Requirement: Overall GPA 3.0; Science GPA 3.0

Healthcare Experience: 1,000 hours

PA Shadowing: Not required

Required Standardized Testing: GRE (302 minimum score)

Letters of Recommendation: Three required; preferred that at least one be from a PA, physician or other health care provider who is familiar with the PA profession

Seat Deposit: $250

RUSH UNIVERSITY

MISSION:

The Rush University PA program mission is to educate advanced health care providers to practice evidence-based medicine with competence, professionalism and compassion driven by academic excellence and service to diverse communities.

CLASS OF 2020

Male: 30%

Female: 70%

Overall GPA: 3.42

Science GPA: 3.37

GRE Total: 309

Average Healthcare Experience: 2,600 hours

Average Age: 27

PANCE SCORES

5-year First Time Pass: 99%

Most Recent First Time Pass: 100%

CURRICULUM STRUCTURE

Didactic: 12 months

Clinical: 18 months

Rotations: 10 mandatory, 2 elective (4 weeks each), 2 advanced practice rotations (15 weeks each)

Master's Research Project: Required for graduation

UNIQUE PROGRAM FEATURES

Advanced Practice Rotations: Students complete 6 months of advanced clinical rotations where they choose a single, focused area of practice to hone their skills and improve patient management prior to graduation.

Community Service: Each class of 30 students on average completes a total of 1,025 hours of community service and medical mission work during their time at Rush.

Admissions Preference: Additional consideration is given to military veterans, underrepresented minorities, persons from economically disadvantaged backgrounds, and those who are the first person to attend a higher education training program in their family.

Southern Illinois University School of Medicine

300 W. Oak St., Mail Code 6516
Carbondale, IL 62901
Phone: 618-453-5527
Email:
paadvisement-L@listserv.siu.edu

PROGRAM HIGHLIGHTS

Accreditation: Continuing

Degree Offered: Master (MSPA)

Start Date: June annually

Program Length: 26 months

Class Capacity: 40 students

Tuition: $70,000 (in-state);
$120,000 (out-of-state)

CASPA Participant: Yes

Supplemental Application: Yes ($50 fee)

Yellow Ribbon: No

Admissions: Rolling

Application Deadline: November 1

PREREQUISITE COURSEWORK

Medical Terminology (or passage of proficiency exam), Chemistry with lab (2 semesters), Psychology (1 semester), Human Physiology (1 semester), Human Anatomy (1 semester), Microbiology with lab (1 semester), General Biology (1 semester), Statistics (1 semester), English Composition (1 semester), Basic Cardiac Life Support. Prerequisites must be completed with a grade "C" or better and by the end of the fall semester prior to matriculation (with the exception of one prerequisite with a grade "A" or "B" and Medical Terminology). Recommended courses: Genetics, Pharmacology, Pathophysiology, Biochemistry.

GPA Requirement: Overall GPA 3.2; Science GPA 3.2; Prerequisite GPA 3.2

Healthcare Experience: Preferred, not required

PA Shadowing: Preferred, not required

Required Standardized Testing: GRE

Letters of Recommendation: Three required; one from a PA

Seat Deposit: $1,000

SOUTHERN ILLINOIS UNIVERSITY

MISSION:

The mission of the Southern Illinois University Physician Assistant Program is to prepare healthcare professionals to provide primary health care to underserved populations in rural and health professional shortage areas. We will enhance this healthcare by preparing graduates who are interdependent medical providers, dedicated to both community and profession. The academic setting, utilizing Problem-Based Learning, will foster creative thinking and communication skills in our pursuit of excellence.

NO CLASS STATISTICS REPORTED

PANCE SCORES

5-year First Time Pass: 100%

Most Recent First Time Pass: 100%

CURRICULUM STRUCTURE

Didactic: 12 months

Clinical: 14 months

Rotations: 8 mandatory, 1 elective, 1 preceptorship (8 weeks)

Master's Project: Required for graduation

UNIQUE PROGRAM FEATURES

Elective Coursework: The program offers both independent study and holistic medicine elective courses.

Problem Based Learning: The program utilizes problem-based learning in didactic and clinical years. The PBL cases are based on real patient problems that are carefully selected by faculty to stimulate students' learning in all relevant areas of basic clinical and behavioral sciences.

Rotations: Students are assigned a hubsite for their clinical rotations in Illinois and may be required to relocate to one of these hubsites during clinical year.

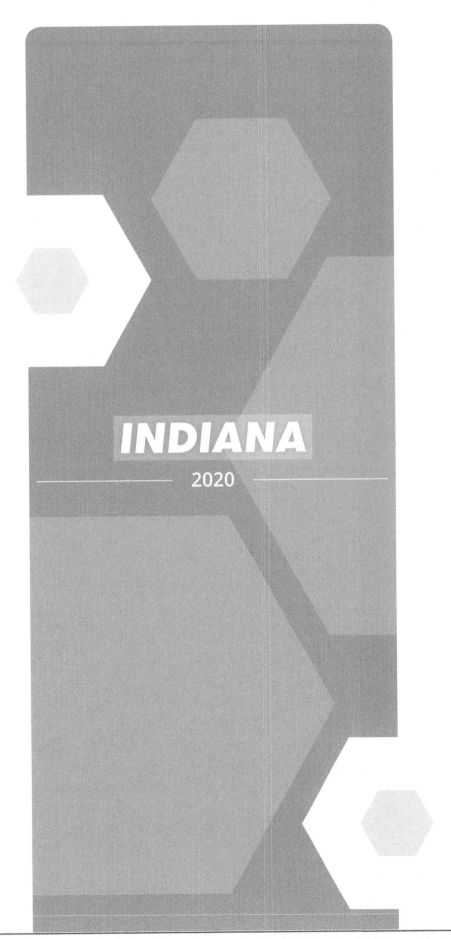

INDIANA

2020

Butler University

4600 Sunset Avenue
Indianapolis, IN 46208
Phone: 317-940-6026
Email: paadmission@butler.edu

PROGRAM HIGHLIGHTS

Accreditation: Continuing
Degree Offered: Master (MPAS)
Start Date: May annually
Program Length: 24 months
Class Capacity: 75 students
Tuition: $89,640

CASPA Participant: Yes
Supplemental Application: No
Yellow Ribbon: No
Admissions: Non-rolling
Application Deadline: August 1

PREREQUISITE COURSEWORK

General Chemistry with lab (2 semesters), Organic Chemistry with lab (1 semester), additional Chemistry course at 300 level or above (1 semester), Biology at 200 level or above (5 semesters), Statistics or Biostatistics (1 semester), Social Sciences (2 semesters). No more than three outstanding prerequisites may be remaining at the time of application, and only one Chemistry or Biology related prerequisite may be outstanding at the time of application. Prerequisites must be completed with a grade "C-" or better. AP exam scores of 4 or 5 may substitute for prerequisite courses. Appropriately earned AP scores may replace no more than two prerequisite courses.

GPA Requirement: Overall GPA 3.2
Healthcare Experience: Preferred, not required
PA Shadowing: Not required
Required Standardized Testing: GRE
Letters of Recommendation: Three required; no one specific
Seat Deposit: $1,000

BUTLER UNIVERSITY

MISSION:

The mission of the Butler University Physician Assistant program is to produce graduates with a foundation in primary care to deliver high quality, patient-centered care in a wide variety of clinical settings.

CLASS OF 2021

Overall GPA: 3.70
GRE Verbal: 157
GRE Quantitative: 156
GRE Analytical: 4.3

PANCE SCORES

5-year First Time Pass: 98%

Most Recent First Time Pass: 96%

CURRICULUM STRUCTURE

Didactic: 12 months
Clinical: 12 months
Rotations: 10 mandatory, 1 elective (each 4 weeks)

UNIQUE PROGRAM FEATURES

SimLab: PA students can practice patient examinations and procedures on standardized patients and mannequins to simulate a variety of illnesses and conditions in the Butler SimLab.

Ultrasound: This is one of the only programs to incorporate ultrasound use and applications longitudinally throughout the program.

Advocacy: Butler PA students and faculty have opportunities to lobby the Indiana General Assembly and U.S. Congress to promote expanded roles in healthcare for PAs.

Admissions Preference: 45 students will be selected for admissions from the Butler University community or alumni pool. This leaves up to 30 students to be admitted through CASPA. Additionally, one seat in the program will be "reserved" for either a veteran or an active military member (Active Duty, Reserve, and National Guard) who meets all minimum application criteria.

Franklin College

101 Branigin Boulevard
Acorn Graduate Health Science Center
Franklin, IN 46131
Phone: 317-738-8095
Email:
paprogram@franklincollege.edu

PROGRAM HIGHLIGHTS

Accreditation: Provisional

Degree Offered: Master (MSPAS)

Start Date: January annually

Program Length: 25 months

Class Capacity: 24 students

Tuition: $85,000

CASPA Participant: Yes

Supplemental Application: No

Yellow Ribbon: Yes

Admissions: Rolling

Application Deadline: September 1

PREREQUISITE COURSEWORK

General Chemistry with lab (2 semesters), Organic Chemistry with lab (1 semester), General Biology with lab (2 semesters), Human Anatomy & Physiology with lab (2 semesters), Microbiology with lab (1 semester), General Psychology (1 semester), additional Behavioral/Social Science (1 semester), Statistics or Biostatistics (1 semester), Composition/Communications (1 semester). Prerequisites must be completed with a grade "C" or better and should be completed by September 1st prior to the year of matriculation (max of 1 course may be completed after this deadline). Chemistry and Biology prerequisites must be completed within the last 7 years. Recommended courses: Medical Terminology, Biochemistry, Bioethics, Cell Biology, Genetics.

GPA Requirement: Overall GPA 3.0; Science GPA 3.0

Healthcare Experience: 200 hours

PA Shadowing: Preferred, not required

Required Standardized Testing: None

Letters of Recommendation: Three required; one from a professor/instructor, one from a physician or other healthcare provider, and one of the applicant's choosing

Seat Deposit: $1,000

FRANKLIN COLLEGE

MISSION:

The Physician Assistant Studies Program trains a new generation of qualified and dedicated advanced practice professionals with a focus on providing safe, patient-centered care to underserved populations in metropolitan and rural settings.

CLASS OF 2021

Male: 11%

Female 89%

Minority: 11%

Overall GPA: 3.60

BCP GPA: 3.44

Science GPA: 3.52

Healthcare Experience: 4,302 hours

Average Age: 24

PANCE SCORES

5-year First Time Pass: N/A

Most Recent First Time Pass: N/A (have not graduated a class yet)

CURRICULUM STRUCTURE

Didactic: 12 months

Clinical: 13 months

Rotations: 7 mandatory, 2 elective (each 5 weeks)

Capstone Community Engagement Project: Required for graduation

UNIQUE PROGRAM FEATURES

Admissions Preference: Applicants who meet any of the following criteria will receive additional consideration in the admissions process for each criterion met, and students must declare on their CASPA application under the Franklin College section that they wish to be considered: graduate of Franklin College's Professional Development Certificate Program; from a medically underserved area or population in Indiana as designated by the Indiana State Department of Health; member of an underrepresented in medicine population as determined by the American Academy of Medical Colleges; current or former member of the US military.

Indiana State University

567 N. 5th Street
Room 230
Terre Haute, IN 47809
Phone: 812-237-3632
Email: isu-pa@indstate.edu

PROGRAM HIGHLIGHTS

Accreditation: Continuing

Degree Offered: Master (MSPAS)

Start Date: January annually

Program Length: 27 months

Class Capacity: 30 students

Tuition: $38,967 (in-state); $76,539 (out-of-state)

CASPA Participant: Yes

Supplemental Application: Yes ($45 fee)

Yellow Ribbon: No

Admissions: Non-rolling

Application Deadline: March 1

PREREQUISITE COURSEWORK

Human Anatomy with lab, Human Physiology with lab, Microbiology with lab, Organic Chemistry I and II with lab, Statistics, Medical Terminology, Two Upper Level Biological Sciences courses. Prerequisites must be completed with a grade "C+" or better and by the end of the summer semester prior to the start of the program. Recommended courses: Cell Biology, Molecular Biology, Genetics, Pharmacology, Embryology, Histology, Immunology.

GPA Requirement: Overall GPA 3.0; Science GPA 3.0

Healthcare Experience: 500 hours (strongly recommended)

PA Shadowing: Not required

Required Standardized Testing: GRE (recommended minimum of 155 in each section and 4 in analytical) or MCAT

Letters of Recommendation: Three required; at least one academic and one professional letter

Seat Deposit: $500

INDIANA STATE UNIVERSITY

MISSION:

The mission of the Indiana State University Physician Assistant Program is to create a student-centered educational environment that engages individuals to become compassionate, competent physician assistants who possess the clinical skills to contribute positively to the dynamic health care needs of rural and underserved populations.

CLASS OF 2022

Overall GPA: 3.43

Science GPA: 3.28

Total GRE: 307

PANCE SCORES

5-year First Time Pass: 94%

Most Recent First Time Pass: 93%

CURRICULUM STRUCTURE

Didactic: 15 months

Clinical: 12 months

Rotations: 9 mandatory, 2 elective (each 4 weeks)

Clinical Project: Required for graduation

UNIQUE PROGRAM FEATURES

Admissions Preference: Preference is given to residents of Indiana, Indiana State University graduates, and those interested in Rural Health Medicine.

Interprofessional Education: PA students interact with physical therapy, nursing, athletic training and medical students throughout their education.

Rural Health Innovation Collaboration: The university participates in RHIC, which expands interprofessional education, training, and deployment of current and future healthcare providers committed to serving rural populations.

Indiana University School of Health and Rehabilitation Sciences

Coleman Hall, Room CF124
1140 W. Michigan Street
Indianapolis, IN 46202
Phone: 317-278-9550
Email: shrsinfo@iupui.edu

PROGRAM HIGHLIGHTS

Accreditation: Continuing

Degree Offered: Master (MPAS)

Start Date: May annually

Program Length: 27 months

Class Capacity: 44 students

Tuition: $59,32 (in-state); $85,565 (out-of-state)

CASPA Participant: Yes

Supplemental Application: Yes ($60 fee)

Yellow Ribbon: Yes

Admissions: Non-rolling

Application Deadline: August 1

PREREQUISITE COURSEWORK

Human Anatomy with lab, Human Physiology, Microbiology with lab, General Chemistry with lab (2 semesters), Statistics or Biostatistics, General Biology I with lab, Upper Level Human Biology (to be satisfied by one of the recommended courses listed below), Organic Chemistry with lab, Introductory Psychology, Medical Terminology (1 credit). Prerequisites must be completed with a grade "C" or better. Only one prerequisite may be outstanding by the application deadline. AP credits are accepted. AP credits are accepted for exam scores 3 or higher. Recommended courses: Genetics, Cell Biology, Molecular Biology, Embryology, Histology, Immunology.

GPA Requirement: Overall GPA 3.0; Science GPA 3.2

Healthcare Experience: Required (no specific number of hours)

PA Shadowing: 10 hours

Required Standardized Testing: None

Letters of Recommendation: Two required; one must be from a PA with whom you have worked or shadowed

Seat Deposit: $500

INDIANA UNIVERSITY SCHOOL OF HEALTH AND REHABILITATION SCIENCES

MISSION:

The mission of the Indiana University Master of Physician Assistant Studies program is to prepare students for physician assistant practice, with a focus on urban and rural underserved communities in the state of Indiana, using an interprofessional team approach to education.

NO CLASS STATISTICS REPORTED

PANCE SCORES

5-year First Time Pass: 96%

Most Recent First Time Pass: 98%

CURRICULUM STRUCTURE

Didactic: 15 months

Clinical: 12 months

Rotations: 9 mandatory, 2 elective, 1 medical/surgical subspecialty (each 2-4 weeks)

Research Project: Required for graduation

UNIQUE PROGRAM FEATURES

Admissions Preference: Indiana residents who live in medically underserved counties as well as military veterans are given preference points added to their total score during application review.

Underserved Rotation: All students complete a clinical rotation at Eskenazi Health Grassy Creek Community Health Center to gain insight and experience working with patients in an underserved population.

Trine University PA Program

1819 Carew Street
Fort Wayne, IN 46805
Phone: 260-702-8060
Email: pa@trine.edu

PROGRAM HIGHLIGHTS

Accreditation: Provisional

Degree Offered: Master (MPAS)

Start Date: August annually

Program Length: 27 months

Class Capacity: 36 students

Tuition: $96,656

CASPA Participant: Yes

Supplemental Application: No

Yellow Ribbon: No

Admissions: Rolling

Application Deadline: March 1

PREREQUISITE COURSEWORK

Microbiology with lab (3 credits), Organic Chemistry with lab (3 credits), Human Anatomy and Physiology with lab (6 credits), Biochemistry (3 credits), Statistics (3 credits), Psychology (3 credits), Medical Terminology (1 credit or certificate). Prerequisites must be completed with grade "C" or better. AP credits are accepted for Psychology and Statistics prerequisites. Recommended courses: Genetics.

GPA Requirement: Overall GPA 3.0; Prerequisite GPA 3.0

Healthcare Experience: Preferred, not required

PA Shadowing: Preferred, not required

Required Standardized Testing: GRE (preference for combined score of 300 and analytical of 3.5)

Letters of Recommendation: Two required; academic or professional preferred

Seat Deposit: $1,000

TRINE UNIVERSITY

MISSION:

The PA Program at Trine University will provide an outstanding educational experience that produces PA graduates capable of delivering safe, appropriate, effective, and cost-efficient medical care in a variety of clinical settings, while also preparing them to succeed, lead, and serve.

NO CLASS STATISTICS REPORTED

PANCE SCORES

5-year First Time Pass: N/A

Most Recent First Time Pass: N/A (have not graduated a class yet)

CURRICULUM STRUCTURE

Didactic: 15 months

Clinical: 12 months

Rotations: 7 mandatory, 2 elective (each 2.5-5 weeks)

Research Project: Required for graduation

UNIQUE PROGRAM FEATURES

Admissions: The program will reserve up to 10 seats for students for the direct entry program. Any of these seats not filled by direct entry students will be available through the regular CASPA admission process.

Interprofessional Education: The PA program participates in the Fort Wayne Area Inter-professional Education Consortium (FWAIPEC) for Graduate Health Care. The consortium includes programs with family medicine residents, medical students, PA students, nursing students, PT students, OT students and pharmacy students. They gather 3 times a year as a collaborative effort to introduce the students to the team concept of health care, strengthen patient outcomes and add value to the community.

Team-Based Learning: The Program has designed a team-based learning (TBL) teaching strategy in the Clinical Application and Reflection Experience (CARE) courses in which small groups of students will work together on clinical cases to apply material learned in other areas of the curriculum. This strategy fosters critical clinical thinking skills.

Stone Family Center for Health Sciences
515 Walnut Street, Room 3001
Evansville, IN 47708
Phone: 812-488-3400
Email: pa@evansville.edu

PROGRAM HIGHLIGHTS

Accreditation: Provisional

Degree Offered: Master (MPAS)

Start Date: January annually

Program Length: 28 months

Class Capacity: 40 students

Tuition: $98,000

CASPA Participant: Yes

Supplemental Application: No

Yellow Ribbon: Yes

Admissions: Non-rolling

Application Deadline: August 1

PREREQUISITE COURSEWORK

General Chemistry with lab (2 semesters), Organic Chemistry with lab (2 semesters), General Biology with lab (1 semester), Microbiology with lab (1 semester), Anatomy and Physiology with lab (2 semesters), Psychology (1 semester), Social Science (1 semester), Medical Terminology. All but three prerequisites must be completed at the time of application. Prerequisites must be completed with a grade "C" or better.

GPA Requirement: Overall GPA 3.0; Prerequisite GPA 3.0

Healthcare Experience: Preferred, not required

PA Shadowing: Preferred, not required

Required Standardized Testing: GRE (minimum combined score of 300) or MCAT, CASPer

Letters of Recommendation: None required

Seat Deposit: $500

UNIVERSITY OF EVANSVILLE

MISSION:

The University of Evansville Physician Assistant Program mission is to educate well-rounded, empathetic, competent physician assistants who possess an understanding and appreciation of civic engagement, life-long learning and are leaders of change within their communities.

CLASS OF 2022

Male: 25%

Female: 75%

Overall GPA: 3.55

Prerequisite GPA: 3.52

GRE Total: 308

Average Healthcare Experience: 2,093 hours

Average Age: 24.4

PANCE SCORES

5-year First Time Pass: 100% (based on one year of data)

Most Recent First Time Pass: 100%

CURRICULUM STRUCTURE

Didactic: 16 months

Clinical: 12 months

Rotations: 10 mandatory, 3 elective (each 2-4 weeks)

UNIQUE PROGRAM FEATURES

Interprofessional Education: Students will spend 2 weeks with another member of the healthcare team that is not a physician, PA or NP. The goal is to learn about professions that are part of the interdisciplinary team and how these members contribute to the health and wellness of patients. Students also share classes with both medical school and physical therapy programs.

Facilities: The program is housed in a new multi-institutional teach facility which provides inter-professional experiences among various health professional students, collaborative learning, and research opportunities. The program offers full cadaver dissection as well.

Admissions: The program accepts 25-40 students each year from their undergraduate direct entry program, leaving 0-15 spots each year for CASPA applicants.

University of Saint Francis

2701 Spring Street
Doermer 069
Fort Wayne, IN 46808
Phone: 260-399-7700
Email: cchapman@sf.edu

PROGRAM HIGHLIGHTS

Accreditation: Continuing

Degree Offered: Master (MSPAS)

Start Date: May annually

Program Length: 27 months

Class Capacity: 25 students

Tuition: $101,045

CASPA Participant: Yes

Supplemental Application: No

Yellow Ribbon: No

Admissions: Rolling

Application Deadline: December 1

PREREQUISITE COURSEWORK

Chemistry (12 credits to include General, Organic, and Biochemistry), Biology (15 credits to include Human Anatomy, Physiology, and Microbiology), Psychology (6 credits). Prerequisites must be completed with a grade "C" or better.

GPA Requirement: No minimum

Healthcare Experience: Required (no specific number of hours)

PA Shadowing: Not required

Required Standardized Testing: GRE (analytical score of 4.0 required)

Letters of Recommendation: Three required; no one specific

Seat Deposit: $1,000

UNIVERSITY OF SAINT FRANCIS (FORT WAYNE)

MISSION:

The Department of Physician Assistant Studies provides education in medical knowledge and skills needed by individuals to serve effectively as mid-level practitioners with a special focus on meeting the needs of underserved populations. The Department prepares students to be clinicians who achieve professional standards and have enhanced critical thinking, clinical, and research skills. We offer an educational environment of mutual respect, personal growth, and professional advancement.

NO CLASS STATISTICS REPORTED

PANCE SCORES

5-year First Time Pass: 98%

Most Recent First Time Pass: 95%

CURRICULUM STRUCTURE

Didactic: 15 months

Clinical: 12 months

Rotations: 8 mandatory, 1 elective, 2 specialty tracks (each 2.5-5 weeks)

UNIQUE PROGRAM FEATURES

Specialty Tracks: Students can choose a specialty track for their clinical rotations, in which they complete a series of rotations in trauma or surgery, hospital-based care, family practice, or internal medicine.

On-campus Labs: PA students have access to a simulation lab, cadaver lab, and a resource lab with exam rooms, high-fidelity simulators (infant, child, and adult patients), and more.

Problem Based Learning: The program uses problem-based learning as the exclusive method of teaching for its medicine and therapeutics courses in the third and fourth semesters of the program.

Dual Track: Up to seven seats may be filled through the dual BS/MS program.

Valparaiso University

LeBien Hall, Annex B
802 LaPorte Avenue
Valparaiso, IN 46383
Phone: 219-464-5611
Email: Jodi.gass@valpo.edu

PROGRAM HIGHLIGHTS

Accreditation: Provisional

Degree Offered: Master (MSPA)

Start Date: August annually

Program Length: 24 months

Class Capacity: Not reported

Tuition: $98,680 (master's portion)

CASPA Participant: No

Supplemental Application: No

Yellow Ribbon: No

Admissions: Non-rolling

Application Deadline: Not reported

PREREQUISITE COURSEWORK

This is a 5-year direct entry program only that requires successful completion of four years of lab science in high school (biology, chemistry, anatomy/physiology, and physics recommended).

GPA Requirement: Overall GPA: 3.3

Healthcare Experience: Not required

PA Shadowing: Recommended, not required

Required Standardized Testing: ACT (minimum 25) or SAT (minimum 1230)

Letters of Recommendation: As per undergraduate application

Seat Deposit: None

VALPARAISO UNIVERSITY

MISSION:

The mission of the Valparaiso University Physician Assistant Program is to create a student-centered educational environment that develops graduates who are compassionate, competent physician assistants who provide excellent patient care and who lead and serve in dynamic health care environments.

NO CLASS STATISTICS REPORTED

PANCE SCORES

5-year First Time Pass: N/A

Most Recent First Time Pass: N/A (have not graduated a class yet)

CURRICULUM STRUCTURE

Didactic: 12 months

Clinical: 12 months

Rotations: 7 mandatory, 2 electives (each 5 weeks)

Graduate Project: Required for graduation

UNIQUE PROGRAM FEATURES

Direct Entry: This is a direct entry program that accepts high school students into a 5 year BSHS/MSPA program. Students can not transfer into the program or apply through CASPA.

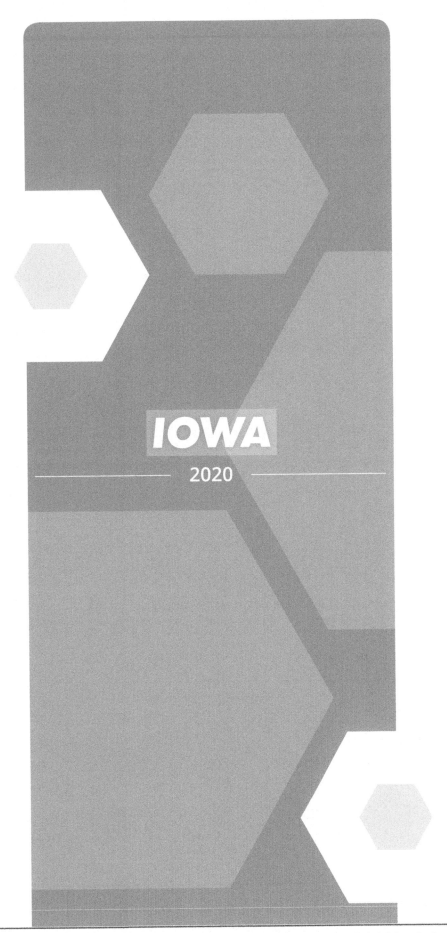

IOWA
2020

PROGRAM HIGHLIGHTS

Accreditation: Continuing

Degree Offered: Master (MSPAS)

Start Date: June annually

Program Length: 25 months

Class Capacity: 50 students

Tuition: $72,296

CASPA Participant: Yes

Supplemental Application: No

Yellow Ribbon: No

Admissions: Rolling

Application Deadline: December 1

PREREQUISITE COURSEWORK

Human Anatomy, Human Physiology, Microbiology, Genetics (total of 16 biology credits with labs when available), Inorganic Chemistry, Organic Chemistry, Biochemistry (total of 15 chemistry credits with labs when available), Psychology (9 credits including Abnormal Psychology), Statistics or Biostatistics, Medical Terminology. Chemistry and Biology prerequisites must be completed within the last 5 years. Prerequisites must be completed with a grade "C" or better. AP credits are not accepted.

GPA Requirement: Overall GPA 2.8

Healthcare Experience: 750 hours

PA Shadowing: Required (no specific number of hours)

Required Standardized Testing: GRE

Letters of Recommendation: Two required; no one specific

Seat Deposit: $500

DES MOINES UNIVERSITY

MISSION:

The mission of the Physician Assistant Program is to develop highly competent and compassionate Physician Assistants who are committed to four core values: 1) Prevention of Disease; 2) Maintenance of Health; 3) Patient Education; and 4) Treatment of Disease.

CLASS OF 2021

Male: 22%

Female: 78%

Overall GPA: 3.71

Science GPA: 3.63

GRE Verbal: 154

GRE Quantitative: 153

Average Age: 23

PANCE SCORES

5-year First Time Pass: 99%

Most Recent First Time Pass: 100%

CURRICULUM STRUCTURE

Didactic: 13 months

Clinical: 12 months

Rotations: 7 mandatory, 1 elective (each 2-12 weeks)

Capstone Project: Required for graduation

UNIQUE PROGRAM FEATURES

Global Health: Students can participate in short medical service trips or extended international rotations through the global health department.

Early Clinical Exposure: Students begin early in the first year to have clinical experiences with preceptors in various settings and also receive experience prior to clinical rotations via simulated teaching tools, Standardized Performance Assessment Lab, and on-site clinic.

Interprofessional Education: PA students study with students from other DMU programs on selected clinical topics.

Northwestern College

101 7th Street SW
Orange City Iowa, 51041
Phone: 712-707-7359
Email:
physician.assistant@nwciowa.edu

PROGRAM HIGHLIGHTS

Accreditation: Provisional

Degree Offered: Master (MSPAS)

Start Date: May annually

Program Length: 27 months

Class Capacity: 32 students

Tuition: $87,000

CASPA Participant: Yes

Supplemental Application:
Yes ($50 fee)

Yellow Ribbon: No

Admissions: Rolling

Application Deadline: October 1

PREREQUISITE COURSEWORK

Human Anatomy (3 credits),
Human Physiology (3 credits),
Microbiology (3 credits), Organic
Chemistry (3 credits), Biochemistry
(3 credits), Psychology (3 credits),
Statistics (3 credits), Genetics (3
credits). Anatomy, Physiology and
Microbiology must be completed
within the last 5 years. Five of the
eight required courses must be
completed by the time of application
and all prerequisites must be
completed with a grade "B-" or
better. AP credits are accepted
for Psychology and Statistics
only. Recommended Courses:
Pharmacology, Physics, Ethics,
Pathophysiology, Immunology,
Embryology.

GPA Requirement: Overall GPA 3.0;
Science GPA 3.0

Healthcare Experience: 500 hours

PA Shadowing: 16 hours

Required Standardized Testing: None

Letters of Recommendation: Two
required; no one specific

Seat Deposit: $500

NORTHWESTERN COLLEGE

MISSION:

The mission of the Northwestern College Physician Assistant Program is to equip students with an exceptional education grounded in a biblical theology of human dignity and flourishing.

NO CLASS STATISTICS REPORTED

PANCE SCORES

5-year First Time Pass: N/A

Most Recent First Time Pass: N/A (have not graduated a class yet)

CURRICULUM STRUCTURE

Didactic: 15 months

Clinical: 12 months

Rotations: 8 mandatory, 2 elective (each 2-8 weeks)

Capstone Project: Required for graduation

UNIQUE PROGRAM FEATURES

Admissions Preference: Any Northwestern College graduate who completes all application materials and meets all admissions criteria will be granted an admission interview.

Master of Physician Assistant Studies
1320 W. Lombard Street
Davenport, IA 52804
Phone: 563-333-5827
Email: pa@sau.edu

PROGRAM HIGHLIGHTS

Accreditation: Probation

Degree Offered: Master (MPAS)

Start Date: June annually

Program Length: 29 months

Class Capacity: 30 students

Tuition: $98,489

CASPA Participant: Yes

Supplemental Application: Yes (no fee)

Yellow Ribbon: No

Admissions: Non-rolling

Application Deadline: November 1

PREREQUISITE COURSEWORK

General Biology with lab (4 credits), Human Anatomy with lab (4 credits), Human Physiology with lab (4 credits), Microbiology with lab (4 credits), General Chemistry with lab (8 credits), Organic Chemistry with lab (4 credits), Biochemistry (3-4 credits), Statistics or Biostatistics (3 credits), General Psychology (3 credits), Abnormal Psychology (3 credits), Lifespan or Developmental Psychology (3 credits), English (6 credits), Medical Terminology. Prerequisites must be completed with a grade "C" or better. AP credits are not accepted. Recommended courses: Oral Communication, Biomedical Ethics.

GPA Requirement: Overall GPA 3.0

Healthcare Experience: 500 hours

PA Shadowing: Not required

Required Standardized Testing: GRE

Letters of Recommendation: Three required; no one specific

Seat Deposit: $200

ST. AMBROSE UNIVERSITY

MISSION:

The mission of the St. Ambrose University Physician Assistant Program is to prepare physician assistants to deliver high quality patient-centered care with compassion and respect. The program provides a supportive environment to assist students as they develop into professionals with the knowledge and skills to contribute to the health and welfare of their communities.

NO CLASS STATISTICS REPORTED

PANCE SCORES

5-year First Time Pass: 93% (based on three years of data)

Most Recent First Time Pass: 83%

CURRICULUM STRUCTURE

Didactic: 14 months

Clinical: 15 months

Rotations: 8 mandatory, 4 elective (each 4 weeks)

UNIQUE PROGRAM FEATURES

Service Learning: All students have opportunities to take part in service learning projects such as volunteering at local parish health fairs and homeless shelters, screening for high blood pressure at soup kitchens, and building homes with Habitat for Humanity.

University of Dubuque

2000 University Ave
PA Program
Dubuque, IA 52001
Phone: 563-589-3664
Email: MPAS@dbq.edu

PROGRAM HIGHLIGHTS

Accreditation: Probation
Degree Offered: Master (MSPAS)
Start Date: July annually
Program Length: 27 months
Class Capacity: 26 students
Tuition: $90,000

CASPA Participant: Yes
Supplemental Application: No
Yellow Ribbon: No
Admissions: Rolling
Application Deadline: November 1

PREREQUISITE COURSEWORK

Mathematics (3 credits), Statistics (3 credits), General Chemistry I and II with lab (8 credits), Organic Chemistry I with lab (4 credits), Organic Chemistry II or Biochemistry with lab (4 credits), General Biology with lab (4 credits), General Microbiology with lab (4 credits), Genetics with lab (4 credits), Human Anatomy and Physiology with lab (8 credits). Up to three prerequisites may be in progress at the time of application but must be completed by June 1st of the year of matriculation. Prerequisites must be completed with a grade "C" or better. Recommended courses: Cell Biology, Histology, Molecular Biology, Medical Terminology, Calculus, Ethics, Immunology, Endocrinology, Neuroscience, Pharmacology.

GPA Requirement: Overall GPA 2.7; Science GPA 2.9

Healthcare Experience: 500 hours

PA Shadowing: Required (no specific number of hours)

Required Standardized Testing: GRE

Letters of Recommendation: Three required; one form an academic professor, one from a supervisor/manager/director in the healthcare workplace, and one character reference

Seat Deposit: $1,000

UNIVERSITY OF DUBUQUE

MISSION:

The mission of the University of Dubuque Physician Assistant Program is to prepare master's level primary care physician assistants who will practice with physicians and other members of the health care team. The program is committed to developing clinicians who are educated in all aspects of healthcare with special emphasis placed on primary healthcare in rural and underserved areas.

CLASS OF 2022

Male: 31%

Female: 69%

Overall GPA: 3.46

Science GPA: 3.48

GRE Total: 310

Average Healthcare Experience: 2,500 hours

Average Age: 24

PANCE SCORES

5-year First Time Pass: 100% (based on one year of data)

Most Recent First Time Pass: 100%

CURRICULUM STRUCTURE

Didactic: 15 months

Clinical: 12 months

Rotations: 9 mandatory, 2 elective (each 4 weeks)

Capstone Project: Required for graduation

UNIQUE PROGRAM FEATURES

Rural Medicine: The program emphasizes rural medicine throughout the curriculum and requires all students to complete a rural medicine clerkship.

Admissions Preference: Students with prior military service and/or UD graduates will be looked at favorably, particularly in the areas of leadership and/or community service that reflect the mission and commitment of the program to the Dubuque area and UD.

University of Iowa

375 Newton Road
1221 Medical Education Research
Facility (MERF)
Iowa City, IA 52242
Phone: 319-335-8922
Email: paprogram@uiowa.edu

PROGRAM HIGHLIGHTS

Accreditation: Continuing

Degree Offered: Master (MPAS)

Start Date: August annually

Program Length: 28 months

Class Capacity: 25 students

Tuition: $49,555 (in-state);
$96,797 (out-of-state)

CASPA Participant: Yes

Supplemental Application: No

Yellow Ribbon: No

Admissions: Rolling

Application Deadline: October 1

PREREQUISITE COURSEWORK

Biology or General Zoology (complete sequence), Physiology (1 semester), 3 Upper Level Biology/Zoology Science Courses, General Chemistry I and II (2 semesters), Organic Chemistry (1 semester), Biochemistry, General Statistics or Biostatistics. The majority of prerequisites, including Biochemistry, must be completed at the time of application. Recommended courses: Cell Biology, Genetics, Immunology, Microbiology, Molecular Biology, Pharmacology, Anatomy, Embryology, Endocrinology, Histology, Neuroscience.

GPA Requirement: Overall GPA 3.0; Science GPA 3.2 (overall or for the most recently completed 40 semester hours)

Healthcare Experience: 1,000 hours

PA Shadowing: Not required

Required Standardized Testing: GRE (25th percentile minimum on each section) or MCAT

Letters of Recommendation: Three required; one academic letter, one healthcare supervisor letter, and one additional professional reference

Seat Deposit: $800

UNIVERSITY OF IOWA

MISSION:

To recruit exemplary individuals from diverse backgrounds and life experiences and to equip them with the knowledge, skills and abilities to provide high quality, compassionate health care to diverse patient populations.

CLASS OF 2020

Overall GPA: 3.71

Science GPA: 3.76

GRE Verbal: 159

GRE Quantitative: 158

GRE Analytical: 4.5

Average Healthcare Experience: 2,478 hours

Average Age: 26

PANCE SCORES

5-year First Time Pass: 100%

Most Recent First Time Pass: 100%

CURRICULUM STRUCTURE

Didactic: 16 months

Clinical: 12 months

Rotations: 7 mandatory plus electives (duration not specified)

Capstone Project: Required for graduation

UNIQUE PROGRAM FEATURES

Interprofessional Education: PA students complete their entire didactic curriculum taking the same coursework as the medical students, fostering the Physician-PA relationship. PA students complete coursework specific to the PA program as well.

Leadership: The program is well known for producing leaders in the field. Various leadership positions that faculty and graduates have held are listed on the program website.

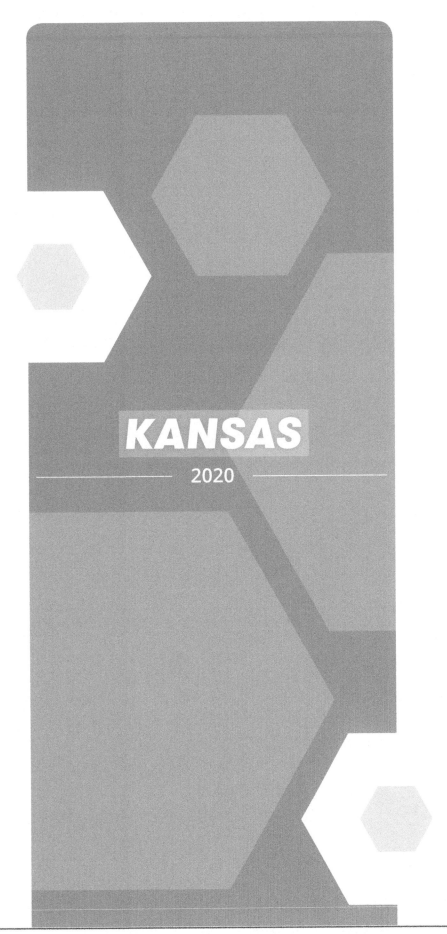

KANSAS

2020

Wichita State University

1845 N Fairmount Street
Box 214
Wichita, KS 67260
Phone: 316-978-3011
Email:
physician.assistant@wichita.edu

PROGRAM HIGHLIGHTS

Accreditation: Probation

Degree Offered: Master (MPA)

Start Date: June annually

Program Length: 26 months

Class Capacity: 48 students

Tuition: $49,700 (in-state, including fees); $89,587 (out-of-state, including fees)

CASPA Participant: Yes

Supplemental Application: Yes ($75 fee)

Yellow Ribbon: Yes

Admissions: Non-rolling

Application Deadline: September 1

PREREQUISITE COURSEWORK

Chemistry with lab (12 credits), Biology (9 credits, to include Microbiology with lab), Human Anatomy and Physiology with lab (5 credits), Statistics (3 credits), Psychology (3 credits), Medical Terminology (1 credit). Science prerequisites must be completed at the time of application. All prerequisites should be completed within the last 10 years and with a grade "C-" or better. Recommended courses: Pharmacology, Genetics, Organic Chemistry, Biochemistry, Pathophysiology, Gerontology, Medical Ethics, Health Care Policy, Epidemiology, Abnormal Psychology, Human Nutrition.

GPA Requirement: Overall GPA 3.0; Science GPA 3.0

Healthcare Experience: Preferred, not required

PA Shadowing: Preferred, not required

Required Standardized Testing: None

Letters of Recommendation: Four required; no one specific

Seat Deposit: $500

WICHITA STATE UNIVERSITY

MISSION:

The mission of the Department of Physician Assistant is to be a learning community dedicated to developing generalist health care professionals by: valuing students; integrating teaching, scholarship, practice, and service; and partnering with the community.

CLASS OF 2020

Overall GPA: 3.70

PANCE SCORES

5-year First Time Pass: 99%

Most Recent First Time Pass: 100%

CURRICULUM STRUCTURE

Didactic: 13 months

Clinical: 13 months

Rotations: 7 mandatory (5-6 weeks), 1 elective (8 weeks)

Capstone Project: Required for graduation

UNIQUE PROGRAM FEATURES

Research Curriculum: The program has arguably the strongest record of student research and publication in the nation with over 40 publications from students working with faculty over the last 5 years.

Service Learning: Every student performs volunteer community service including: Senior Mentor Program; Give-Kids-a-Smile fluoride varnish clinic; United Way Homeless Count; Ready Set Fit health education for elementary children; Sports Physicals provided for free at a socioeconomically disadvantaged rural county; and many others.

Primary Care and Rural/Underserved Focus: Every student gets to know their community by completing at least 18 weeks of rotations in primary care and 12 weeks in rural areas.

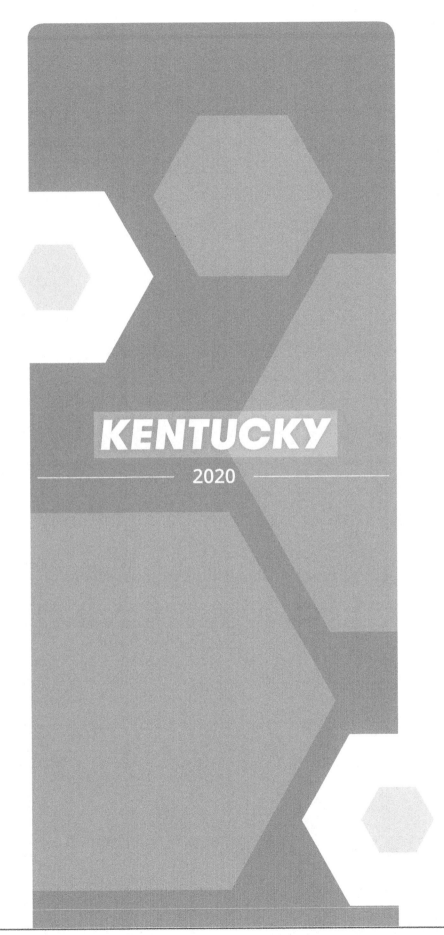

KENTUCKY

2020

Sullivan University

2100 Gardiner Lane
Suite 349
Louisville, KY 40205
Phone: 502-413-8939
Email: PAProgram@sullivan.edu

PROGRAM HIGHLIGHTS

Accreditation: Continuing

Degree Offered: Master (MSPA)

Start Date: May annually

Program Length: 24 months

Class Capacity: 48 students

Tuition: $88,155

CASPA Participant: Yes

Supplemental Application: Yes ($100 fee)

Yellow Ribbon: No

Admissions: Non-rolling

Application Deadline: August 1

PREREQUISITE COURSEWORK

Human Anatomy and Physiology (6 credits), Microbiology (3 credits), General Chemistry I and II with lab (8 credits), Organic Chemistry or Biochemistry (3 credits), Statistics (3 credits), Introduction to Psychology or Developmental Psychology or Abnormal Psychology (3 credits), English Composition (3 credits), Medical Terminology (1-3 credits). Up to two courses may be in progress at the time of application, but all must be completed by April 1st of the year of matriculation. Prerequisites must be completed with a grade "C" or better. AP credits are not accepted. Recommended courses: Organic Chemistry I and II, Biochemistry, Molecular and Cellular Biology.

GPA Requirement: Overall GPA 3.0; Math/Science Prerequisite GPA 3.0

Healthcare Experience: 500 hours

PA Shadowing: 25 hours

Required Standardized Testing: None

Letters of Recommendation: Three required; one must be from a physician or PA

Seat Deposit: $1,000

SULLIVAN UNIVERSITY

MISSION:

The mission of Sullivan University's Physician Assistant Program is to educate medical professionals to provide ethical, high quality healthcare as part of an interprofessional team. We will educate students to become life-long learners that remain dedicated to serving diverse communities with compassion and promoting the profession.

CLASS OF 2021

Male: 44%

Female: 56%

Minority: 13%

Overall GPA: 3.53

Prerequisite GPA: 3.56

Average Healthcare Experience: 1,513 hours

Average Shadowing Experience: 143 hours

PANCE SCORES

5-year First Time Pass: 92% (based on four years of data)

Most Recent First Time Pass: 91%

CURRICULUM STRUCTURE

Didactic: 12 months

Clinical: 12 months

Rotations: 7 mandatory, 1 elective (each 6 weeks)

Capstone Project: Required for graduation

UNIQUE PROGRAM FEATURES

Curriculum Variety: The curriculum uses a variety of teaching methodologies including asynchronous learning, case-based learning, early clinical exposure, problem based learning, and hybrid courses.

Admissions Preference: Some consideration is given to first generation college students, students from medically underserved areas and veterans of the US Armed Forces.

149

PROGRAM HIGHLIGHTS

Accreditation: Continuing

Degree Offered: Master (MSPAS)

Start Date: January annually

Program Length: 29 months

Class Capacity: 56 students

Tuition: $56,730 (in-state);
$104,828 (out-of-state)

CASPA Participant: Yes

Supplemental Application: Yes ($125 fee)

Yellow Ribbon: No

Admissions: Rolling

Application Deadline: July 15

PREREQUISITE COURSEWORK

General Chemistry I and II with lab (2 semesters), Organic Chemistry I with lab (1 semester), Human Anatomy and Physiology I and II (2 semesters), General Biology with lab (1 semester), Microbiology with lab (1 semester), Statistics (1 semester), Psychology (1 semester), Developmental Psychology (1 semester), Anthropology or Sociology (1 semester), Medical Terminology (1 semester). At most two prerequisites may be in progress at the time of application. Prerequisites must be completed with a grade "C" or better. AP credits may be accepted. Applicants must also be Basic Life Support certified.

GPA Requirement: Overall GPA 2.75

Healthcare Experience: Required (no specific number of hours)

PA Shadowing: Preferred, not required

Required Standardized Testing: GRE

Letters of Recommendation: Three required; one from a physician or PA, one from an academic professor or advisor, and one medical or academic letter

Seat Deposit: $300 (in-state); $600 (out-of-state)

UNIVERSITY OF KENTUCKY

MISSION:

The mission of the University of Kentucky Physician Assistant Studies program is to improve the health and well-being of the people in the Commonwealth of Kentucky by graduating competent and compassionate physician assistants who will become transformative leaders in their practices and communities.

CLASS OF 2022

Overall GPA: 3.60

Science GPA: 3.50

Prerequisite GPA: 3.64

Last 60 Credit GPA: 3.69

GRE Verbal: 153

GRE Quantitative: 152

GRE Writing: 4.0

Average Healthcare Experience: 4,463 hours

Average Shadowing Experience: 108 hours

PANCE SCORES

5-year First Time Pass: 95%

Most Recent First Time Pass: 93%

CURRICULUM STRUCTURE

Didactic: 17 months

Clinical: 12 months

Rotations: 8 mandatory, 1 selective, 1 elective (each 4-8 weeks)

Master's Graduate Project: Required for graduation

UNIQUE PROGRAM FEATURES

Two Campuses: This program operates with 40 students at the Lexington Campus and 16 students at the Morehead State site. Students complete the same requirements for graduation and have dedicated faculty members at each location.

International Rotations: The program offers rotations in various countries including Kenya, Swaziland, and England, as well as opportunities to travel on shorter trips to Ecuador and Mexico.

Interprofessional Education: All students complete the UK Interprofessional Collaboration and Team Skills (iCATS) curriculum with other health professions students.

University of the Cumberlands

6191 College Station Drive
Williamsburg, KY 40769
Phone: 606-539-4398
Email: pa@ucumberlands.edu

PROGRAM HIGHLIGHTS

Accreditation: Provisional

Degree Offered: Master (MSPAS)

Start Date: January

Program Length: 27 months

Class Capacity: 30 students

Tuition: $81,550

CASPA Participant: Yes

Supplemental Application: Yes ($30 fee)

Yellow Ribbon: No

Admissions: Non-rolling

Application Deadline: August 1

PREREQUISITE COURSEWORK

Anatomy with lab (3 credits), Physiology with lab (3 credits), Microbiology with lab (3 credits), Medical Terminology, Upper Level Biology (6 credits), General Chemistry I and II with lab (6 credits), Organic Chemistry I or Biochemistry, Psychology (3 credits), Statistics (3 credits). The majority of coursework should be completed prior to application and within the last 10 years. Prerequisites must be completed with a grade "C" or better. Recommended courses: Genetics, Molecular Biology, Histology, Immunology, Abnormal Psychology, Developmental Psychology.

GPA Requirement: Overall GPA 3.0; Science GPA 3.0; Prerequisite GPA 3.0

Healthcare Experience: 500 hours

PA Shadowing: 50 hours (counts towards healthcare experience)

Required Standardized Testing: PA-CAT

Letters of Recommendation: Three required; acceptable references include physician, PA, NP, and academic advisors

Seat Deposit: $1,000

UNIVERSITY OF THE CUMBERLANDS

MISSION:

The mission of the Physician Assistant Program is to educate and prepare competent, compassionate, and committed Physician Assistant leaders who, as integral members of the modern professional healthcare team, are driven by academic excellence and will be servant leaders in their communities. The faculty and staff of the Physician Assistant Program will provide academic and clinical excellence in an environment of compassion and team cooperation, seeking to prepare clinicians for a lifelong commitment to continuing education, leadership, and medical service.

NO CLASS STATISTICS REPORTED

PANCE SCORES

5-year First Time Pass: 98% (based on two years of data)

Most Recent First Time Pass: 96%

CURRICULUM STRUCTURE

Didactic: 15 months

Clinical: 12 months

Rotations: 9 mandatory, 1 elective (each 4 weeks)

Capstone Project: Required for graduation

UNIQUE PROGRAM FEATURES

Appalachian Students: The program recruits students from the underserved Appalachian region and 37% of the first two cohorts were from this area, while 39% were from within 100 miles of campus.

University of the Cumberlands

410 Meijer Drive
Florence, KY 41042
Phone: 859-980-7912
Email: nkypa@ucumberlands.edu

PROGRAM HIGHLIGHTS

Accreditation: Provisional

Degree Offered: Master (MSPAS)

Start Date: August

Program Length: 27 months

Class Capacity: 30 students

Tuition: $81,550

CASPA Participant: Yes

Supplemental Application: Yes ($30 fee)

Yellow Ribbon: No

Admissions: Non-rolling

Application Deadline: March 1

PREREQUISITE COURSEWORK

Anatomy with lab (3 credits), Physiology with lab (3 credits), Microbiology with lab (3 credits), Medical Terminology, Upper Level Biology (6 credits), General Chemistry I and II with lab (6 credits), Organic Chemistry I or Biochemistry, Psychology (3 credits), Statistics (3 credits). The majority of coursework should be completed prior to application and within the last 10 years. Prerequisites must be completed with a grade "C" or better. Recommended courses: Genetics, Molecular Biology, Histology, Immunology, Abnormal Psychology, Developmental Psychology.

GPA Requirement: Overall GPA 3.0; Science BCP GPA 3.0

Healthcare Experience: 500 hours

PA Shadowing: 50 hours (counts towards healthcare experience)

Required Standardized Testing: GRE (total score > 50th percentile is considered competitive)

Letters of Recommendation: Three required; at least one should be from a physician or PA

Seat Deposit: $1,000

UNIVERSITY OF THE CUMBERLANDS - NORTHERN KENTUCKY

MISSION:

The mission of the Physician Assistant Program is to educate and prepare competent, compassionate, and committed Physician Assistant leaders who, as integral members of the modern professional healthcare team, are driven by academic excellence and will be servant leaders in their communities. The faculty and staff of the Physician Assistant Program will provide academic and clinical excellence in an environment of compassion and team cooperation, seeking to prepare clinicians for a lifelong commitment to continuing education, leadership, and medical service.

NO CLASS STATISTICS REPORTED

PANCE SCORES

5-year First Time Pass: N/A

Most Recent First Time Pass: N/A (have not graduated a class yet)

CURRICULUM STRUCTURE

Didactic: 17 months

Clinical: 10 months

Rotations: 9 mandatory, 1 elective (each 4 weeks)

Capstone Project: Required for graduation

UNIQUE PROGRAM FEATURES

None reported

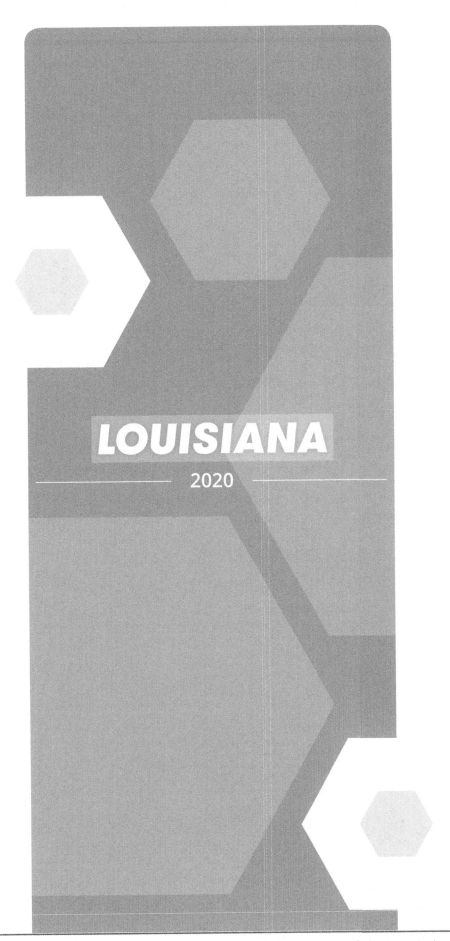

LOUISIANA

2020

Franciscan Missionaries of Our Lady University

5414 Brittany Drive
Baton Rouge, LA 70808
Phone: 225-490-16550
Email: pa@franu.edu

PROGRAM HIGHLIGHTS

Accreditation: Continuing

Degree Offered: Master (MMS)

Start Date: January annually

Program Length: 28 months

Class Capacity: 30 students

Tuition: $89,166 (including fees)

CASPA Participant: Yes

Supplemental Application: Yes ($25 fee)

Yellow Ribbon: No

Admissions: Rolling

Application Deadline: August 1

PREREQUISITE COURSEWORK

Human Anatomy with lab, Human Physiology, Microbiology, Organic Chemistry I, Organic Chemistry II or Biochemistry, General Psychology, Statistics, Genetics, Medical Terminology. All prerequisites must be completed within the last 7 years. Completion of all prerequisites with a grade "B" or better is considered competitive.

GPA Requirement: Overall GPA 3.0; Science GPA 3.0; Prerequisite GPA 3.0

Healthcare Experience: 80 hours (recommended)

PA Shadowing: Preferred, not required

Required Standardized Testing: GRE (minimum combined score of 290 and 3.5 on analytical)

Letters of Recommendation: Three required; letters from former professors, employers or healthcare workers are preferred

Seat Deposit: $1,000

FRANCISCAN MISSIONARIES OF OUR LADY UNIVERSITY

MISSION:

Guided by the tradition of compassionate health care exemplified by the Franciscan Missionaries of Our Lady, the Physician Assistant Program will develop graduates who will provide evidence based, patient centered medical care in diverse settings, and who are committed to serving all God's people.

CLASS OF 2020

Overall GPA: 3.50

Prerequisite GPA: 3.46

GRE Verbal: 152

GRE Quantitative: 152

GRE Analytical: 3.9

PANCE SCORES

5-year First Time Pass: 94%

Most Recent First Time Pass: 100%

CURRICULUM STRUCTURE

Didactic: 16 months

Clinical: 12 months

Rotations: 8 mandatory, 2 elective (each 4 weeks)

Master's Project: Required for graduation

UNIQUE PROGRAM FEATURES

PA Student Organization: The PASO started in 2016 and students participated in several community service projects and won the AAPA PA week photo contest. Students and faculty combined completed nearly 318 hours of community service this past year.

Early Admissions: Early admission will be considered for students enrolled in, and in good standing, in Franciscan University's 3+2 Biology degree program. All 3+2 applicants must meet all other PA program criteria.

Admissions Preference: Applicants with military service, who are graduates of the university, or who are from medically underserved areas are given additional admissions consideration.

Louisiana State University Health Science Center

411 South Prieur St.
New Orleans, LA 70112
Phone: 504-556-3420
Email: PAProgram@lsuhsc.edu

PROGRAM HIGHLIGHTS

Accreditation: Continuing

Degree Offered: Master (MPAS)

Start Date: January annually

Program Length: 29 months

Class Capacity: 30 students

Tuition: $54,000 (in-state, including fees); $106,000 (out-of-state, including fees)

CASPA Participant: Yes

Supplemental Application: No

Yellow Ribbon: No

Admissions: Non-rolling

Application Deadline: August 1

PREREQUISITE COURSEWORK

Biological Sciences (8 credits of upper level coursework), Microbiology or Bacteriology with lab (4 credits), Chemistry I and II with lab (8 credits), Anatomy with lab (4 credits), Physiology with lab (4 credits), Statistics (3 credits), Genetics (3 credits), Organic Chemistry or Biochemistry with lab (4 credits), Behavioral Sciences (6 credits), College Algebra or higher (3 credits). Prerequisites must be completed within the last 10 years and with a grade "C" or better. Current CPR certification is required. Recommended courses: Immunology, Bacteriology, Histology, Parasitology, Nutrition, Molecular Biology, Cell Biology, Embryology.

GPA Requirement: Overall GPA 3.0; Science GPA 3.0

Healthcare Experience: 80 hours (recommended)

PA Shadowing: Preferred, not required

Required Standardized Testing: GRE (recommended minimum 153 quantitative, 144 verbal, and 3.5 analytical)

Letters of Recommendation: Three required; one must be from a PA and the other two should come from doctors shadowed, current or former professors, and current or former employers

Seat Deposit: $500

LOUISIANA STATE UNIVERSITY - NEW ORLEANS

MISSION:

The Mission of the LSUHSC-New Orleans Master of Physician Assistant Studies Program is to recruit and educate individuals of the highest quality from diverse backgrounds to provide evidence-based, patient-centered healthcare to the people of Louisiana.

CLASS OF 2021

Overall GPA: 3.65

Science GPA: 3.60

Average Healthcare Experience: 1,894 hours

PANCE SCORES

5-year First Time Pass: 95%

Most Recent First Time Pass: 90%

CURRICULUM STRUCTURE

Didactic: 17 months

Clinical: 12 months

Rotations: 7 mandatory, 1 elective, 1 preceptorship (each 4-8 weeks)

Capstone Project: Required for graduation

UNIQUE PROGRAM FEATURES

Admissions Preference: The school has preference for applicants who are Louisiana residents. Typically 90% of the incoming class resides in Louisiana.

LSUHSC PA Program

1501 Kings Highway
Shreveport, LA 71103
Phone: 318-813-2920
Email:
PAProgramShreveport@lsuhsc.edu

PROGRAM HIGHLIGHTS

Accreditation: Continuing

Degree Offered: Master (MPAS)

Start Date: May annually

Program Length: 27 months

Class Capacity: 40 students

Tuition: $39,000 (in-state); $66,000 (out-of-state)

CASPA Participant: Yes

Supplemental Application: Yes ($50 fee)

Yellow Ribbon: No

Admissions: Rolling

Application Deadline: October 1

PREREQUISITE COURSEWORK

Anatomy with lab (4 credits), Physiology (3 credits), Microbiology with lab (4 credits), Chemistry with lab (8 credits), Upper Level Biology (8 credits), Statistics (3 credits), Medical Terminology (3 credits). Courses can be in progress at the time of application. Prerequisites must be completed with a grade "C" or better. Recommended courses: Advanced Anatomy, Advanced Physiology, Cell Biology, Genetics, Immunology, Parasitology, Virology.

GPA Requirement: Overall GPA 3.0; Science GPA 3.0

Healthcare Experience: 80 hours

PA Shadowing: Preferred, not required (counts towards healthcare experience)

Required Standardized Testing: GRE (minimum verbal 143, quantitative 145, analytical 3.0)

Letters of Recommendation: Three required; no one specific

Seat Deposit: $150

LOUISIANA STATE UNIVERSITY - SHREVEPORT

MISSION:

The mission of the PA Program is to provide a primary care curriculum to prepare competent Physician Assistant health care providers for Louisiana.

CLASS OF 2020

Overall GPA: 3.75

Science GPA: 3.72

GRE Verbal: 152

GRE Quantitative: 153

GRE Analytical: 4.0

Average Healthcare Experience: 1,769 hours

Average Shadowing Experience: 177 hours

PANCE SCORES

5-year First Time Pass: 99%

Most Recent First Time Pass: 100%

CURRICULUM STRUCTURE

Didactic: 12 months

Clinical: 15 months

Rotations: 9 mandatory, 3 elective, 1 preceptorship (each 4-8 weeks)

Master's Project: Required for graduation

UNIQUE PROGRAM FEATURES

Admissions Preference: The school gives preference to Louisiana residents, and can only take up to 20% of each class from out-of-state.

Xavier University of Louisiana

Department of Physician Assistant Studies
1 Drexel Drive
New Orleans, LA 70125
Phone: 504-520-5119
Email: paprogram@xula.edu

PROGRAM HIGHLIGHTS

Accreditation: Provisional

Degree Offered: Master (MHS)

Start Date: January

Program Length: 28 months

Class Capacity: 40 students

Tuition: $84,000

CASPA Participant: Yes

Supplemental Application: No

Yellow Ribbon: Yes

Admissions: Rolling

Application Deadline: October 1

PREREQUISITE COURSEWORK

General Biology I and II with lab (8 credits), General Chemistry I and II with lab (8 credits), Human Anatomy and Physiology I and II with lab (8 credits), Organic Chemistry I (3-4 credits), Organic Chemistry II or Biochemistry (3-4 credits), Microbiology with lab (4 credits), Genetics (3 credits), Upper Level Biology Electives (3-8 credits), English Composition (3 credits), General Psychology (3 credits), Statistics (3 credits), Pre-Calculus or Calculus (3 credits), Sociology (3 credits), Medical Terminology (1-3 credits). Prerequisites do not expire and must be completed with a grade "C" or better. AP credits are accepted as long as classes appear on a college transcript with assigned credits. Recommended courses: Cell Biology, Molecular Biology, Embryology, Histology, Parasitology, Virology, Immunology, Medical Ethics.

GPA Requirement: Overall GPA 3.0; Science GPA 3.0; Prerequisite GPA 3.0

Healthcare Experience: 80 hours

PA Shadowing: Preferred, not required

Required Standardized Testing: GRE (total score > 290 and 3 on analytical section required)

Letters of Recommendation: Three required; one must be from a PA or physician

Seat Deposit: $1,000

XAVIER UNIVERSITY OF LOUISIANA

MISSION:

The mission of the Xavier University Physician Assistant Program is to educate physician assistants to become ethical, competent, and compassionate physician assistants who are dedicated to providing superior quality healthcare that contributes to the promotion of a more just and humane society by improving the healthcare of the diverse communities we serve.

NO CLASS STATISTICS REPORTED

PANCE SCORES

5-year First Time Pass: N/A

Most Recent First Time Pass: N/A (have not graduated a class yet)

CURRICULUM STRUCTURE

Didactic: 12 months

Clinical: 16 months

Rotations: 7 mandatory,4 elective (each 3-4 weeks)

Capstone Project: Required for graduation

UNIQUE PROGRAM FEATURES

Rotations: Xavier University of Louisiana has partnered with Ochsner Health System, one of the leading hospital systems in the Gulf South and the largest health system in metro New Orleans. Students will complete many rotations within this health network.

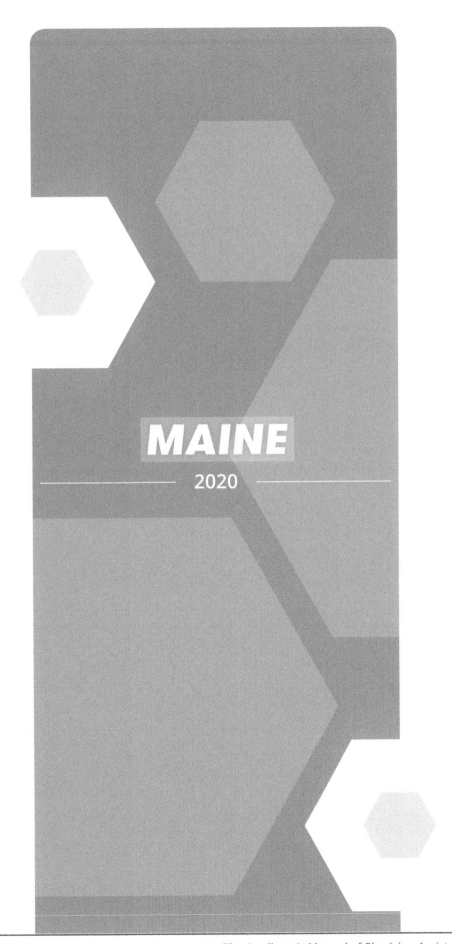

MAINE
2020

University of New England

716 Stevens Avenue
Hersey Hall-Graduate Admissions Office
Portland, ME 04103
Phone: 207-221-4529
Email: agrindell@une.edu

PROGRAM HIGHLIGHTS

Accreditation: Continuing

Degree Offered: Master (MS)

Start Date: June annually

Program Length: 24 months

Class Capacity: 50 students

Tuition: $99,090 (including fees)

CASPA Participant: Yes

Supplemental Application: No

Yellow Ribbon: No

Admissions: Rolling

Application Deadline: October 1

PREREQUISITE COURSEWORK

Biology with lab (8 credits), General Chemistry with lab (8 credits), Human Anatomy and Physiology with lab (8 credits), Psychology or Sociology (6 credits), English (6 credits), Statistics (3 credits). Prerequisites may be in-progress or planned at the time of application, but must be completed by December 31st of the application year. Anatomy and Physiology must be completed within 7 years of matriculation. Prerequisites must be completed with a grade "C" or better. Up to 3 AP credits are accepted for the English prerequisite only. Recommended courses: Advanced Physiology, Pathophysiology, Microbiology, Physics, Biochemistry.

GPA Requirement: Overall GPA 3.0; Science GPA 3.0

Healthcare Experience: 500 hours

PA Shadowing: 20 hours

Required Standardized Testing: None

Letters of Recommendation: Three required; from individuals who can speak to your academic abilities and/or professional experience

Seat Deposit: $1,000

UNIVERSITY OF NEW ENGLAND

MISSION:

The mission of the University of New England Physician Assistant Program is to prepare master's level primary care physician assistants to be highly skilled members of the interprofessional healthcare teams. The program is committed to developing clinicians who will provide compassionate, competent and evidence-based patient centered health care to people of all backgrounds and cultures throughout their lifespans. The program places special emphasis on training clinicians who are knowledgeable about the healthcare needs of our aging population and have the skills and passion to provide health care to people in underserved rural and urban communities.

CLASS OF 2021

Overall GPA: 3.55

PANCE SCORES

5-year First Time Pass: 93%

Most Recent First Time Pass: 87%

CURRICULUM STRUCTURE

Didactic: 12 months

Clinical: 12 months

Rotations: 5 mandatory, 1 primary care selective, 1 inpatient selective, 1 other elective (each 6 weeks)

Research Project: Required for graduation

UNIQUE PROGRAM FEATURES

Community Service: Students have the opportunity to participate in many community service activities, including a mobile health van, partnering with the local Boys and Girls Club, working at community health fairs, and mission trips to Ghana.

Interprofessional Education: Throughout the PA program students participate in interprofessional education experiences in clinical settings and the simulation lab that prepares for working with other healthcare professionals.

Facilities: The Harold Alfond Center for Health Sciences is a state-of-the-art laboratory and educational facility. This three-story building houses labs and lecture halls for our College of Osteopathic Medicine and other health professions. It places UNE at the national forefront of health and life sciences education. As a PA student you study anatomy in the center's Gross Anatomy Lab.

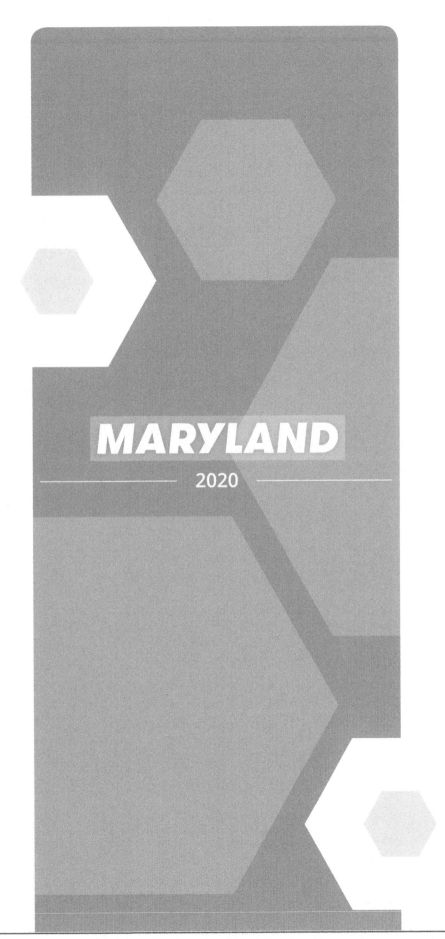

MARYLAND
2020

Anne Arundel Community College

101 College Parkway
Arnold, MD 21012
Phone: 410-777-1888
Email: paadmissions@aacc.edu

PROGRAM HIGHLIGHTS

Accreditation: Continuing

Degree Offered: Certificate, Master (MSHS)

Start Date: May annually

Program Length: 25 months

Class Capacity: 40 students

Tuition: $50,522 (in-county); $60,412 (out-of-county); $83,096 (out-of-state)

CASPA Participant: Yes

Supplemental Application: Yes ($25 fee)

Yellow Ribbon: Yes

Admissions: Non-rolling

Application Deadline: September 1

PREREQUISITE COURSEWORK

General Microbiology with lab (4 credits), Anatomy and Physiology I and II with lab (8 credits), General Chemistry I or General Chemistry II or Organic Chemistry or Biochemistry with lab (4 credits), Introduction to Psychology or Developmental Psychology or Human Growth and Development (3 credits), Elementary Statistics or Statistics in Social and Behavioral Sciences or Biostatistics (3 credits). Prerequisites must be completed with a grade "B" or better. Anatomy and Physiology must be completed within the last 7 years. AP scores of 4 or 5 are accepted for Psychology, Statistics and General Chemistry prerequisites. Recommended courses: Biochemistry, Medical Terminology, Developmental Psychology.

GPA Requirement: Overall GPA 3.0; Prerequisite GPA 3.0

Healthcare Experience: 1,400 hours (recommended)

PA Shadowing: Not required

Required Standardized Testing: GRE

Letters of Recommendation: Three required; no one specific

Seat Deposit: $500

ANNE ARUNDEL COMMUNITY COLLEGE

MISSION:

The mission of the program is to promote excellence in education in order to produce competent, ethical and compassionate primary care providers. Together we recognize and promote the value of diversity, lifelong learning, research and scholarship.

CLASS OF 2021

Male: 22%

Female: 78%

Overall GPA: 3.55

Science GPA: 3.50

Average Healthcare Experience: 4,256 hours

Average Age: 28

PANCE SCORES

5-year First Time Pass: 96%

Most Recent First Time Pass: 97%

CURRICULUM STRUCTURE

Didactic: 12 months

Clinical: 13 months

Rotations: 9 total (specific details not reported)

Capstone Project: Required for graduation

UNIQUE PROGRAM FEATURES

University of Maryland: AACC has a partnership with the University of Maryland, allowing students to take courses from both colleges to obtain the PA certificate and Master's degree in 25 months. University of Maryland courses are taken online during clinical year.

Primary Care Focus: The coursework is based in primary care and approximately 40% of graduates enter into the field.

Frostburg State University

101 Braddoc Road
Pullen Hall 141
Frostburg, MD 21532
Phone: 310-687-7053
Email: brsmolko@frostburg.edu

PROGRAM HIGHLIGHTS

Accreditation: Provisional

Degree Offered: Master (MMS)

Start Date: May annually

Program Length: 24 months

Class Capacity: 25 students

Tuition: $60,372 (in-state); $72,072 (regional); $87,750 (out-of-state)

CASPA Participant: Yes

Supplemental Application: Yes ($45 fee)

Yellow Ribbon: No

Admissions: Rolling

Application Deadline: December 1

PREREQUISITE COURSEWORK

Anatomy and Physiology I and II (8 credits), Microbiology with lab (4 credits), Medical Terminology (1-3 credits), Chemistry with lab (4 credits), Biochemistry with lab or Organic Chemistry with lab (4 credits), Abnormal or Development Psychology (3 credits), Statistics. Prerequisites, with the exception of one required non-science prerequisite course, must be completed with a grade of "C" or better and at the time of application. Prerequisites must be completed within the last 10 years, with the exception of Anatomy, Physiology and Microbiology, which must be completed within the last 5 years. AP credits are accepted. Recommended courses: Genetics, Physics.

GPA Requirement: Overall GPA 3.0; Prerequisite GPA 3.0

Healthcare Experience: 500 hours

PA Shadowing: Preferred, not required

Required Standardized Testing: GRE

Letters of Recommendation: Three required; acceptable references include MD, DO, PA, or NP, academic advisor or faculty member able to verify your potential for academic success, and individuals (professional or academic) who can attest to your commitment to leadership and service

Seat Deposit: Not reported

FROSTBURG STATE UNIVERSITY

MISSION:

The Mission of the Frostburg State University's Physician Assistant Program is to educate students in compassionate patient-centered care. Students will learn best practices, use innovative technology, and work in interprofessional teams to deliver quality care, particularly in rural and medically underserved areas in Maryland and beyond. Frostburg State University Physician Assistant graduates will have a commitment to excellence, inclusivity, and community service.

NO CLASS STATISTICS REPORTED

PANCE SCORES

5-year First Time Pass: N/A

Most Recent First Time Pass: N/A (have not graduated a class yet)

CURRICULUM STRUCTURE

Didactic: 13 months

Clinical: 11 months

Rotations: 7 mandatory, 3 electives (3-4 weeks)

Capstone Course: Required for graduation

UNIQUE PROGRAM FEATURES

Admissions Preference: The program gives admissions preference to students with a western Maryland Heritage (FSU alumni, resident of western Maryland regional area (100 mile radius of FSU), one or more parent is a resident of western Maryland regional area, graduate from high school or college/university other than FSU located in regional area, those with heritage of living in a rural or medically underserved area, and veterans.

Rotations: The program will strive to assure that students are placed in one to three sites considered to be a rural area or which serves a large population of medically underserved patients.

Towson University

8000 York Road
Towson, MD 21252
Phone: 410-840-1159
Email: paprogram@towson.edu

PROGRAM HIGHLIGHTS

Accreditation: Continuing

Degree Offered: Certificate, Master (MSPAS)

Start Date: June annually

Program Length: 26 months

Class Capacity: 36 students

Tuition: $40,758 (in-county); $49,236 (out-of-county); $82,608 (out-of-state)

CASPA Participant: Yes

Supplemental Application: Yes ($95 fee)

Yellow Ribbon: No

Admissions: Non-rolling

Application Deadline: August 1

PREREQUISITE COURSEWORK

Human Anatomy and Physiology I and II with lab (8 credits), Microbiology with lab (4 credits), Biochemistry (3 credits), Statistics (3 credits), Medical Terminology (2-3 credits). Prerequisites must be completed with a grade "B" or better. All prerequisites must be completed at the time of application and within the past 10 years (preferably within the last 5).

GPA Requirement: Overall GPA 3.0; Science GPA 3.0

Healthcare Experience: 800 hours (1,600 preferred)

PA Shadowing: Not required

Required Standardized Testing: None

Letters of Recommendation: Three required; preferably from PAs or from physicians who work with PAs

Seat Deposit: $2,750

TOWSON UNIVERSITY CCBC - ESSEX

MISSION:

The Towson University - CCBC Essex Physician Assistant Program provides a generalist foundation with a broad range of knowledge and skills to prepare competent PAs for practice in diverse medical settings.

CLASS OF 2021

Male: 20%

Female: 80%

Overall GPA: 3.50

Science GPA: 3.50

Prerequisite GPA: 3.70

Average Age: 28

PANCE SCORES

5-year First Time Pass: 96%

Most Recent First Time Pass: 95%

CURRICULUM STRUCTURE

Didactic: 12 months

Clinical: 14 months

Rotations: 6 mandatory, 1 primary care preceptorship (duration not specified)

Research Project: Required for graduation

UNIQUE PROGRAM FEATURES

Towson University: The CCBC program collaborates with Towson University so that students can be awarded a Certificate as a PA and Master's degree (from Towson) upon graduation. Students take 36 graduate level credits from Towson during the program.

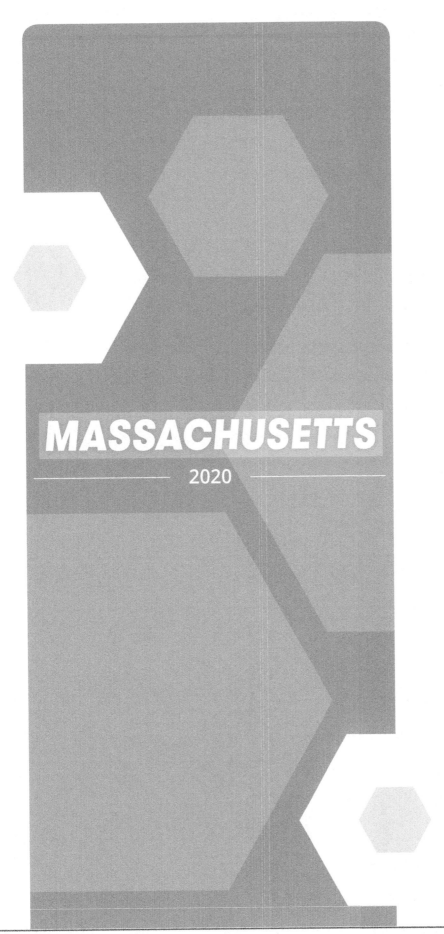

MASSACHUSETTS
2020

PROGRAM HIGHLIGHTS

Accreditation: Continuing

Degree Offered: Master (MSPAS)

Start Date: June annually

Program Length: 24 months

Class Capacity: 30 students

Tuition: $108,000 (including fees)

CASPA Participant: Yes

Supplemental Application: Yes ($60 fee)

Yellow Ribbon: Yes

Admissions: Non-rolling

Application Deadline: October 1

PREREQUISITE COURSEWORK

Biological Sciences (15 credits, to include Human Anatomy and Physiology I and II with lab and Microbiology), Chemical/Physical Sciences (15 credits, to include Organic or Biological Chemistry), Statistics (3 credits), Ethics (3 credits). At most two prerequisites may be in progress at the time of application. Prerequisites must have been completed within 10 years of matriculation and with a grade "C" or better. AP credits are not accepted.

GPA Requirement: Overall GPA 3.0; Prerequisite GPA: 3.0

Healthcare Experience: 500 hours

PA Shadowing: 24 hours

Required Standardized Testing: None

Letters of Recommendation: Three required; no one specific

Seat Deposit: $750

BAY PATH UNIVERSITY

MISSION:

The Bay Path University Physician Assistant Program educates a diverse student body to develop compassionate, culturally aware healthcare providers who advocate for their patients, maintain the highest quality and ethical standards of care, and recognize their obligation to care for the underserved, and fosters the advancement of and leadership in the Physician Assistant profession.

CLASS OF 2021

Male: 30%

Female: 70%

Overall GPA: 3.50

Prerequisite GPA: 3.60

Average Healthcare Experience: 6,790 hours

Average Age: 25

PANCE SCORES

5-year First Time Pass: 93%

Most Recent First Time Pass: 90%

CURRICULUM STRUCTURE

Didactic: 12 months

Clinical: 12 months

Rotations: 10 mandatory, 1 elective (each 4-5 weeks)

Capstone Project: Required for graduation

UNIQUE PROGRAM FEATURES

Facilities: The program is located in a 58,000 square foot state-of-the-art facility that includes laboratories, classrooms, study areas, and a student wellness center.

Public Health: The curriculum includes public health seminar courses designed to identify public health issues, develop interventions, assess outcomes and overcome burdens associated with intervention.

Boston University

72 East Concord Street, Suite L805
Boston, MA 02118
Phone: 617-358-9589
Email: paoffice@bu.edu

PROGRAM HIGHLIGHTS

Accreditation: Probation

Degree Offered: Master (MMSc)

Start Date: April annually

Program Length: 28 months

Class Capacity: 36 students

Tuition: $109,039

CASPA Participant: Yes

Supplemental Application: Yes ($45 fee)

Yellow Ribbon: Yes

Admissions: Non-rolling

Application Deadline: October 1

PREREQUISITE COURSEWORK

General Biology or Zoology with lab (1 semester), Human or Animal Physiology (1 semester), General Chemistry with lab (1 semester), Organic Chemistry with lab (1 semester), Biochemistry (1 semester), 3 upper level Biology courses (1 semester each). Online courses do not count towards prerequisite course requirements. Prerequisites may be in progress at the time of e-submission to CASPA but must be completed by the October 1st deadline.

GPA Requirement: Science GPA 3.0

Healthcare Experience: Preferred, not required

PA Shadowing: Not required

Required Standardized Testing: GRE (scores must be above the 50th percentile)

Letters of Recommendation: Three required; one from a PA or MD, one from a former professor, and one from a former employer

Seat Deposit: $550

BOSTON UNIVERSITY SCHOOL OF MEDICINE

MISSION:

The mission of the Boston University School of Medicine PA Program is to educate physician assistants who will provide exceptional care for diverse populations of patients, including those from vulnerable communities, and to cultivate leaders. We value integrity, social justice, service, and are committed to developing a successful model for interprofessional education and clinical practice.

CLASS OF 2020

Male: 53%

Female: 47%

Overall GPA: 3.50

Science GPA: 3.46

GRE: Verbal: 75th percentile

GRE Quantitative: 69th percentile

GRE Analytical: 74th percentile

Average Healthcare Experience: 4,280 hours

PANCE SCORES

5-year First Time Pass: 100% (based on four years of data)

Most Recent First Time Pass: 100%

CURRICULUM STRUCTURE

Didactic: 12 months

Clinical: 16 months

Rotations: 9 mandatory, 5 elective (each 4 weeks)

Thesis: Required for graduation

UNIQUE PROGRAM FEATURES

Interprofessional Education: PA students complete much of the didactic curriculum with medical students and the two programs are beginning to integrate clinical rotation experiences. Students also are starting to participate in a longitudinal primary care clinic with medical, social work, and nutrition students. Additionally, students receive oral health training from dentists and dental students.

International Rotations: There are several international rotations available, which can be taken as electives.

Leadership: Students are encouraged to pursue leadership roles with AAPA, MAPA, and other organizations under the mentorship of PA faculty. Several students attend advocacy events in Washington, DC each year while others attend the AAPA or PAEA conference.

179 Longwood Avenue
Boston, MA 02115
Phone: 617-732-2918
Email: admissions@mcphs.edu

PROGRAM HIGHLIGHTS

Accreditation: Continuing

Degree Offered: Master (MPAS)

Start Date: September annually

Program Length: 30 months

Class Capacity: 100 students

Tuition: $129,875

CASPA Participant: Yes

Supplemental Application: Yes

Yellow Ribbon: Yes

Admissions: Rolling

Application Deadline: October 1

PREREQUISITE COURSEWORK

General Biology I (3 credits), General Biology II with lab (4 credits), Anatomy and Physiology I and II (6 credits), Microbiology with lab (4 credits), Chemistry (10 credits with one lab and one upper level course), Psychology (3 credits), Statistics (3 credits). Math and science courses must be completed no more than 10 years prior to the anticipated date of matriculation. At most two prerequisites may be outstanding at the time of application. Prerequisites must be completed with a grade "C" or better.

GPA Requirement: Overall GPA 3.2; Science GPA 3.2; Prerequisite GPA 3.2

Healthcare Experience: 250 hours

PA Shadowing: Not required

Required Standardized Testing: None

Letters of Recommendation: Two required; must be professional references

Seat Deposit: $500

MCPHS UNIVERSITY - BOSTON

MISSION:

The mission of MCPHS University Boston-PA Program is to provide each student with the knowledge and skills to provide quality and compassionate medical care, function as a highly valued member of a health care team, and serve as a patient advocate.

NO CLASS STATISTICS REPORTED

PANCE SCORES

5-year First Time Pass: 97%

Most Recent First Time Pass: 96%

CURRICULUM STRUCTURE

Didactic: 18 months

Clinical: 12 months

Rotations: 7 mandatory, 2 elective (each 5 weeks)

UNIQUE PROGRAM FEATURES

Summer Break: The didactic part of the curriculum spans two years, and students have the summer off following completion of the first year.

Facilities: A state-of-the-art patient assessment laboratory featuring the latest equipment and simulators is available for students to learn physical exam skills.

Admissions Preference: MCPHS University gives priority interview consideration to students currently in their Premedical and Health Studies Pathway Program.

19 Foster Street
Worcester, MA 01608
Phone: 508-373-5607
Email:
admissions.worcester@mcphs.edu

PROGRAM HIGHLIGHTS

Accreditation: Continuing

Degree Offered: Master (MPAS)

Start Date: January annually

Program Length: 24 months

Class Capacity: 70 students

Tuition: $99,000

CASPA Participant: Yes

Supplemental Application: No

Yellow Ribbon: Yes

Admissions: Rolling

Application Deadline: March 1

PREREQUISITE COURSEWORK

Human Anatomy and Physiology I and II with lab (8 credits), Microbiology with lab (4 credits), General Chemistry I with lab (4 credits), Organic Chemistry I with lab (4 credits), Biochemistry (3 credits), Psychology (3 credits), Statistics (3 credits). Math and science courses must be completed no more than 10 years prior to the anticipated date of matriculation. Prerequisites must be completed with a grade "C" or better.

GPA Requirement: Overall GPA 3.0; Science GPA 3.2 (recommended)

Healthcare Experience: Preferred, not required (250-500 hours)

PA Shadowing: Preferred, not required

Required Standardized Testing: None

Letters of Recommendation: Two required; no one specific

Seat Deposit: $500

MCPHS UNIVERSITY - WORCESTER

MISSION:

The program educates and inspires the future generation of Physician Assistants to become compassionate clinicians who demonstrate professionalism; practice collaborative, evidence-based medicine and advocate for patients and their communities.

NO CLASS STATISTICS REPORTED

PANCE SCORES

5-year First Time Pass: 93%

Most Recent First Time Pass: 88%

CURRICULUM STRUCTURE

Didactic: 12 months

Clinical: 12 months

Rotations: 8 mandatory, 1 elective (each 5 weeks)

Capstone Project: Required for graduation

UNIQUE PROGRAM FEATURES

Two Campuses: Lectures are provided on both Worcester and Manchester, NH campuses through state-of-the-art simultaneous video distance education to the students in each cohort split between the two campuses.

International Rotations: Several international rotations are available to students in Belize and Bolivia.

Articulation Agreements: The program has articulation agreements with 11 colleges and universities with respect to the admission of a specified number of students from each of them to the program.

Community Service: Events recently have included Rebuilding Worcester, BeTheMatch Event, Collection for the Homeless Fundraiser Event, Dental Supply Drive for a local shelter, Acupuncture and Infertility Awareness Event, Red Nose Day Fundraiser Event for Children in Poverty, Health Professions Awareness Event for local Elementary School children.

MGH Institute of Health Professions

MGH Institute of Health Professions

34 First Avenue
Charlestown, MA 02129
Phone: 617-726-1839
Email: pa@mghihp.edu

PROGRAM HIGHLIGHTS

Accreditation: Probation
Degree Offered: Master (MPAS)
Start Date: May annually
Program Length: 26 months
Class Capacity: 46 students
Tuition: $100,800

CASPA Participant: Yes
Supplemental Application: No
Yellow Ribbon: Yes
Admissions: Non-rolling
Application Deadline: August 1

PREREQUISITE COURSEWORK

Human Anatomy and Physiology I
and II with lab (8 credits), Biology
with lab (4 credits), Microbiology
with lab (4 credits), Chemistry
with lab (8 credits), Psychology
(3 credits), Statistics (3 credits).
Prerequisites must be completed
with a grade "B-" or better.
There may be no more than two
outstanding prerequisites at the
time of application. Recommended
courses: Organic Chemistry,
Biochemistry.

GPA Requirement: Prerequisite GPA
3.0 (recommended)

Healthcare Experience: 1,000 hours

PA Shadowing: Not required

Required Standardized Testing: GRE
or MCAT

Letters of Recommendation: Three
required; no one specific

Seat Deposit: $500

MGH INSTITUTE OF HEALTH PROFESSIONS

MISSION:

The Master of Physician Assistant Studies Program (MPAS) at MGH Institute of Health Professions will prepare PA graduates to provide compassionate and highly competent medical care for patients across the lifespan.

AVERAGE FOR LAST 4 CLASSES

Male: 30%

Female: 70%

Overall GPA: 3.33

Science GPA: 3.27

Prerequisite GPA: 3.44

GRE Verbal: 58th percentile

GRE Quantitative: 44th percentile

GRE Analytical: 59th percentile

Average Healthcare Experience: 4,542 hours

Average Age: 28

PANCE SCORES

5-year First Time Pass: 91% (based on three years of data)

Most Recent First Time Pass: 86%

CURRICULUM STRUCTURE

Didactic: 13 months

Clinical: 13 months

Rotations: 7 mandatory, 2 elective (each 5 weeks)

Capstone Project: Required for graduation

UNIQUE PROGRAM FEATURES

Team-Based Learning: TBL is used throughout the didactic curriculum as class time is spent working through clinical problems and scenarios in small groups with a faculty member. Students also work in small interprofessional collaborative teams with students representing a variety of disciplines.

IMPACT: The MGH Institute's new IMPACT Practice Center brings together students from nursing, occupational therapy, physical therapy, physician assistant studies, speech-language pathology, and genetic counseling to learn and practice in teams and to deliver essential free care to the community. Students provide care to a variety of clients, under the direct supervision of Institute faculty.

Rotations: The program is partnered with New England's largest healthcare organization, offering unparalleled access to Harvard Medical School affiliated medical centers.

175

Northeastern University

360 Huntington Avenue
202 Robinson Hall
Boston, MA 02115
Phone: 617-373-3195
Email: paprogram@northeastern.edu

PROGRAM HIGHLIGHTS

Accreditation: Continuing

Degree Offered: Master (MSPAS)

Start Date: August annually

Program Length: 24 months

Class Capacity: 52 students

Tuition: $93,318

CASPA Participant: Yes

Supplemental Application: Yes ($75 fee)

Yellow Ribbon: Yes

Admissions: Non-rolling

Application Deadline: August 1

PREREQUISITE COURSEWORK

Anatomy and Physiology (2 semesters), Biology (2 semesters) with 1 semester of lab, Chemistry (2 semesters) with 1 semester of lab, Statistics (1 semester). Prerequisites must be completed with a grade "B" or better, by the application deadline, and within the last 10 years. Basic Life Support Certification is required before matriculation. AP credits are not accepted.

GPA Requirement: Overall GPA 3.0; Science GPA 3.0

Healthcare Experience: 1,000 hours (recommended)

PA Shadowing: Preferred, not required

Required Standardized Testing: None

Letters of Recommendation: Three required; two should be from individuals that the applicant worked with while obtaining health care experience

Seat Deposit: $500

NORTHEASTERN UNIVERSITY

MISSION:

The mission of the Northeastern University Physician Assistant Program is to educate and inspire compassionate clinicians prepared to be leaders in all aspects of healthcare.

NO CLASS STATISTICS REPORTED

PANCE SCORES

5-year First Time Pass: 98%

Most Recent First Time Pass: 100%

CURRICULUM STRUCTURE

Didactic: 12 months

Clinical: 12 months

Rotations: 8 mandatory, 1 elective (each 5 weeks)

Capstone Project: Required for graduation

UNIQUE PROGRAM FEATURES

Facilities: Classroom facilities include spacious theater-style seating, conference rooms for small group interactive learning, the cadaver lab for anatomy, and the state-of-the-art Arnold S. Goldstein Simulation Laboratories Suite. In addition, new high-tech classrooms have been added to the Snell Library for special classes such as team-based learning (TBL).

Interprofessional Education: Students work with other medical professions students in the health sciences to analyze patient cases throughout the didactic curriculum.

Dual Degree: A dual PA/MPH and PA/MSHI degree option is available and adds an additional 6 months to the duration of the program.

Springfield College

263 Alden Street
Springfield, MA 01109-3797
Phone: 413-748-3554
Email:
lsaloio@springfieldcollege.edu

PROGRAM HIGHLIGHTS

Accreditation: Continuing

Degree Offered: Master (MSPAS)

Start Date: January annually

Program Length: 27 months

Class Capacity: 35 students

Tuition: $124,468

CASPA Participant: No

Supplemental Application: Yes ($50 application fee)

Yellow Ribbon: No

Admissions: Rolling

Application Deadline: June 1 (preferred April 1)

PREREQUISITE COURSEWORK

Biology I and II (8 credits), General Chemistry I and II (8 credits), Human Anatomy and Physiology I and II (8 credits), Biochemistry (3 credits), Organic Chemistry (4 credits), Microbiology (3 credits), Pre-Calculus (3 credits), Statistics (3 credits). Prerequisites must be completed with a grade "C+" or better.

GPA Requirement: Overall GPA 3.0; Prerequisite GPA 3.0

Healthcare Experience: 470 hours

PA Shadowing: 30 hours

Required Standardized Testing: None

Letters of Recommendation: Three required; no one specific

Seat Deposit: $200

SPRINGFIELD COLLEGE

MISSION:

The mission of the Springfield College Physician Assistant Program is to educate students in spirit, mind, and body for leadership in clinical, community, and academic service to humanity by building upon its foundations of Humanics and academic excellence.

NO CLASS STATISTICS REPORTED

PANCE SCORES

5-year First Time Pass: 97%

Most Recent First Time Pass: 100%

CURRICULUM STRUCTURE

Didactic: 15 months

Clinical: 12 months

Rotations: 7 mandatory, 1 elective (each 6 weeks)

Research Project: Required for graduation

UNIQUE PROGRAM FEATURES

Program Entry: There are two different entry points to the program, as a freshman college student (6 year program) or as a graduate student (2 year program). Freshmen students have priority, often leaving few if any spots open to graduate students.

Medical Simulation: The state-of-the-art Medical Simulation Lab features high fidelity 3G adult and baby patient simulator mannequins that respond to treatment as human patients would, allowing students to experience realistic, hands-on training, and complicated medical techniques without fear of error.

Rotations: A six-week international medical Spanish elective rotation in Costa Rica is now available.

PROGRAM HIGHLIGHTS

Accreditation: Continuing

Degree Offered: Master (MMS)

Start Date: January annually

Program Length: 25 months

Class Capacity: 50 students

Tuition: $97,860

CASPA Participant: Yes

Supplemental Application: No

Yellow Ribbon: No

Admissions: Rolling

Application Deadline: August 1

PREREQUISITE COURSEWORK

Human Anatomy and Physiology I and II (2 semesters), General Biology I and II with lab (2 semesters), General Chemistry I and II with lab (2 semesters), Microbiology with lab (1 semester), Statistics (1 semester). All prerequisites must be completed at the time of application and within the last 10 years. Prerequisites must be completed with a grade "C" or better. Recommended courses: Medical Terminology, Biochemistry, Psychology. AP credits are accepted but students must taken higher level courses in the same department to fulfill the prerequisite requirement.

GPA Requirement: Science GPA 3.0; Prerequisite GPA 3.0

Healthcare Experience: 1,000 hours

PA Shadowing: Preferred, not required

Required Standardized Testing: GRE or MCAT

Letters of Recommendation: Three required; at least one should be from a supervisor of a direct patient care experience and should substantiate the applicant's experience and performance

Seat Deposit: $1,000

TUFTS UNIVERSITY

MISSION:

The Tufts PA program mission is to promote human health by providing excellent education to future physician assistants so that they are prepared to become integral members of the health care team. We fulfill this mission in a dynamic learning environment that emphasizes rigorous fundamentals, innovative delivery of the curriculum, and compassionate care to diverse patient populations. Our graduates will be prepared to participate in all aspects of the health care continuum, including disease management, health promotion and maintenance, and palliative care.

CLASS OF 2021

Male: 31%

Female: 69%

Overall GPA: 3.62

Prerequisite GPA: 3.61

GRE Verbal: 72nd percentile

GRE Quantitative: 61st percentile

MCAT: 507

Average Healthcare Experience: 3,182 hours

Average Age: 24.2

PANCE SCORES

5-year First Time Pass: 100%

Most Recent First Time Pass: 100%

CURRICULUM STRUCTURE

Didactic: 12 months

Clinical: 13 months

Rotations: 10 mandatory, 1 elective (each 4-5 weeks)

Capstone Project: Required for graduation

UNIQUE PROGRAM FEATURES

Dual Degree: The program offers a 3 year combined PA/MPH option to students.

Community Service: The Sharewood Project is a free health care organization serving the medically underserved populations of the greater Boston area. Physician Assistant students have the opportunity to volunteer in the clinic alongside medical students and physicians.

Facilities: Tufts has a state-of-the-art anatomy lab and clinical skills and simulation center where students work with human cadavers and can gain hands on experience with new procedures before attempting them on a real patient.

577 Western Ave.
Westfield, MA 01086
Phone: 413-572-8149
Email: PAstudies@westfield.ma.edu

PROGRAM HIGHLIGHTS

Accreditation: Provisional

Degree Offered: Master (MSPAS)

Start Date: January annually

Program Length: 24 months

Class Capacity: 30 students

Tuition: $83,400

CASPA Participant: Yes

Supplemental Application: Yes ($50 fee)

Yellow Ribbon: No

Admissions: Non-rolling

Application Deadline: July 15

PREREQUISITE COURSEWORK

30 credits of Biological, Chemical, and Physical Sciences (to include Human Anatomy and Physiology I and II with lab, Microbiology, Genetics, and Biochemistry), Statistics, Ethics, Psychology. Science coursework must be completed within the last 10 years. Up to two prerequisites may be outstanding at the time of application. Prerequisites must be completed with a grade "C" or better.

GPA Requirement: Overall GPA 3.0

Healthcare Experience: 500 hours

PA Shadowing: Preferred, not required

Required Standardized Testing: None

Letters of Recommendation: Three required; no one specific

Seat Deposit: $1,000

WESTFIELD STATE UNIVERSITY

MISSION:

The Westfield State University Physician Assistant Program seeks excellence in educating a diverse student body of compassionate, culturally aware healthcare providers who are prepared to practice in a patient centered team assuring care to all citizens of the Commonwealth of Massachusetts and beyond.

CLASS OF 2020:

Overall GPA 3.57

Average Healthcare Experience: 6,552 hours

PANCE SCORES

5-year First Time Pass: N/A

Most Recent First Time Pass: N/A (have not graduated a class yet)

CURRICULUM STRUCTURE

Didactic: 12 months

Clinical: 12 months

Rotations: 10 mandatory, 1 elective (each 4 weeks)

Capstone Project: Required for graduation

UNIQUE PROGRAM FEATURES

Admissions Preference: Preference is given to Massachusetts residents and those with a Bachelor's degree from a Massachusetts public institution. An interview will be granted for all students who have graduated from a Massachusetts public four-year institution if the following criteria are met: overall GPA 3.5, prerequisite GPA 3.5, a recommendation from a PA or MD indicating support for consideration of the applicant, 500 hours of patient care experience, and successful completion of all other admissions requirements.

Rotations: Unique to this program, all students complete an addiction medicine rotation.

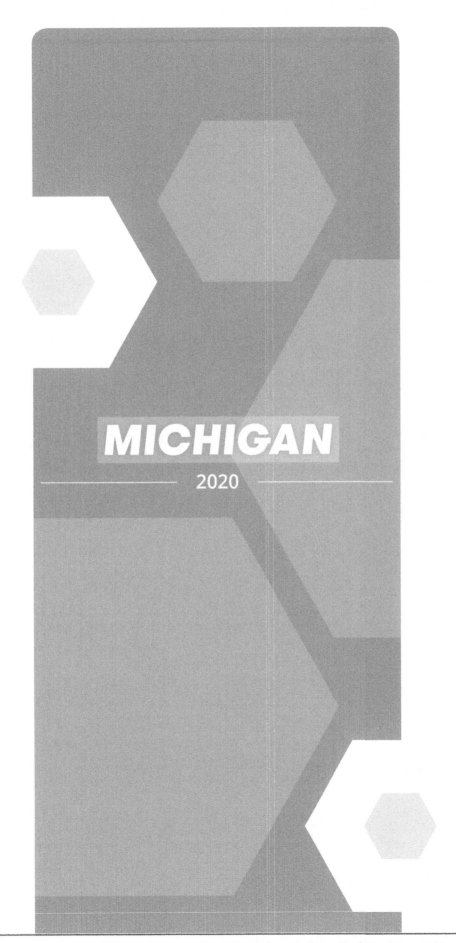

MICHIGAN

2020

Central Michigan University

Health Professions 1223
Mount Pleasant, MI 48859
Phone: 989-774-1730
Email: chpgradadm@cmich.edu

PROGRAM HIGHLIGHTS

Accreditation: Continuing

Degree Offered: Master (MSPA)

Start Date: May annually

Program Length: 27 months

Class Capacity: 40 students

Tuition: $82,810

CASPA Participant: Yes

Supplemental Application: Yes ($50 fee)

Yellow Ribbon: No

Admissions: Non-rolling

Application Deadline: September 1

PREREQUISITE COURSEWORK

Anatomy with lab, Physiology with lab, Pathophysiology, Microbiology, Biochemistry, Developmental Psychology. At most two prerequisites may be in progress at the time of application but must be completed by December 31st of the application year. Prerequisites must be completed within the last 6 years. AP credits may be accepted and are subject to the PA Program Director's approval.

GPA Requirement: Overall GPA 3.0; Prerequisite GPA 3.0

Healthcare Experience: 500 hours

PA Shadowing: Not required

Required Standardized Testing: PA-CAT

Letters of Recommendation: Three required; no one specific

Seat Deposit: $1,000

CENTRAL MICHIGAN UNIVERSITY

MISSION:

The mission of the Central Michigan University Physician Assistant Program is to produce well-educated and highly-trained Physician Assistants who provide evidence-based medical services within the interdisciplinary primary care environment, with an emphasis on diversity and service to medically underserved populations in rural or urban communities.

NO CLASS STATISTICS REPORTED

PANCE SCORES

5-year First Time Pass: 96%

Most Recent First Time Pass: 97%

CURRICULUM STRUCTURE

Didactic: 15 months

Clinical: 12 months

Rotations: 7 mandatory, 1 elective (each 5 weeks)

UNIQUE PROGRAM FEATURES

Early Clinical Exposure: In their first year, students spend one day per week seeing patients with a primary care preceptor for approximately 7 months. This allows them to hone their clinical skills and apply didactic information to patients as it is learned.

Fundamental Critical Care Support: The students complete the FCCS curriculum at the end of didactic year, which provides them with procedural skills but also gives them the chance to take a specialty exam for certification in critical care medicine.

Articulation Agreement: The program agrees to admit up to four suitably-qualified and duly-enrolled full-time students from Northern Michigan University (NMU) to the PA Program who satisfy all of the criteria. The admission of these candidates shall occur on a non-competitive basis with respect to the applicant pool as a whole.

Eastern Michigan University

222 Rackham Building
Ypsilanti, MI 48197
Phone: 734-487-2843
Email: chhs_paprogram@emich.edu

PROGRAM HIGHLIGHTS

Accreditation: Continuing

Degree Offered: Master (MSPAS)

Start Date: May annually

Program Length: 24 months

Class Capacity: 30 students

Tuition: $87,089 (in-state, including fees); $150,177 (out-of-state, including fees)

CASPA Participant: Yes

Supplemental Application: Yes ($45 fee)

Yellow Ribbon: No

Admissions: Non-rolling

Application Deadline: September 1

PREREQUISITE COURSEWORK

Human Anatomy, Human Physiology, General Chemistry with lab, Organic Chemistry with lab or Biochemistry with lab, Microbiology with lab, Lifespan Psychology, Statistics. Five out of seven must be completed at the time of the application and all must be completed within the last 10 years. Prerequisites must be completed with a grade "B-" or better. AP credits are not accepted.

GPA Requirement: Overall GPA 3.0

Healthcare Experience: Preferred, not required

PA Shadowing: Not required

Required Standardized Testing: GRE

Letters of Recommendation: Two required; no one specific

Seat Deposit: $1,000

EASTERN MICHIGAN UNIVERSITY

MISSION:

The Eastern Michigan University Physician Assistant Program mission is to identify, train and support a diverse population of graduate students to become highly respected ambassadors of the profession and extraordinary healthcare providers with a strong foundation in primary care medicine and interdisciplinary practice.

CLASS OF 2021

Male: 30%

Female: 70%

Overall GPA: 3.80

GRE Total: 315

Average Age: 24.7

PANCE SCORES

5-year First Time Pass: 100% (based on four years of data)

Most Recent First Time Pass: 100%

CURRICULUM STRUCTURE

Didactic: 12 months

Clinical: 12 months

Rotations: 7 mandatory, 2 elective, 1 preceptorship (each 4-6 weeks)

UNIQUE PROGRAM FEATURES

Multiple Teaching Styles: The program utilizes traditional lectures, problem-based learning, practical training, out of classroom learning and high fidelity medical simulation.

Facilities: There are newly renovated facilities for PA students including a human anatomy lab and advanced medical simulation center, as well as clinical skills laboratories, small group rooms, physical exam laboratory, advanced patient exam suites, a computer room, and a student lounge.

Simulation: Students hone their skills through advanced medical simulation experiences as part of the regular schedule of courses each semester.

Grand Valley State University

301 Michigan Street
Suite 200
Grand Rapids, MI 49315
Phone: 616-331-5700
Email: pas@gvsu.edu

PROGRAM HIGHLIGHTS

Accreditation: Continuing
Degree Offered: Master (MPAS)
Start Date: August annually
Program Length: 28 months
Class Capacity: 48 students
Tuition: $75,499

CASPA Participant: Yes
Supplemental Application: Yes ($30 fee)
Yellow Ribbon: No
Admissions: Non-rolling
Application Deadline: September 1

PREREQUISITE COURSEWORK

General Biology, General Chemistry, Genetics, Organic Chemistry, Biochemistry, Human Anatomy, Human Physiology, Statistics, Psychology, Microbiology, Physics. Human Anatomy, Human Physiology, Biochemistry and Microbiology must be completed within the last 5 years and by the application deadline. Organic Chemistry must also be complete by the application deadline. Prerequisites must be completed with a grade "C" or better. Recommended courses: Immunology, Medical Ethics, Pharmacology, Pathophysiology, Nutrition, Cadaver Lab.

GPA Requirement: Overall GPA 3.0; Prerequisite GPA 3.0; Last 60 Credit GPA 3.0

Healthcare Experience: 500 hours

PA Shadowing: Preferred, not required (counts towards healthcare experience)

Required Standardized Testing: GRE

Letters of Recommendation: Two required; one should be from a health care professional

Seat Deposit: None

GRAND VALLEY STATE UNIVERSITY

MISSION:

The mission of the program is to educate individuals to become competent Physician Assistants, who possess the skills necessary for interprofessional medical practice.

CLASS OF 2021

Overall GPA: 3.76

Prerequisite GPA: 3.82

Last 60 Credit GPA: 3.77

GRE Verbal: 153

GRE Quantitative: 154

GRE Analytical: 4.25

Average Healthcare Experience: 2,529 hours

PANCE SCORES

5-year First Time Pass: 100%

Most Recent First Time Pass: 100%

CURRICULUM STRUCTURE

Didactic: 16 months

Clinical: 12 months

Rotations: 10 mandatory, 2 elective (each 4 weeks)

UNIQUE PROGRAM FEATURES

One Program, Two Locations: The program accepts up to 36 students at its Grand Rapids campus and 12 students at its Traverse City campus. The Traverse City students interact with the Grand Rapids lecturers and students through video conferencing.

Academic Medical Center: The main campus is located in the center of a growing health complex which includes a medical school, pharmacy school, 1000 bed hospital system with level 1 trauma center, cancer center, heart center, world class children's hospital and an international research institute.

Hospital Community Experience: This course exposes students to patients in their first year. Learning opportunities may include, but are not limited to, long-term care, clinical job shadowing, public health, research, and virtual and simulated patient experiences.

185

PROGRAM HIGHLIGHTS

Accreditation: Continuing

Degree Offered: Master (MS)

Start Date: August annually

Program Length: 24-36 months
(full/part-time option)

Class Capacity: 60 students

Tuition: $98,622

CASPA Participant: Yes

Supplemental Application: No

Yellow Ribbon: Yes

Admissions: Non-rolling

Application Deadline: January 15

PREREQUISITE COURSEWORK

Nutrition, Medical Ethics, Statistics, Advanced Physiology, Microbiology, Developmental Psychology. Prerequisites must be completed within the last 6 years and by the application deadline.

GPA Requirement: Overall GPA 3.0; Prerequisite GPA 3.0

Healthcare Experience: 1,000 hours

PA Shadowing: Not required

Required Standardized Testing: GRE (minimum combined score of 291)

Letters of Recommendation: Two required; one should be from a PA or physician

Seat Deposit: $500

UNIVERSITY OF DETROIT - MERCY

MISSION:

The University of Detroit Mercy Physician Assistant Program is dedicated to the education of clinically competent medical professionals thoroughly prepared to deliver quality patient care in the context of a dynamic health care delivery system.

NO CLASS STATISTICS REPORTED

PANCE SCORES

5-year First Time Pass: 98%

Most Recent First Time Pass: 100%

CURRICULUM STRUCTURE

Didactic: 12 months

Clinical: 12 months

Rotations: 8 mandatory (each 2-5 weeks), 1 elective (2 weeks), 1 preceptorship (8 weeks)

UNIQUE PROGRAM FEATURES

Part-Time Program: Students who wish to continue working during their training can enter the part-time track, which is completed over 36 months. The didactic curriculum is divided into 2 years. Students then complete their rotations afterwards.

Admissions Preference: UDM undergraduates, applicants from underserved communities and underrepresented minorities in the profession may be given additional consideration in the application process.

Community Service: Students are active in the community in several projects including collecting Christmas donations, volunteer cancer screenings, among other projects.

3+2 Track: Detroit Mercy's five-year accelerated track in the Physician Assistant program accepts a select number of highly-qualified entering freshmen to complete a combined Bachelor of Science degree in Biology and a Master of Science degree in Physician Assistant Studies in 5 years.

Wayne State University

259 Mack Avenue, Suite 2590
Detroit, MI 48201
Phone: 313-577-3707
Email: paadmit@wayne.edu

PROGRAM HIGHLIGHTS

Accreditation: Continuing

Degree Offered: Master (MSPAS)

Start Date: May annually

Program Length: 24 months

Class Capacity: 50 students

Tuition: $46,178 (in-state); $86,411 (out-of-state)

CASPA Participant: Yes

Supplemental Application: Yes ($50 fee)

Yellow Ribbon: No

Admissions: Non-rolling

Application Deadline: September 1

PREREQUISITE COURSEWORK

Human Anatomy (1 course), Human Physiology (1 course), Upper Level Physiology (1 course, can be fulfilled by Exercise Physiology, Human Physiology, Comparative Physiology, Genetics, Cell Biology, Endocrinology, Pathophysiology, Immunology, Neurophysiology, or Histology), Microbiology with lab (1 course), Chemistry (2 courses, one must be Organic Chemistry or Biochemistry), Nutrition (1 course), Developmental Psychology (1 course), Basic Statistics (1 course), English Composition (2 courses), Medical Terminology (1 course). Anatomy, Physiology, Microbiology and Chemistry prerequisites must be completed within the last 6 years. All must be completed by the application deadline and with a grade "B" or better. Applicants may request that their last 60 undergraduate credit hours be used to calculate the cumulative GPA.

GPA Requirement: Overall GPA 3.0; Prerequisite GPA 3.0

Healthcare Experience: 500 hours (obtained within the last 2 years)

PA Shadowing: Not required

Required Standardized Testing: GRE (minimum combined score of 285 and 3.5 analytical)

Letters of Recommendation: Three required; one should be from a work supervisor who can comment on the direct patient care that you provide, and one from a PA/MD/DO

Seat Deposit: $1,000

WAYNE STATE UNIVERSITY

MISSION:

The mission of the Wayne State University Physician Assistant Studies program is to develop highly competent and passionate physician assistants who are deeply committed to the practice of medicine in a range of urban and underserved health care settings. The program exemplifies excellence and innovation in health care delivery and service to the community.

CLASS OF 2020

Male: 28%

Female: 72%

Overall GPA: 3.75

Prerequisite GPA: 3.86

GRE Verbal: 153

GRE Quantitative: 154

GRE Analytical: 4.2

PANCE SCORES

5-year First Time Pass: 99%

Most Recent First Time Pass: 98%

CURRICULUM STRUCTURE

Didactic: 12 months

Clinical: 12 months

Rotations:
7 mandatory
(each 4-12 weeks),
1 preceptorship
(4 weeks)

UNIQUE PROGRAM FEATURES

Community Service: The program has an extensive history of community service working with medically underserved populations, Detroit public schools, Special Olympics Detroit, WSU Health Education for Longevity and Prevention Clinic, and other organizations selected by current students.

Scholarships: The program offers three different scholarships to PA students. More information can be found on the program's website.

Hands-on Experience: The program has a commitment to hands-on learning evidenced in its utilization of standardized patients for clinical skills testing, human dissection in anatomy course, and interaction with patients starting early in the program.

187

Western Michigan University

1903 W. Michigan Ave.
Kalamazoo, MI 49008
Phone: 269-387-5311
Email: pa-info@wmich.edu

PROGRAM HIGHLIGHTS

Accreditation: Continuing

Degree Offered: Master (MS)

Start Date: September annually

Program Length: 24 months

Class Capacity: 40 students

Tuition: $64,759 (in-state);
$84,694 (out-of-state)

CASPA Participant: Yes

Supplemental Application: Yes ($50 fee)

Yellow Ribbon: No

Admissions: Non-rolling

Application Deadline: December 1

PREREQUISITE COURSEWORK

Human Anatomy, Human Physiology (upper level), Microbiology with lab, Biochemistry (upper level), Developmental/Lifespan Psychology, Introductory Statistics. Prerequisites must be completed with a grade "C" or better and by December 31st of the application year. Students completing an Anatomy and Physiology I and II series must complete an additional upper level human physiology course.

GPA Requirement: Last 60 Credit GPA 3.0

Healthcare Experience: 1,000 hours

PA Shadowing: Not required

Required Standardized Testing: None

Letters of Recommendation: Three required; no one specific

Seat Deposit: $750

WESTERN MICHIGAN UNIVERSITY

MISSION:

The WMU Department of Physician Assistant is dedicated to educating competent, caring physician assistants to practice primary care medicine in all areas of society.

NO CLASS STATISTICS REPORTED

PANCE SCORES

5-year First Time Pass: 95%

Most Recent First Time Pass: 97%

CURRICULUM STRUCTURE

Didactic: 12 months

Clinical: 12 months

Rotations: 7 mandatory (each 4-8 weeks), 2 electives

Research Project: Required for graduation

UNIQUE PROGRAM FEATURES

Community Service: Students participate in several local, state, and national projects including Girls on the Run, Adopt a Family, Relay for Life, WC SAFE, Angel House and Goodwill Inn Homeless Shelter.

Scholarships: There are several scholarships available to incoming students. More information can be found on the program website.

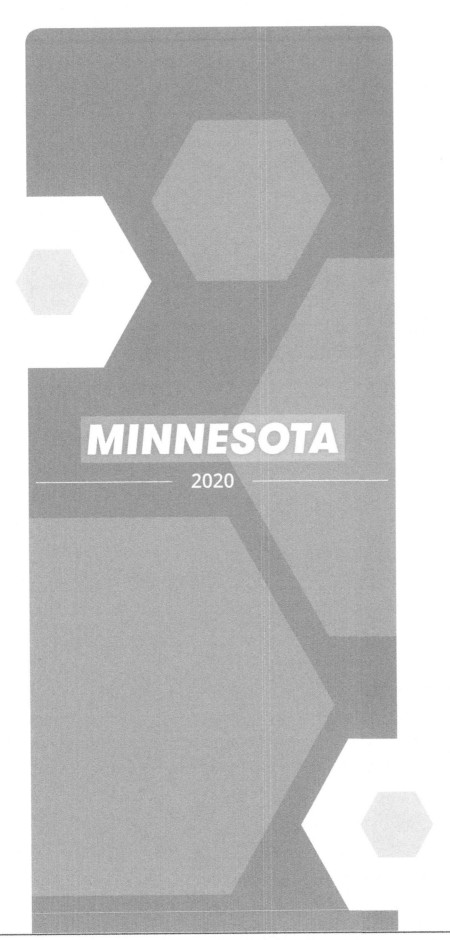

MINNESOTA

2020

PROGRAM HIGHLIGHTS

Accreditation: Probation

Degree Offered: Master (MSPAS)

Start Date: May annually

Program Length: 27 months

Class Capacity: 33 students

Tuition: $92,500

CASPA Participant: Yes

Supplemental Application: Yes ($50 fee)

Yellow Ribbon: No

Admissions: Non-rolling

Application Deadline: August 1

PREREQUISITE COURSEWORK

Physiology (3-4 credits), Microbiology (3-4 credits), Biochemistry (3-4 credits), Psychology (3-4 credits), Statistics (3-4 credits), Medical Terminology (1-3 credits). Labs are strongly recommended but not required. Prerequisites must be completed within 10 years of the program start date and with a grade "B" or better. AP credits are not accepted. Recommended courses: Anatomy, Biomedical Ethics, Cell Biology, Immunology, Genetics, Health Policy, Sociology, Research Methods.

GPA Requirement: Overall GPA 3.0; Science GPA 3.0

Healthcare Experience: 2,000 hours (recommended)

PA Shadowing: Preferred, not required

Required Standardized Testing: None

Letters of Recommendation: Three required; one should be from an employer/colleague (a professional reference), one from a professor or adviser (an academic reference), and one from a person of your choice

Seat Deposit: $1,000

AUGSBURG UNIVERSITY

MISSION:

The mission of the Augsburg University Physician Assistant Studies Program is based on a foundation of respect and sensitivity to persons of all cultures and backgrounds and oriented towards providing care to underserved populations. Students are well educated in current medical theory and practice, and graduates are encouraged to work in primary care settings. The program promotes dedication to excellence in performance, with the highest standards of ethics and integrity, and commitment to lifelong personal and professional development.

NO CLASS STATISTICS REPORTED

PANCE SCORES

5-year First Time Pass: 99%

Most Recent First Time Pass: 100%

CURRICULUM STRUCTURE

Didactic: 15 months

Clinical: 12 months

Rotations: 7 mandatory, 1 elective (each 5 weeks), 1 preceptorship (8 weeks)

Master's Project: Required for graduation

UNIQUE PROGRAM FEATURES

Primary Care Focus: This program has a focus on providing primary care to underserved populations. 72% of graduates report practicing in primary care after graduation.

Admissions Preference: The PA program favors applicants whose experience demonstrates a commitment to underserved communities, disadvantaged, minority, or under-represented populations. Applicants should have a strong record of commitment to the community.

Elective Master's Project: During the second summer of the program, students have the option to enroll in an elective course offered through another Augsburg department or independently research a clinical topic in-depth. Students complete a clinical research paper based on the course content or specific research question.

International Rotations: There are opportunities for students to complete international rotations and complete their Master's research project through an international experience. Currently the program has approved international clinical sites in Belize, Ecuador and South Africa.

191

Bethel University

3900 Bethel Drive
St. Paul, MN 55112
Phone: 651-638-6242
Email: physician-assistant@bethel.edu

PROGRAM HIGHLIGHTS

Accreditation: Continuing

Degree Offered: Master (MSPA)

Start Date: June annually

Program Length: 27 months

Class Capacity: 32 students

Tuition: $93,632

CASPA Participant: Yes

Supplemental Application: Yes ($50 fee)

Yellow Ribbon: Yes

Admissions: Non-rolling

Application Deadline: August 1

PREREQUISITE COURSEWORK

Human Anatomy (3 credits), Human Physiology (3 credits), Organic Chemistry (3 credits), Biochemistry (3 credits), Microbiology (3 credits), Genetics (3 credits), Psychology (3 credits), Statistics (3 credits). Anatomy, Physiology, and Microbiology must be completed within the last 5 years. Up to three prerequisites may be in progress at the time of application but must be completed by March 1st of the year of matriculation. Prerequisites must be completed with a grade "B-" or better. AP scores of 4 or 5 may be accepted for the Psychology and Statistics requirements only. Recommended courses: Ethics, Pathophysiology, Physics, Pharmacology.

GPA Requirement: Overall GPA 3.25; Science GPA 3.25

Healthcare Experience: 250 hours

PA Shadowing: Preferred, not required

Required Standardized Testing: None

Letters of Recommendation: Three required; no one specific

Seat Deposit: $500

BETHEL UNIVERSITY

MISSION:

Boldly motivated by the Christian faith and in the spirit of Bethel University's academic excellence and ministry focus, the Bethel Physician Assistant program will educate students to become physician assistants who develop the skills for competent and excellent medical practice, live out ethical principles and Bethel's academic excellence, serve their community and all cultures, and possess integrity and compassion.

AVERAGE CLASS STATISTICS

Male: 23%

Female: 77%

Overall GPA: 3.80

Science GPA: 3.77

Average Healthcare Experience: 1,954 hours

PANCE SCORES

5-year First Time Pass: 98%

Most Recent First Time Pass: 97%

CURRICULUM STRUCTURE

Didactic: 15 months

Clinical: 12 months

Rotations: 7 mandatory, 2 elective (each 4-8 weeks)

Evidence-Based Medicine/ Thesis Project: Required for graduation

UNIQUE PROGRAM FEATURES

Christian Tradition: The professors embrace a holistic approach to medical care that takes into account the mind, body, and spirit connection in medicine and how to integrate it with Christian faith in patient treatment.

Facilities: You will learn in a state-of-the-art training facility that uses patient simulators, video-monitored clinics, and other technologies to enhance learning.

Admissions: Any candidate meeting all application requirements with a bachelor's degree or master's degree from Bethel University or U.S. Military veteran will be granted an interview.

College of St. Scholastica

1200 Kenwood Ave.
Duluth, MN 55811
Phone: 218-625-4823
Email: ceickman@css.edu

PROGRAM HIGHLIGHTS

Accreditation: Provisional

Degree Offered: Master (MSPAS)

Start Date: August annually

Program Length: 24 months

Class Capacity: 30 students

Tuition: $95,765

CASPA Participant: Yes

Supplemental Application: No

Yellow Ribbon: Yes

Admissions: Non-rolling

Application Deadline: September 1

PREREQUISITE COURSEWORK

Organic Chemistry I and II, Biochemistry, Anatomy and Physiology I and II, Microbiology, Lifespan Developmental Psychology, Medical Terminology, Statistics. Prerequisites must be completed with a grade "C" or better and within the last 10 years. AP credits are not accepted.

GPA Requirement: Overall GPA 3.0; Prerequisite GPA 3.0

Healthcare Experience: 750 hours (strongly recommended)

PA Shadowing: Preferred, not required

Required Standardized Testing: GRE (preferred minimum verbal 146, quantitative 144 and analytical 4.0)

Letters of Recommendation: Three required; no one specific

Seat Deposit: $500

COLLEGE OF SAINT SCHOLASTICA

MISSION:

In accordance with our Benedictine values, the College of St. Scholastica's Master of Physician Assistant Studies program's mission is to educate physician assistant students within a comprehensive, interprofessional and innovative curriculum to provide high-quality care across the lifespan and meet the healthcare needs of our region.

NO CLASS STATISTICS REPORTED

PANCE SCORES

5-year First Time Pass: N/A

Most Recent First Time Pass: N/A (have not graduated a class yet)

CURRICULUM STRUCTURE

Didactic: 12 months

Clinical: 12 months

Rotations: 10 mandatory (each 4 weeks), 2 elective (each 2 weeks)

Capstone Project: Required for graduation

UNIQUE PROGRAM FEATURES

Interprofessional Education: Students will interact and learn with students from the Physical Therapy, Occupational Therapy, Social Work, Health Information Management, Athletic Training, Exercise Physiology and Nursing programs.

Facilities: Classes are held in a state-of-the-art building featuring the latest in simulation, telehealth and technology-supported patient care equipment.

Curriculum: The curriculum incorporates medical simulation software and online textbooks in addition to traditional classroom-based learning.

Admissions Preference: Preference is given to factors such as connections to the region, student hometown, undergraduate institution, and veteran's status.

Saint Catherine University

2004 Randolph Avenue
Saint Paul, MN 55105
Phone: 651-690-7827
Email: mpas@stkate.edu

PROGRAM HIGHLIGHTS

Accreditation: Continuing

Degree Offered: Master (MPAS)

Start Date: September annually

Program Length: 28 months

Class Capacity: 32 students

Tuition: $92,620

CASPA Participant: Yes

Supplemental Application: No

Yellow Ribbon: Yes

Admissions: Non-rolling

Application Deadline: July 15

PREREQUISITE COURSEWORK

Human or Vertebrate Anatomy (4 credits), Human or Vertebrate Physiology (4 credits), Organic Chemistry with Lab (8 credits), Biochemistry (3-4 credits), Microbiology (3-4 credits), Pre-calculus or higher math (3-4 credits), Statistics (3-4 credits), General Psychology (3-4 credits), Lifespan Developmental Psychology or Abnormal Psychology (3-4 credits), Medical Terminology (1 course). At the time of application, no more than three courses may be in progress or yet to be taken. Biochemistry and Microbiology must be completed within the last 10 years. Prerequisites must be completed with a grade "C" or better. AP credits are accepted for Pre-Calculus, Statistics and Psychology.

GPA Requirement: Overall GPA 3.2; Prerequisite GPA 3.0

Healthcare Experience: 1,000 hours

PA Shadowing: Not required

Required Standardized Testing: GRE

Letters of Recommendation: Two required; one should be from a healthcare provider and the other can be from a professor or employer

Seat Deposit: $1,000

SAINT CATHERINE UNIVERSITY

MISSION:

Influenced by Catholic intellectual tradition, the MPAS program is committed to preparing competent and compassionate Physician Assistant scholar practitioners who possess the knowledge, clinical acumen and critical thinking skills necessary to practice exemplary, ethical, patient-centered care, and who will lead and influence with grace emphasizing global responsibility, social justice and the preservation of human dignity.

CLASS OF 2021

Overall GPA: 3.64

Prerequisite GPA: 3.67

GRE Verbal: 155

GRE Quantitative: 156

GRE Analytical: 4.25

PANCE SCORES

5-year First Time Pass: 99%

Most Recent First Time Pass: 100%

CURRICULUM STRUCTURE

Didactic: 14 months

Clinical: 14 months

Rotations:
10 mandatory,
2 elective
(each 4 weeks)

Professional Portfolio Presentation: Required for graduation

UNIQUE PROGRAM FEATURES

International Experience: Students have traveled for clinical rotations and medical mission trips to Haiti, Cuba, the Dominican Republic, South Korea, and Guatemala and have participated in activities ranging from depression screenings to orthopedics care.

Curriculum Delivery: Though much of the content is delivered through lecture format, the program also focuses on small group clinical reasoning sessions and using educational technology throughout to enhance the student experience.

Interprofessional Education: There are opportunities for interprofessional education with nursing, occupational therapy, physical therapy and public health students within the Henrietta Schmoll School of Health.

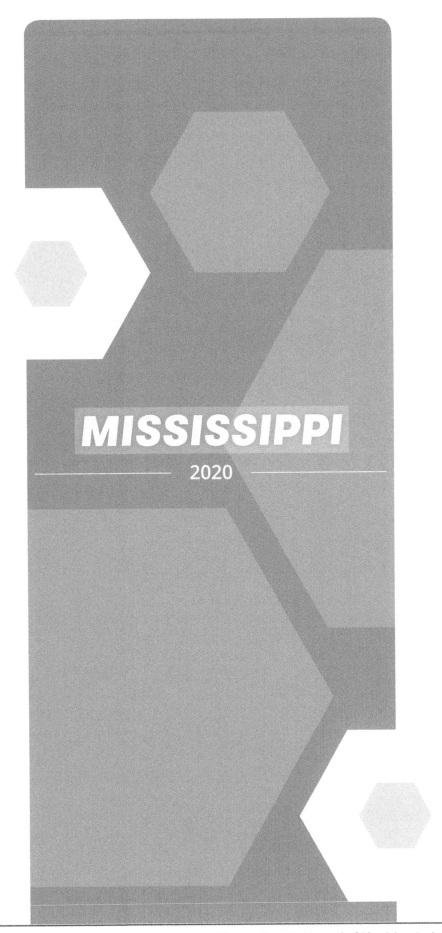

MISSISSIPPI

2020

Mississippi College

200 S. Capitol Street, Box 4053
Clinton, MS 39056
Phone: 601-925-7371
Email: jrkendrick@mc.edu

PROGRAM HIGHLIGHTS

Accreditation: Continuing

Degree Offered: Master (MSM)

Start Date: May annually

Program Length: 30 months

Class Capacity: 30 students

Tuition: $85,200

CASPA Participant: Yes

Supplemental Application: No

Yellow Ribbon: No

Admissions: Rolling

Application Deadline: March 1

PREREQUISITE COURSEWORK

Human Anatomy and Physiology I and II with lab (8 credits), Microbiology with lab (4 credits), General Chemistry I and II with lab (8 credits), Organic Chemistry with lab (4 credits), Statistics (3 credits). At most two prerequisites may be in progress at the time of application and all should be completed within the last 10 years. Prerequisites must be completed with a grade "C" or better. AP credits are not accepted.

GPA Requirement: Overall GPA 3.0; BCP GPA 3.0

Healthcare Experience: 1,000 hours (recommended)

PA Shadowing: Preferred, not required

Required Standardized Testing: GRE (minimum verbal 146, quantitative 141, and analytical 2.5)

Letters of Recommendation: Three required; one should be from a clinician with personal knowledge of the applicant's character and work habits

Seat Deposit: None

MISSISSIPPI COLLEGE

MISSION:

The primary mission of the Mississippi College's Department of Physician Assistant Studies is to help students acquire core competencies, as well as specialized knowledge and skills necessary to perform effectively as physician assistants and to prepare them to provide primary health care services in medically underserved areas of Mississippi and surrounding states. Secondary missions are to prepare graduates for roles in surgery and as hospitalists.

CLASS OF 2020

Male:	37%
Female:	63%
Minority:	13%
Overall GPA:	3.54
Science GPA:	3.44
Average Age:	26.1

PANCE SCORES

5-year First Time Pass: 96%

Most Recent First Time Pass: 93%

CURRICULUM STRUCTURE

Didactic: 16 months

Clinical: 14 months

Rotations: 7 mandatory, 1 elective (each 6 weeks), 1 advanced clerkship (12 weeks)

UNIQUE PROGRAM FEATURES

Advanced Clerkship: This 12-week rotation allows students to choose one of three areas of concentration for their final semester of training (primary care, critical care, or surgery) and to spend the entire semester at one training site.

Admissions Preference: The program gives preference to Mississippi residents. 50% of the class at a minimum is reserved for Mississippi residents.

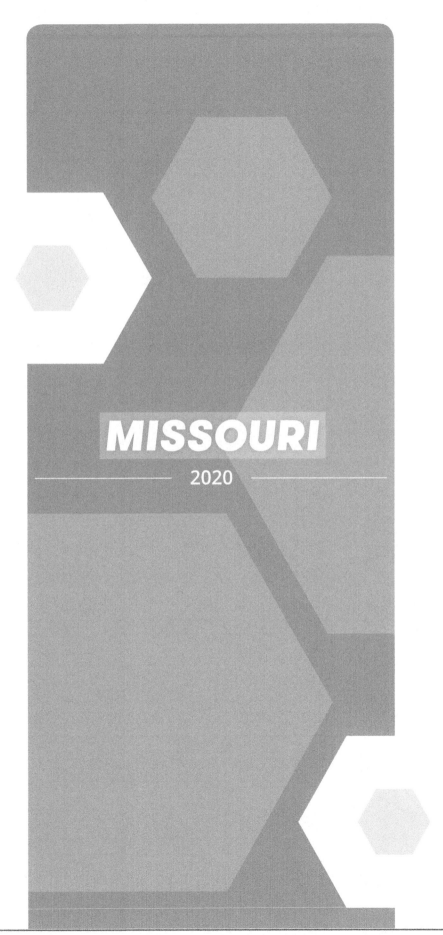

MISSOURI
2020

Missouri State University

901 S. National Avenue
OCHS 200
Springfield, MO 65897
Phone: 417-836-6151
Email:
PhysicianAsstStudies@missouristate.edu

PROGRAM HIGHLIGHTS

Accreditation: Continuing

Degree Offered: Master (MSPAS)

Start Date: January annually

Program Length: 24 months

Class Capacity: 30 students

Tuition: $44,751 (in-state, including fees);
$70,242 (out-of-state, including fees)

CASPA Participant: Yes

Supplemental Application: Yes ($35 fee)

Yellow Ribbon: No

Admissions: Non-rolling

Application Deadline: July 15

PREREQUISITE COURSEWORK

Anatomy and Physiology with lab (8 credits),
Microbiology (3 credits), Genetics (3 credits),
General Chemistry with lab (8 credits), Organic
Chemistry or Biochemistry (4 credits), Statistics
(3 credits), General or Introductory Psychology
(3 credits), additional Social Science (3 credits).
It is preferred that applicants complete courses
within the last 5 years. Prerequisites must
be completed with a grade "C" or better. AP
credits are not accepted. Recommended
courses: Cell Biology/Physiology, Embryology,
Endocrinology, Histology, Virology, Immunology,
Molecular Biology, Neurobiology, Bacteriology,
Pathophysiology, Epidemiology, Developmental
Psychology, Abnormal Psychology, Sociology,
Health Care Ethics, Death and Dying, Medical
Terminology.

GPA Requirement: Overall GPA 3.0; Last 60
Credit GPA 3.0; Prerequisite GPA 3.0

Healthcare Experience: 500 hours

PA Shadowing: 24 hours (recommended)

Required Standardized Testing: GRE or MCAT

Letters of Recommendation: Three required;
from individuals who can attest to your
potential as a physician assistant

Seat Deposit: $500

MISSOURI STATE UNIVERSITY

MISSION:

The Missouri State University Physician Assistant Program
seeks to prepare highly competent physician assistant
graduates to practice primary care medicine in the context
of team delivered care in a rapidly evolving health care
arena. Using the resources of the College of Health and
Human Services and affiliated clinical sites, the Program
seeks to provide a comprehensive didactic and clinical
educational experience for its students that incorporates
the principles of scientific inquiry, self-directed study,
critical analysis and problem-solving, all within the context
of holistic care.

CLASS OF 2020

Overall GPA: 3.70

Science GPA: 3.70

Last 60 Hour GPA: 3.80

GRE Total: 306

Average Healthcare
Experience: >5,000
hours

PANCE SCORES

5-year First Time Pass:
96%

Most Recent First Time
Pass: 97%

CURRICULUM STRUCTURE

Didactic: 12 months

Clinical: 12 months

Rotations: 7 mandatory,
1 elective (each
6 weeks)

Research Project:
Required for graduation

UNIQUE PROGRAM FEATURES

Underserved Populations:
All students are required to
do at least one underserved
or rural population rotation.

Admissions Preference:
The program has a
preference for Missouri
residents and those with
significant national, regional
or local public service
activities, with leadership
experience, who possess a
strong motivation to practice
in rural/underserved areas
after graduation, and who
possess characteristics
likely to fulfill the program's
mission and vision.

Facilities: The O'Reilly
Clinical Health Science
Center was completed in
2015 and houses the PA
program. It includes a large
classroom, laboratory for
clinical skills training, state-
of-the-art clinical simulation
facility, and dedicated
graduate student study
areas.

PROGRAM HIGHLIGHTS

Accreditation: Continuing

Degree Offered: Master (MMS)

Start Date: August annually

Program Length: 27 months

Class Capacity: 46 students

Tuition: $88,370

CASPA Participant: Yes

Supplemental Application: Yes ($45 fee)

Yellow Ribbon: Yes

Admissions: Rolling

Application Deadline: November 1

PREREQUISITE COURSEWORK

Medical Terminology (1-3 credits), Statistics (3 credits), Chemistry I and II (8 credits), Organic Chemistry I and II (6-8 credits), Microbiology (3-4 credits), Vertebrate or Human Anatomy (3-4 credits), Vertebrate or Human Physiology (3-4 credits), Genetics (3-4 credits). Prerequisites must be completed by the May prior to matriculation and within 7 years of application. Prerequisites must be completed with a grade of "C" or better.

GPA Requirement: Overall GPA 3.0; Science GPA 3.0

Healthcare Experience: 500 hours

PA Shadowing: Preferred, not required

Required Standardized Testing: None

Letters of Recommendation: Three required; should be from people who know the applicant well, either professionally or academically, such as a job supervisor, professor or academic adviser

Seat Deposit: $1,000

SAINT LOUIS UNIVERSITY

MISSION:

The primary mission of the Saint Louis University Physician Assistant Program is to educate men and women to become competent, compassionate physician assistants dedicated to excellence in healthcare and the service of humanity.

NO CLASS STATISTICS REPORTED

PANCE SCORES

5-year First Time Pass: 98%

Most Recent First Time Pass: 94%

CURRICULUM STRUCTURE

Didactic: 15 months

Clinical: 12 months

Rotations: 8 mandatory, 1 elective (each 4-6 weeks)

Research Project: Required for graduation

UNIQUE PROGRAM FEATURES

Student Clinic: All students are required to complete community service and can volunteer in the student-operated free health clinic, which includes days for adults, pediatrics, women, cardiology, diabetes, asthma, allergy, and homeless patients.

Facilities: The educational facilities available to PA students provide an exceptional learning environment and include a medical library, classrooms, a computer laboratory, a lecture hall, a 300-seat auditorium and a simulated medical office with eight exam rooms.

Stephens College

1200 East Broadway
Columbia, MO 65215
Phone: 572-876-2310
Email: ejohnson@stephens.edu

PROGRAM HIGHLIGHTS

Accreditation: Provisional

Degree Offered: Master (MPAS)

Start Date: August annually

Program Length: 27 months

Class Capacity: 30 students

Tuition: $87,200

CASPA Participant: Yes

Supplemental Application: No (but supplemental $50 fee)

Yellow Ribbon: No

Admissions: Rolling

Application Deadline: November 1

PREREQUISITE COURSEWORK

Medical Terminology (1 credit), Psychology (3 credits), Statistics (3 credits), Chemistry I and II (6 credits), Organic Chemistry or Biochemistry (3 credits), Microbiology (3 credits), Human Anatomy (3 credits), Human Physiology (3 credits), Genetics (3 credits), Cell/Molecular Biology (3 credits). At most 3 prerequisites may be pending as of December 31st of the year prior to matriculation. Anatomy and Physiology must be completed within the last 7 years. Prerequisites must be completed with a grade "C" or better. Recommended Courses: Immunology, Molecular Biology, Biochemistry, Pharmacology, Embryology, Endocrinology, Gerontology, Virology, Pathophysiology, Molecular Pathology, Evolution, Histology, Medical Ethics, Nutrition, Epidemiology.

GPA Requirement: Overall GPA 2.75; Science GPA 3.0; Last 60 Hour GPA 3.0; Prerequisite GPA 3.0

Healthcare Experience: 500 hours

PA Shadowing: 16 hours (8 must be PA shadowing, the other 8 can be with a PA, MD or DO)

Required Standardized Testing: GRE

Letters of Recommendation: Three required; no one specific

Seat Deposit: $750

STEPHENS COLLEGE

MISSION:

The mission of the Stephens College Physician Assistant Program is to educate and prepare clinically astute, compassionate, and patient-centered physician assistants who will become leaders in their profession, while remaining dedicated to meeting the needs of the medically underserved. Graduates will be ethical professionals, committed members of the healthcare team, practitioners of evidence-based medicine, and providers of quality healthcare for those they serve.

CLASS OF 2020

Male: 26%

Female: 74%

Overall GPA: 3.53

Science GPA: 3.48

Last 60 Credit GPA: 3.70

Average Healthcare Experience: 5,144 hours

PANCE SCORES

5-year First Time Pass: 100% (based on one year of data)

Most Recent First Time Pass: 100%

CURRICULUM STRUCTURE

Didactic: 13 months

Clinical: 14 months

Rotations: 7 mandatory, 1 elective, 1 leadership rotation (each 4-6 weeks)

Capstone Project: Required for graduation

UNIQUE PROGRAM FEATURES

PA Leadership Rotation: All students complete a four-week rotation during clinical year where they learn about leadership in the PA profession.

Facilities: The Center for Health Science features a state-of-the-art facility featuring an anatomy lab, high-tech classrooms, student study and gathering spaces, and a suite of faculty offices.

PROGRAM HIGHLIGHTS

Accreditation: Continuing

Degree Offered: Master (MMS)

Start Date: January annually

Program Length: 29 months

Class Capacity: 20 students

Tuition: $74,145 (in-state); $88,094 (out-of-state)

CASPA Participant: Yes

Supplemental Application: Yes ($50 fee)

Yellow Ribbon: Yes

Admissions: Non-rolling

Application Deadline: August 1

PREREQUISITE COURSEWORK

Biology with lab (1 semester), Anatomy with lab (1 semester), Physiology with lab (1 semester), Microbiology with lab (1 semester), General Chemistry I and II with lab (2 semesters), Organic Chemistry with lab (1 semester), Biochemistry (1 semester), Statistics (1 semester), Medical Terminology (1 course). Two prerequisites may be planned or in progress at the time of application and it is preferred that all be completed within 7 years of the application deadline. Prerequisites must be completed with a grade "C" or better. AP credits are accepted for Biology, General Chemistry and Statistics requirements.

GPA Requirement: Overall GPA 3.0; Prerequisite GPA 3.0

Healthcare Experience: Preferred, not required

PA Shadowing: 8 hours

Required Standardized Testing: GRE or MCAT

Letters of Recommendation: Three required; no one specific

Seat Deposit: $400

UNIVERSITY OF MISSOURI - KANSAS CITY

MISSION:

To educate competent, compassionate, and culturally-aware Physician Assistants who are prepared to meet the healthcare needs of our community. Graduates will advance the Physician Assistant profession through clinical excellence, service, and dedication to professional stewardship.

CLASS OF 2016-2021

Male: 31%

Female: 69%

Minority: 12%

Overall GPA: 3.66

Prerequisite GPA: 3.63

GRE Total: 308

Average Shadowing Experience: 38 hours

PANCE SCORES

5-year First Time Pass: 100% (based on four years of data)

Most Recent First Time Pass: 100%

CURRICULUM STRUCTURE

Didactic: 17 months

Clinical: 12 months

Rotations: 10 mandatory, 2 elective (each 4 weeks)

Capstone Project: Required for graduation

UNIQUE PROGRAM FEATURES

Admissions Preference: Missouri residents are preferred in the admissions process with the goal of 80% of each class being from Missouri.

Early Clinical Exposure: Students begin a weekly clinical experience in the first semester of the program under the supervision of a preceptor where they develop interviewing, physical exam and written/oral presentation skills.

Free Clinic: PA students complete experiences at Sojourner Clinic, a student run free clinic providing outpatient care to the homeless and underprivileged population.

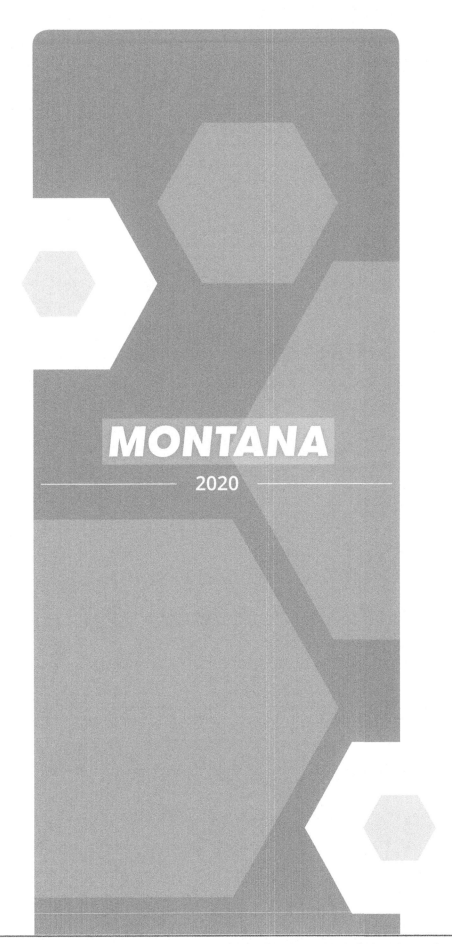

MONTANA
2020

Rocky Mountain College

1511 Poly Drive
Billings, MT 59101
Phone: 406-657-1190
Email: sharon.klem@rocky.edu

PROGRAM HIGHLIGHTS

Accreditation: Continuing
Degree Offered: Master (MPAS)
Start Date: July annually
Program Length: 26 months
Class Capacity: 36 students
Tuition: $103,457 (including fees)

CASPA Participant: Yes
Supplemental Application: No (but $45 fee)
Yellow Ribbon: No
Admissions: Rolling
Application Deadline: October 1

PREREQUISITE COURSEWORK

Human Anatomy and Physiology with lab (8 credits), Microbiology with lab (3 credits), Genetics (3 credits), Medical Terminology (1-2 credits), Mathematics (3 credits), Statistics (3 credits), Psychology (3 credits), Social Science (3 credits), English Composition (3 credits), Organic Chemistry (2 courses) or Biochemistry (1 course) and Organic Chemistry (1 course). Prerequisites must be completed with a grade "C" or better. AP credits are not accepted. Recommended courses: Developmental or Abnormal Psychology, Physics.

GPA Requirement: Overall GPA 3.0; Science GPA 3.0

Healthcare Experience: 1,500 hours

PA Shadowing: 40 hours (recommended)

Required Standardized Testing: GRE (minimum score 291)

Letters of Recommendation: Three required; one must be from a healthcare provider (preferably a PA)

Seat Deposit: $1,000

ROCKY MOUNTAIN COLLEGE

MISSION:

The mission of the Rocky Mountain College Master of Physician Assistant Studies Program (MPAS) is to educate primary care providers who embody a combination of academic talents of evidence-based medicine, clinical skills, and professionalism while providing compassionate health care services, particularly to those in rural and underserved areas of this region. Our graduates distinguish themselves through an emphasis on patient safety and quality improvement.

NO CLASS STATISTICS REPORTED

PANCE SCORES

5-year First Time Pass: 98%

Most Recent First Time Pass: 94%

CURRICULUM STRUCTURE

Didactic: 14 months

Clinical: 12 months

Rotations: 7 mandatory, 1 elective (each 6 weeks)

Capstone Project: Required for graduation

UNIQUE PROGRAM FEATURES

Admissions Preference: Applicants from Montana, Wyoming, Colorado, North Dakota, South Dakota, Utah or Idaho are given preference points in the admissions process, as are those who graduated high school in a rural area.

Rotations: One rotation must be performed in a rural area.

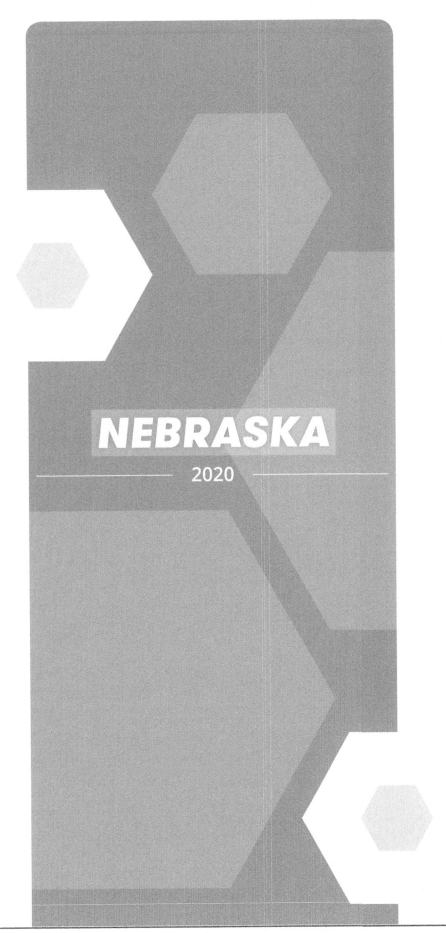

NEBRASKA

2020

College of Saint Mary

7000 Mercy Road
Omaha, NE 68106
Phone: 402-399-2477
Email: PA@csm.edu

PROGRAM HIGHLIGHTS

Accreditation: Probation

Degree Offered: Master (MSPAS)

Start Date: August annually

Program Length: 24 months

Class Capacity: 40 students

Tuition: $81,000

CASPA Participant: Yes

Supplemental Application: No

Yellow Ribbon: No

Admissions: Non-rolling

Application Deadline: October 1

PREREQUISITE COURSEWORK

Human Anatomy and Physiology with lab (8 credits), Microbiology with lab, Upper Level Biology Course with lab, General Chemistry I and II with lab (8 credits), Organic Chemistry I with lab (4 credits), Biochemistry with lab, Abnormal Psychology, Developmental/Lifespan Development Psychology, Statistics, Medical Terminology. Prerequisites must be completed within 7 years of matriculation into the program and with a grade "C" or better.

GPA Requirement: Overall GPA 3.0; Prerequisite GPA 3.0

Healthcare Experience: 300 hours

PA Shadowing: Not required

Required Standardized Testing: GRE (25th percentile or above in each section), CASPer

Letters of Recommendation: Three required; one academic and one employer/supervisor

Seat Deposit: $150

COLLEGE OF SAINT MARY

MISSION:

The mission of the College of Saint Mary Physician Assistant Program is to establish an educational environment fostering academic excellence and leadership, which prepares students to become competent Physician Assistants who possess the knowledge, compassion and clinical skills necessary to provide high quality medical care to all patient populations, including those that are underserved.

NO CLASS STATISTICS REPORTED

PANCE SCORES

5-year First Time Pass: 92% (based on two years of data)

Most Recent First Time Pass: 88%

CURRICULUM STRUCTURE

Didactic: 12 months

Clinical: 12 months

Rotations: 8 mandatory, 3 elective (each 4 weeks)

Research Project: Required for graduation

UNIQUE PROGRAM FEATURES

Admissions Preference: This program has a pre-PA pipeline for undergraduate students (5 year track) and there are typically around 10 spots open for graduate students to enter into the program through traditional admissions. CSM alumni, previous Master's degree, first generation and fluency in a second language will receive special consideration on the application evaluation.

Rotations: All students will complete a rotation in a rural or underserved setting.

Creighton University

2500 California Plaza
Hixson Lied Science Building,
Suite 202
Omaha, NE 68178
Phone: 402-280-4531
Email: pa.admissions@creighton.edu

PROGRAM HIGHLIGHTS

Accreditation: Provisional

Degree Offered: Master (MPAS)

Start Date: August annually

Program Length: 28 months

Class Capacity: 28 students

Tuition: $83,155

CASPA Participant: Yes

Supplemental Application: Yes ($50 fee)

Yellow Ribbon: No

Admissions: Rolling

Application Deadline: September 1

PREREQUISITE COURSEWORK

Human Anatomy with lab (4 credits), Physiology
with lab (4 credits), Microbiology with lab (4
credits), Organic Chemistry with lab (4 credits),
Biochemistry (3 credits), Abnormal Psychology
(3 credits), Statistics (3 credits), Medical
Terminology (1 credit). Prerequisites must
be completed with a grade "C" or better. No
more than 16 semester hours of prerequisite
coursework may be outstanding at the time
of application submission. AP credits are not
accepted. Recommended courses: Immunology,
Genetics.

GPA Requirement: Overall GPA 3.0

Healthcare Experience: 250 hours

PA Shadowing: Preferred, not required

Required Standardized Testing: GRE (25th
percentile or above in each section)

Letters of Recommendation: Three required; no
one specific

Seat Deposit: $500

CREIGHTON UNIVERSITY

MISSION:

The Creighton University physician assistant
program mission is to foster a tradition of excellence
by transforming learners into compassionate
physician assistants who are dedicated to exemplary
patient care. Rooted in our Ignatian heritage, we
empower students to realize their full potential
through a commitment to professional growth and
service to humanity.

CLASS OF 2021

Overall GPA: 3.70

Science GPA: 3.65

Faculty to Student Ratio: 1:6

PANCE SCORES

5-year First Time Pass: N/A

Most Recent First Time Pass: N/A (have not
graduated a class yet)

CURRICULUM STRUCTURE

Didactic: 12 months

Clinical: 16 months

Rotations: 8 mandatory, 1 selective, 3 electives (each
4-8 weeks)

UNIQUE PROGRAM FEATURES

Rotations: All students complete a selective
rotation in a medically underserved area.

Union College

3800 South 48th Street
Lincoln, NE 68506
Phone: 402-486-2527
Email: paprog@ucollege.edu

PROGRAM HIGHLIGHTS

Accreditation: Continuing

Degree Offered: Master (MPAS)

Start Date: August annually

Program Length: 33 months

Class Capacity: 30 students

Tuition: $101,040

CASPA Participant: Yes

Supplemental Application: No

Yellow Ribbon: No

Admissions: Non-rolling

Application Deadline: October 1

PREREQUISITE COURSEWORK

General Biology I and II with lab (8 credits), Microbiology with lab (4 credits), Human Anatomy with lab (4 credits), Human Physiology with lab (4 credits), General Chemistry I and II with labs (4-8 credits), Organic Chemistry I and II with labs (4-8 credits), Biochemistry (3-4 credits), Medical Terminology (1 credit), Elementary Statistics and Probability (3 credits), Developmental/ Lifespan Psychology (3 credits). Biochemistry, Anatomy and Physiology must be completed within the last 7 years. Prerequisites must be completed with a grade "C" or better.

GPA Requirement: Overall GPA 3.0; Science GPA 3.0

Healthcare Experience: 480 hours (at least 240 completed at the time of application)

PA Shadowing: Required (no specific number of hours)

Required Standardized Testing: None

Letters of Recommendation: Three required; one should be from an employer/healthcare supervisor, one from a professor, and one from someone who knows your character (i.e., clergyman)

Seat Deposit: $650

UNION COLLEGE

MISSION:

To equip PA students, through rigorous training and caring mentorship in a quality program within a Christian atmosphere, to work in a team environment, demonstrate academic excellence, practice clinical acumen, show a high degree of professionalism, and exhibit servanthood.

CLASS OF 2021

Male: 29%

Female: 71%

Overall GPA: 3.53

Science GPA: 3.42

PANCE SCORES

5-year First Time Pass: 96%

Most Recent First Time Pass: 89%

CURRICULUM STRUCTURE

Didactic: 21 months

Clinical: 12 months

Rotations: 10 mandatory, 1 elective (each 4 weeks)

Capstone Project: Required for graduation

UNIQUE PROGRAM FEATURES

Christian Influence: This school has a Seventh-day Adventist heritage and students must adhere to a lifestyle agreement dedicated to the high ethical and moral values of Christian living as a condition for acceptance at the program.

Early Clinical Exposure: Students begin helping patients early in the curriculum through volunteering at foot clinics, community kitchens, and other outreach programs.

University of Nebraska

984300 Nebraska Medical Center
Omaha, NE 68198
Phone: 402-559-6673
Email: jodie.babcock@unmc.edu

PROGRAM HIGHLIGHTS

Accreditation: Continuing

Degree Offered: Master (MPAS)

Start Date: August annually

Program Length: 28 months

Class Capacity: 66 students

Tuition: $48,040 (in-state); $124,865 (out-of-state)

CASPA Participant: Yes

Supplemental Application: Yes ($60 fee)

Yellow Ribbon: No

Admissions: Non-rolling

Application Deadline: September 1

PREREQUISITE COURSEWORK

General Biology with lab, Human Anatomy with lab, Human Physiology with lab, Microbiology with lab, General or Inorganic Chemistry I and II with lab, Organic Chemistry with lab, Biochemistry, General Psychology, Abnormal Psychology, Life Span/Developmental Psychology, Statistics, Medical Terminology, English Composition, Writing Intensive course. Courses may be in progress at the time of application. Prerequisites must be completed with a grade "C" or better. AP credits are not accepted. Recommended courses: Immunology, Genetics, Algebra.

GPA Requirement: Overall GPA 3.0

Healthcare Experience: Preferred, not required

PA Shadowing: Preferred, not required

Required Standardized Testing: None

Letters of Recommendation: Three required; at least one academic letter and one from a health professional

Seat Deposit: $500

UNIVERSITY OF NEBRASKA

MISSION:

The mission of the Physician Assistant Program at the University of Nebraska Medical Center is to be innovative leaders in physician assistant education, developing diverse clinicians who practice evidence-based medicine and provide exceptional, team-based care to all individuals and communities.

CLASS OF 2021

Male: 20%

Female: 80%

Overall GPA: 3.75

Science GPA: 3.65

Average Age: 24

PANCE SCORES

5-year First Time Pass: 100%

Most Recent First Time Pass: 100%

CURRICULUM STRUCTURE

Didactic: 13 months

Clinical: 15 months

Rotations: 9 mandatory, 6 elective (each 4 weeks)

UNIQUE PROGRAM FEATURES

Two Campuses: This program operates with 66 students total split between the University of Nebraska Medical Center at Omaha and University of Nebraska Kearney Campuses.

Admissions Preference: The admissions committee gives preference to applicants with an overall and science GPA of 3.20 or greater, GRE scores at 50th percentile or greater, those with strong motivation to practice in medically underserved area, prior work or volunteer direct patient care experience and shadowing, significant extracurricular, professional, or service organization activity, and Nebraska or contiguous state residents.

Dual Degree: A dual PA/MPH program is offered with a specialization in Community-Oriented Primary Care within the Department of Health Promotion, and it takes just over three years to complete.

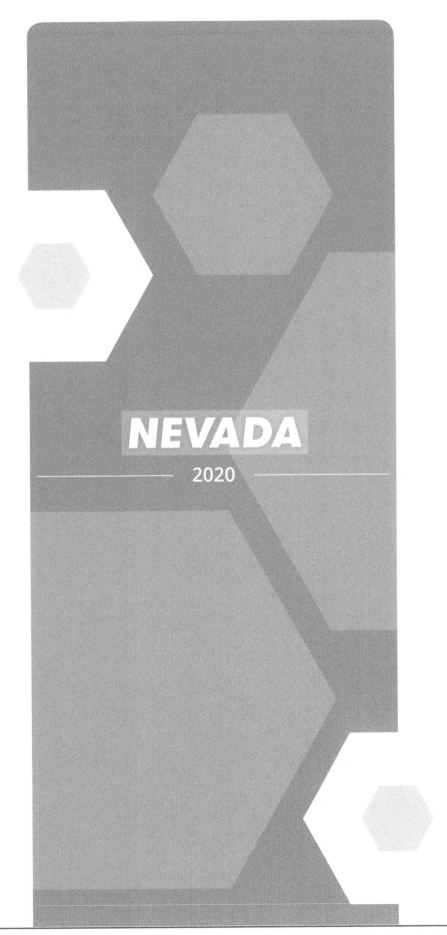

NEVADA

2020

Touro University

874 American Pacific Drive
Henderson, NV 89014
Phone: 702-777-1750
Email: admissions@tun.touro.edu

PROGRAM HIGHLIGHTS

Accreditation: Continuing

Degree Offered: Master (MPAS)

Start Date: July annually

Program Length: 28 months

Class Capacity: 70 students

Tuition: $98,700

CASPA Participant: Yes

Supplemental Application: Yes ($75 fee)

Yellow Ribbon: Yes

Admissions: Rolling

Application Deadline: September 1

PREREQUISITE COURSEWORK

Human Anatomy and Physiology (8 credits), Organic Chemistry (4 credits), Biochemistry (3 credits), Microbiology (3 credits). At most two prerequisites may be in progress at the time of application and all must be completed within the last 7 years except Organic Chemistry. Prerequisites must be completed with a grade "C" or better. Recommended courses: General Psychology, Statistics.

GPA Requirement: Overall GPA 3.0; Science GPA 3.0

Healthcare Experience: 500 hours

PA Shadowing: Not required

Required Standardized Testing: GRE

Letters of Recommendation: Two required; one must be from a PA, NP or physician

Seat Deposit: $1,000

TOURO UNIVERSITY - NEVADA

MISSION:

The Master of Physician Assistant Studies Program is committed to the education of highly qualified compassionate Physician Assistants who are part of the health care team and are responsive to the developing health needs of their communities as culturally competent clinicians, educators, facilitators, and leaders.

CLASS OF 2020

Science GPA: 3.35

Average Age: 27

Healthcare Experience: 3,357 hours

PANCE SCORES

5-year First Time Pass: 93%

Most Recent First Time Pass: 95%

CURRICULUM STRUCTURE

Didactic: 16 months

Clinical: 12 months

Rotations: 10 mandatory, 2 elective (each 4 weeks)

UNIQUE PROGRAM FEATURES

Interprofessional Education: As the program is offered on campus with osteopathy, physical therapy, and nursing students, PA program students learn to work with all health care team members and also complete a service-learning course that prepares graduates to be culturally sensitive and advocates for the community.

University of Nevada Reno

18600 Wedge Parkway
Nell J. Redfield Bldg. A, Ste. 104
Reno, NV 89511
Phone: 775-784-4843
Email: paprogram@med.unr.edu

PROGRAM HIGHLIGHTS

Accreditation: Provisional

Degree Offered: Master (MPAS)

Start Date: July annually

Program Length: 25 months

Class Capacity: 24 students

Tuition: $87,698 (including fees)

CASPA Participant: Yes

Supplemental Application: No

Yellow Ribbon: No

Admissions: Rolling

Application Deadline: September 1

PREREQUISITE COURSEWORK

Human Anatomy and Physiology I and II (6 credits), Biology (3 credits), Chemistry (3 credits), Statistics (3 credits). Prerequisites must be complete with a grade of "B-" or better. It is strongly recommended that prerequisites be completed within the last 7 years. AP credits are not accepted. Recommended courses: Microbiology, Biochemistry, Genetics, Immunology, Medical Terminology, Spanish, Abnormal Psychology, Public Health.

GPA Requirement: Overall GPA 2.75

Healthcare Experience: 2,000 hours

PA Shadowing: Preferred, not required

Required Standardized Testing: None

Letters of Recommendation: Three required; recommended that at least one be from a PA with whom you have worked with or shadowed

Seat Deposit: $1,000

UNIVERSITY OF NEVADA RENO

MISSION:

The mission of the University of Nevada, Reno School of Medicine Physician Assistant (PA) Studies Program is to train flexible and committed primary care clinicians dedicated to strengthening health care in their communities.

CLASS OF 2021

Male: 25%

Female: 75%

Minority: 25%

Overall GPA: 3.56

Science GPA: 3.51

Healthcare Experience: 7,712 hours

Average Age: 28

PANCE SCORES

5-year First Time Pass: N/A

Most Recent First Time Pass: N/A (have not graduated a class yet)

CURRICULUM STRUCTURE

Didactic: 13 months

Clinical: 12 months

Rotations: 8 mandatory, 2 selective, 2 elective (each 4 weeks)

Capstone Project: Required for graduation

UNIQUE PROGRAM FEATURES

Admissions Preference: Preference is given to Nevada residents, Veterans, and rural residents.

Rotations: All students complete a rotation working with medically underserved populations.

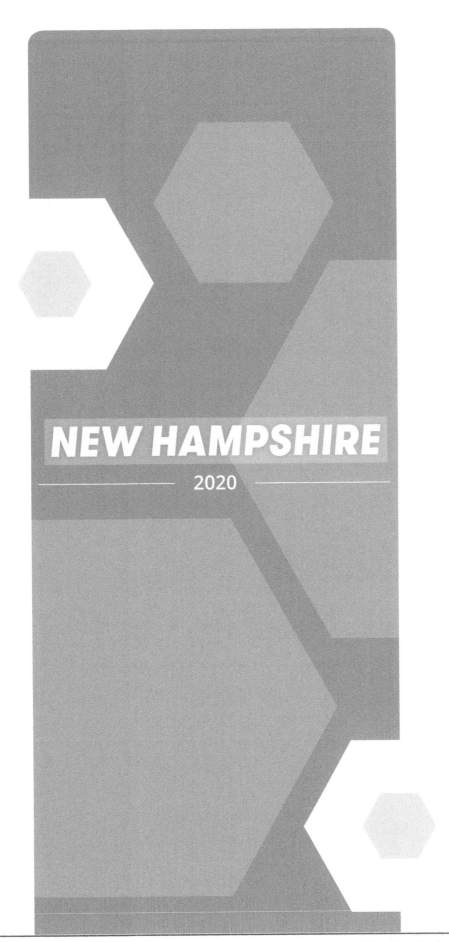

NEW HAMPSHIRE

2020

Franklin Pierce University

24 Airport Road, Suite 20
West Lebanon, NH 03784
Phone: 603-298-6617
Email:
paprogram@franklinpierce.edu

PROGRAM HIGHLIGHTS

Accreditation: Continuing

Degree Offered: Master (MPAS)

Start Date: November annually

Program Length: 27 months

Class Capacity: 24 students

Tuition: $101,975

CASPA Participant: Yes

Supplemental Application: Yes (no fee)

Yellow Ribbon: No

Admissions: Rolling

Application Deadline: November 1

PREREQUISITE COURSEWORK

Anatomy and Physiology I and II with lab (8 credits), Chemistry I and II with lab (8 credits), Biology with lab (4 credits), Microbiology with lab (4 credits), Statistics (3 credits), Psychology (3 credits). Prerequisites must be completed with a grade "C" or better. At most two prerequisites may be outstanding at the time of application, but they must be completed with a grade "B" or better before matriculation. AP credits are not accepted. Recommended courses: Genetics, Immunology, Organic Chemistry, Biochemistry, Cell Biology, Nutrition, Sociology.

GPA Requirement: Overall GPA 3.0; Science GPA 3.0

Healthcare Experience: Preferred, not required

PA Shadowing: 20 hours

Required Standardized Testing: None

Letters of Recommendation: Three required; no one specific

Seat Deposit: $500

FRANKLIN PIERCE UNIVERSITY

MISSION:

The mission of the Franklin Pierce University Physician Assistant Program is to graduate competent and compassionate physician assistants who possess the requisite knowledge, skills, and attitudes to provide high quality, patient-centered primary care.

NO CLASS STATISTICS REPORTED

PANCE SCORES

5-year First Time Pass: 94%

Most Recent First Time Pass: 100%

CURRICULUM STRUCTURE

Didactic: 14 months

Clinical: 13 months

Rotations: 8 mandatory (each 6 weeks), 1 elective (4 weeks)

Case Presentation and Community Service Project: Required for graduation

UNIQUE PROGRAM FEATURES

Student Demographics: The program strives to accept at least 40-50% of NH/VT residents for each class.

Rural Focus: 69% of graduates report working in rural and underserved areas after graduation.

MCPHS University

1260 Elm Street
Manchester, NH 03101
Phone: 888-441-0931
Email:
admissions.manchester@mcphs.edu

PROGRAM HIGHLIGHTS

Accreditation: Continuing

Degree Offered: Master (MPAS)

Start Date: January annually

Program Length: 24 months

Class Capacity: 55 students

Tuition: $99,000

CASPA Participant: Yes

Supplemental Application: No

Yellow Ribbon: Yes

Admissions: Rolling

Application Deadline: March 1

PREREQUISITE COURSEWORK

Human Anatomy and Physiology I and II with lab (8 credits), Microbiology with lab (4 credits), General Chemistry I with lab (4 credits), Organic Chemistry I with lab (4 credits), Biochemistry (3 credits), Psychology (3 credits), Statistics (3 credits). Math and science courses must be completed no more than 10 years prior to the anticipated date of matriculation. Prerequisites must be completed with a grade "C" or better.

GPA Requirement: Overall GPA 3.0; Science GPA 3.2 (recommended)

Healthcare Experience: Preferred, not required (250-500 hours)

PA Shadowing: Preferred, not required

Required Standardized Testing: None

Letters of Recommendation: Two required; no one specific

Seat Deposit: $500

MCPHS UNIVERSITY - MANCHESTER

MISSION:

The program educates and inspires the future generation of Physician Assistants to become compassionate clinicians who demonstrate professionalism; practice collaborative, evidence-based medicine and advocate for patients and their communities.

NO CLASS STATISTICS REPORTED

PANCE SCORES

5-year First Time Pass: 93%

Most Recent First Time Pass: 88%

CURRICULUM STRUCTURE

Didactic: 12 months

Clinical: 12 months

Rotations: 8 mandatory, 1 elective (each 5 weeks)

Capstone Project: Required for graduation

UNIQUE PROGRAM FEATURES

Two Campuses: Lectures are provided on both Worcester and Manchester, NH campuses through state-of-the-art simultaneous video distance education to the students in each cohort split between the two campuses.

International Rotations: Several international rotations are available to students in Belize and Bolivia.

Articulation Agreements: The program has articulation agreements with 11 colleges and universities with respect to the admission of a specified number of students from each of them to the program.

Community Service: Recent events include American Heart Association Fundraiser Event, American Lung Association Fundraiser Event, Habitat for Humanity Fundraiser Event, DEA Prevention Awareness Day, DEA Drug Take Back Day, Dempsey Challenge Cycle Fundraiser Event for Cancer, Canned Food Drive for the homeless, Red Nose Day Fundraiser for Children in Poverty, Health Professions Awareness Event for local Elementary School children

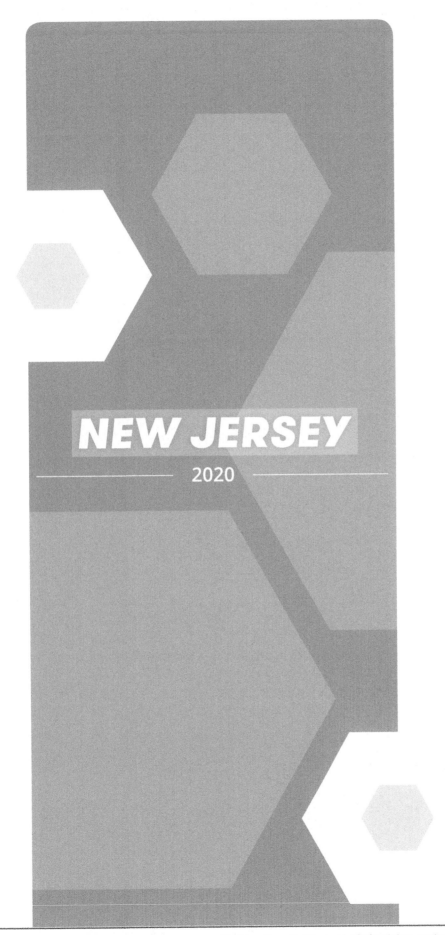

NEW JERSEY

2020

College of Saint Elizabeth

2 Convent Road
Morristown, NJ 07960
Phone: 973-290-4154
Email: kbooth@cse.edu

PROGRAM HIGHLIGHTS

Accreditation: Provisional

Degree Offered: Master (MS)

Start Date: October annually

Program Length: 27 months

Class Capacity: Not reported

Tuition: $104,104

CASPA Participant: Yes

Supplemental Application: Yes ($35 fee)

Yellow Ribbon: No

Admissions: Rolling

Application Deadline: March 1

PREREQUISITE COURSEWORK

English Composition (3 credits), General Psychology (3 credits), Statistics (3 credits), Medical Terminology (1 credit), General Biology with lab (4 credits), Genetics (3 credits), Anatomy and Physiology I and II with lab (8 credits), Microbiology with lab (4 credits), General Chemistry I and II with lab (8 credits), Biochemistry (3 credits). Anatomy, Physiology and Microbiology must be completed within the last 10 years. Two prerequisites may be outstanding at the time of application. Prerequisites must be completed with a grade "B-" or better.

GPA Requirement: Overall GPA 3.0; Prerequisite GPA 3.2

Healthcare Experience: 300 hours

PA Shadowing: 16 hours

Community Service: 50 hours

Required Standardized Testing: None

Letters of Recommendation: Three required; one letter must be from a professor attesting to academic capability and at least one must be from a physician or PA attesting to professional capacity

Seat Deposit: $500

COLLEGE OF SAINT ELIZABETH

MISSION:

The mission of the MS PA Program at the College of Saint Elizabeth is to provide a collaborative, respectful, and spiritually enriched learning environment that educates PAs who are competent and ethical medical providers committed to high-quality patient care as responsible members of the healthcare team. Our graduates will promote the dignity and diversity of all patients, in the spirit of service, social justice, and leadership to the community and the PA profession.

NO CLASS STATISTICS REPORTED

PANCE SCORES

5-year First Time Pass: N/A

Most Recent First Time Pass: N/A (have not graduated a class yet)

CURRICULUM STRUCTURE

Didactic: 15 months

Clinical: 12 months

Rotations: 7 mandatory, 2 elective (each 5 weeks)

Capstone: Required for graduation

UNIQUE PROGRAM FEATURES

Didactic Curriculum: The didactic component includes specific coursework regarding social determinants of health, patient education, patient advocacy, and public health.

Simulation Center: The Simulation Center uses virtual and simulated patients, high, medium, and low fidelity manikins, human subjects, skill trainers, and sophisticated video technology to enhance learning. The facility can mimic medical settings including hospital wards, physician offices, and clinics. All lab facilities are fully equipped to practice clinical skills in real life simulations.

Monmouth University

400 Cedar Avenue
West Long Branch, NJ 07764
Phone: 732-923-4505
Email: paprogram@monmouth.edu

PROGRAM HIGHLIGHTS

Accreditation: Probation

Degree Offered: Master (MS)

Start Date: September annually

Program Length: 36 months (with summers off)

Class Capacity: 30 students

Tuition: $117,135

CASPA Participant: Yes

Supplemental Application: Yes ($50 fee)

Yellow Ribbon: No

Admissions: Rolling

Application Deadline: January 15

PREREQUISITE COURSEWORK

Human Anatomy with lab (4 credits), Human Physiology with lab (4 credits), Chemistry I and II with lab (8 credits), Biology I with lab (4 credits), Microbiology with lab (4 credits), General Psychology (3 credits), Medical Terminology (1-3 credits), Pre-calculus or Calculus or Statistics (3 credits). Prerequisites must be completed with a grade "C" or better and should be completed within the last 10 years. AP credits are accepted.

GPA Requirement: Overall GPA 3.0; Prerequisite GPA 3.0

Healthcare Experience: 200 hours

PA Shadowing: No requirement, but shadowing hours can be counted towards healthcare experience

Required Standardized Testing: GRE

Letters of Recommendation: Three required; no one specific

Seat Deposit: $350

MONMOUTH UNIVERSITY

MISSION:

The mission of the Monmouth University Physician Assistant Program is to educate physician assistants to provide compassionate, patient-centered quality health care in a variety of settings. Program graduates will possess clinical skills to serve a diverse patient population and have the ability to advance the profession through leadership and research.

CLASS OF 2021

Overall GPA: 3.60

Prerequisite GPA: 3.60

PANCE SCORES

5-year First Time Pass: 97% (based on three years of data)

Most Recent First Time Pass: 93%

CURRICULUM STRUCTURE

Didactic: 10.5 months

Clinical: 16 months

Rotations: 10 mandatory, 2 elective (each 4-8 weeks)

UNIQUE PROGRAM FEATURES

Scholarship: Graduate scholarships are offered by the University to students on the basis of their undergraduate GPA. Award values range from $2,400 to $5,100 per semester.

Location: Classes are held at a satellite campus with classrooms and clinical skills laboratories dedicated for PA student use.

Admissions Preference: Preference will be given to students enrolled in Monmouth's biology and health studies programs who meet the admission criteria.

Rutgers University

675 Hoes Lane West
Piscataway, NJ 08854
Phone: 732-235-4445
Email: pa-info@shrp.rutgers.edu

PROGRAM HIGHLIGHTS

Accreditation: Continuing

Degree Offered: Master (MS)

Start Date: August annually

Program Length: 33 months

Class Capacity: 50 students

Tuition: $76,680 (in-state);
$106,380 (out-of-state)

CASPA Participant: Yes

Supplemental Application: Yes ($25 fee)

Yellow Ribbon: No

Admissions: Rolling

Application Deadline: September 1

PREREQUISITE COURSEWORK

General Psychology (3 credits), English Composition (3 credits), Statistics (3 credits), Human Anatomy (3-4 credits), Physiology (3-4 credits), Microbiology (3-4 credits), Biochemistry (3 credits), Upper Level Biology (6-8 credits). Prerequisites must be completed with a grade "C" or better and by the end of the spring semester prior to the program start date. Recommended courses: Genetics, Microbiology, Immunology, Cell Biology, Biochemistry.

GPA Requirement: Overall GPA 3.2; Science GPA 3.2

Healthcare Experience: Required (no specific number of hours)

PA Shadowing: Required (no specific number of hours)

Required Standardized Testing: None

Letters of Recommendation: Three required; no one specific

Seat Deposit: $700

RUTGERS UNIVERSITY

MISSION:

The Rutgers University Physician Assistant Program enhances the delivery of humanistic patient care and advances the PA profession through a dynamic blend of educational programs, research, and service. Carefully crafted curricula and thoughtful mentorship of students develops collaborative, caring, and competent healthcare providers.

CLASS OF 2019

Minority: 38%

Overall GPA: 3.64

Science GPA: 3.61

PANCE SCORES

5-year First Time Pass: 99%

Most Recent First Time Pass: 100%

CURRICULUM STRUCTURE

Didactic: 17 months

Clinical: 16 months

Rotations: 9 mandatory, 2 elective (each 3-8 weeks)

Capstone Project: Required for graduation

UNIQUE PROGRAM FEATURES

Combined Program: Rutgers offers a combined BA/MS track through one of their affiliated universities (see website for qualifying schools).

Dual Degree: Students can earn a dual MS/MPH in four years (including summers).

Part-time Option: Students can complete the program part-time, which adds around an extra year to the curriculum.

Interprofessional Education: Students participate in interprofessional education groups that include many other healthcare professional students including medical students, nursing students and other health profession students.

Admissions Preference: There is special emphasis on the recruitment of: traditionally underrepresented minorities in medicine and health professions, those who speak a foreign language (especially Spanish), individuals who come from economically and/or environmentally disadvantaged backgrounds, and veterans of the US Military.

PROGRAM HIGHLIGHTS

Accreditation: Continuing

Degree Offered: Master (MSPA)

Start Date: August annually

Program Length: 33 months (with summers off)

Class Capacity: 60 students

Tuition: $129,600

CASPA Participant: No

Supplemental Application: Yes ($75 fee)

Yellow Ribbon: No

Admissions: Not reported

Application Deadline: December 15

PREREQUISITE COURSEWORK

General Biology I and II with lab (8 credits), General Chemistry I and II with lab (8 credits), Human Anatomy and Physiology I and II with lab (8 credits), Microbiology with lab (4 credits), Psychology (3 credits), Math (3 credits). Prerequisites must be completed with a grade "C" or better and within the last 10 years. All prerequisites must be completed by June 1st prior to matriculation. AP credits are not accepted.

GPA Requirement: Overall GPA 3.2; Prerequisite GPA 3.2

Healthcare Experience: 250 hours

PA Shadowing: 25 hours (counts towards healthcare experience)

Required Standardized Testing: GRE

Letters of Recommendation: Three required; academic reference, PA, and other healthcare provider preferred

Seat Deposit: $500

SETON HALL UNIVERSITY

MISSION:

The mission of the Physician Assistant Program at Seton Hall University is to prepare primary care PAs who practice in diverse settings. The program provides the foundation for graduates to become critical thinkers who practice evidence-based, patient-centered medicine.

NO CLASS STATISTICS REPORTED

PANCE SCORES

5-year First Time Pass: 99%

Most Recent First Time Pass: 98%

CURRICULUM STRUCTURE

Didactic: 12 months

Clinical: 16 months

Rotations: 8 mandatory, 3 elective (each 4-12 weeks)

Research Project: Required for graduation

UNIQUE PROGRAM FEATURES

Early Clinical Exposures: Interactions with patients begin in the first semester so students can practice their history and physical exam skills and begin to build their clinical acumen.

Teaching Style: A blend of traditional lectures, online coursework and problem-based learning is used throughout the year to ensure that new knowledge can be practically applied.

PROGRAM HIGHLIGHTS

Accreditation: Continuing

Degree Offered: Master (MSPAS)

Start Date: July annually

Program Length: 25 months

Class Capacity: 34 students

Tuition: $92,500

CASPA Participant: Yes

Supplemental Application: No

Yellow Ribbon: No

Admissions: Rolling

Application Deadline: November 1

PREREQUISITE COURSEWORK

Chemistry with lab (8 credits),
Biology with lab (8 credits), Anatomy
and Physiology with lab (8 credits),
Microbiology with lab (4 credits),
College Writing (3 credits), Statistics or
Mathematics (3 credits), Psychology (3
credits), Medical Terminology (1 credit).
Prerequisites must be completed with
a grade "C" or better and within the
last 10 years. AP credits are accepted
if the credit is documented on your
college transcript. Recommended
courses: Abnormal and Developmental
Psychology, Organic Chemistry,
Biochemistry, Genetics.

GPA Requirement: Overall GPA 3.25;
Science GPA 3.25

Healthcare Experience: 200 hours (must
be completed at the time of application)

PA Shadowing: Preferred, not required

Required Standardized Testing: None

Letters of Recommendation: Three
required; Jefferson highly suggests one
academic, one patient care and one
additional academic or patient care

Seat Deposit: $2,000

THOMAS JEFFERSON UNIVERSITY - NEW JERSEY CAMPUS

MISSION:

The mission of the Thomas Jefferson University Physician Assistant Program is to provide students with the foundation of knowledge, technical skills and critical thinking necessary to competently perform the functions of the physician assistant profession in an ethical, empathetic manner working with a licensed practicing physician. A secondary focus is to prepare students to provide comprehensive medical services to diverse under-served patient populations in inner-city and rural locations.

CLASS OF 2018

Overall GPA: 3.55

Science GPA: 3.51

Average Healthcare Experience: 2,400 hours

PANCE SCORES

5-year First Time Pass: 96%

Most Recent First Time Pass: 97%

CURRICULUM STRUCTURE

Didactic: 12 months

Clinical: 13 months

Rotations: 8 mandatory, 1 med/surg selective, 1 elective (each 5 weeks)

UNIQUE PROGRAM FEATURES

Admissions Preference: Graduates from Jefferson and Stockton University are granted preferential admissions.

Two Campuses: Thomas Jefferson now has two campuses for the Physician Assistant Studies program - one at Thomas Jefferson, East Falls, PA and one in Voorhees, NJ. There is also a separate second program offered in Philadelphia.

Pre-PA Track: Available for interested high school seniors. These students will gain a B.S. in Health Sciences and an M.S. in Physician Assistant Studies in 5 years.

Rotations: The program places students in a variety of medically underserved clinical locations in the urban Philadelphia area, as well as sites in New Jersey in Camden, Atlantic County, and Trenton. Additionally, students may have the opportunity to do a rotation in rural Mississippi in a variety of medical specialties. Mission trips are scheduled annually and 5th year students travel to Honduras with members of the faculty.

Facilities: The program has a brand new physical diagnosis/clinical skills lab with medical simulators, a 12 station full-dissection cadaver lab, administrative offices, break out areas and study spaces.

229

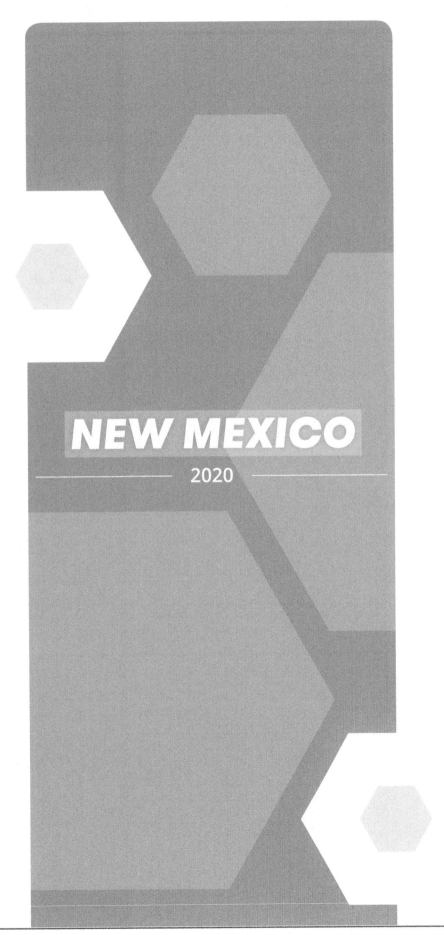

NEW MEXICO

2020

University of New Mexico

2710 Frontier Avenue NE
Albuquerque, NM 87131
Phone: 505-272-9864
Email: PAProgram@salud.unm.edu

PROGRAM HIGHLIGHTS

Accreditation: Continuing

Degree Offered: Master (MSPAS)

Start Date: June annually

Program Length: 27 months

Class Capacity: 17 students

Tuition: $60,702 (in-state); $86,479 (out-of-state)

CASPA Participant: Yes

Supplemental Application: Yes ($64 fee)

Yellow Ribbon: No

Admissions: Non-rolling

Application Deadline: August 1

PREREQUISITE COURSEWORK

General Biology or Molecular Cell Biology with lab (4 credits), General Chemistry I and II with lab (8 credits), Human Anatomy and Physiology I and II with lab (8 credits), Psychology (3 credits), Statistics (3 credits), English (6 credits). Science courses must be completed in the last 10 years. Prerequisites must be completed with a grade "C" or better. One prerequisite may be outstanding at the time of application but it must be completed with a grade "B" or better and by December of the application year. AP credits are accepted for the English requirement only. Recommended courses: Microbiology, Virology, Organic Chemistry, Biochemistry, Genetics, Immunology, Nutrition, Foreign Language.

GPA Requirement: Overall GPA 3.0; Science GPA 3.0

Healthcare Experience: 500 hours

PA Shadowing: Preferred, not required

Required Standardized Testing: GRE

Letters of Recommendation: Three required; one personal reference and two clinical references (preferably an MD/DO or PA/NP) who have known you for six months or longer and can speak to your ability to be a PA; specifically, your clinical abilities, and your problem solving, critical thinking and interpersonal skills

Seat Deposit: $250

UNIVERSITY OF NEW MEXICO

MISSION:

The mission of the University of New Mexico Physician Assistant Program is to educate Physician Assistant students to be competent providers of primary care medicine, with a special focus on the medically underserved and rural populations of New Mexico.

CLASS OF 2021

Male: 35%

Female: 65%

Minority: 30%

Overall GPA: 3.72

Science GPA: 3.77

GRE Verbal: 153

GRE Quantitative: 150

GRE Analytical: 3.9

Average Healthcare Experience: 4,496 hours

Average Age: 28

PANCE SCORES

5-year First Time Pass: 93%

Most Recent First Time Pass: 88%

CURRICULUM STRUCTURE

Didactic: 15 months

Clinical: 12 months

Rotations: 8 mandatory, 1 elective (each 4-6 weeks)

UNIQUE PROGRAM FEATURES

Problem Based Learning: On average six hours per week are devoted to PBL in small groups where students are exposed to pathophysiology, behavioral medicine, and population health.

Admissions Preference: The program prefers applicants who are residents of New Mexico. 88% of students from the class of 2021 are New Mexico residents. Higher consideration is also given to those who have served in the US Military.

Graduate Practice: Approximately 50% of graduates go on to practice primary care in rural and underserved populations within New Mexico.

University of St. Francis

1500 N. Renaissance Blvd NE
Albuquerque, NM 87107
Phone: 505-266-5565
Email: acarter1@stfrancis.edu

PROGRAM HIGHLIGHTS

Accreditation: Continuing
Degree Offered: Master (MSPAS)
Start Date: January annually
Program Length: 27 months
Class Capacity: 40 students
Tuition: $85,500

CASPA Participant: Yes
Supplemental Application: No
Yellow Ribbon: No
Admissions: Rolling
Application Deadline: October 1

PREREQUISITE COURSEWORK

Biology with lab (8 credits), Anatomy and Physiology (8 credits), Chemistry with lab (8 credits), Microbiology, Genetics, Statistics. Prerequisites must be completed within 7 years of admission to the program for applicants with an undergraduate degree and 10 years for applicants with a graduate degree or higher. All should be completed prior to application. AP credits are accepted.

GPA Requirement: Overall GPA 3.0; Science GPA 3.0; Prerequisite GPA 3.0

Healthcare Experience: 500 hours

PA Shadowing: Not required (counts towards healthcare experience)

Required Standardized Testing: GRE (competitive score is 300 total and 4.0 analytical)

Letters of Recommendation: Three required; appropriate references are supervisors, instructors/ professors, academic advisors, or colleagues

Seat Deposit: $650

UNIVERSITY OF ST. FRANCIS

MISSION:

The mission of the USF PA program is to educate highly qualified Physician Assistants preparing them to become competent, compassionate and comprehensive health care providers for practice in primary care fields.

CLASS OF 2020

Overall GPA: 3.57

Science GPA: 3.51

Prerequisite GPA: 3.60

Average Healthcare Experience: 3,400 hours

PANCE SCORES

5-year First Time Pass: 94%

Most Recent First Time Pass: 83%

CURRICULUM STRUCTURE

Didactic: 15 months

Clinical: 12 months

Rotations: 7 mandatory, 1 elective (each 6 weeks)

Research Project: required for graduation

UNIQUE PROGRAM FEATURES

Rural Focus: All students must complete at least two rural rotations during the clinical year.

Community Service: Faculty and students participate in community service together throughout the program. Recent projects have included food banks, 5k runs, a teddy bear drive, nursing home visits, school supply drives, care packages, flu vaccination clinics and providing Christmas presents to underprivileged kids, among others.

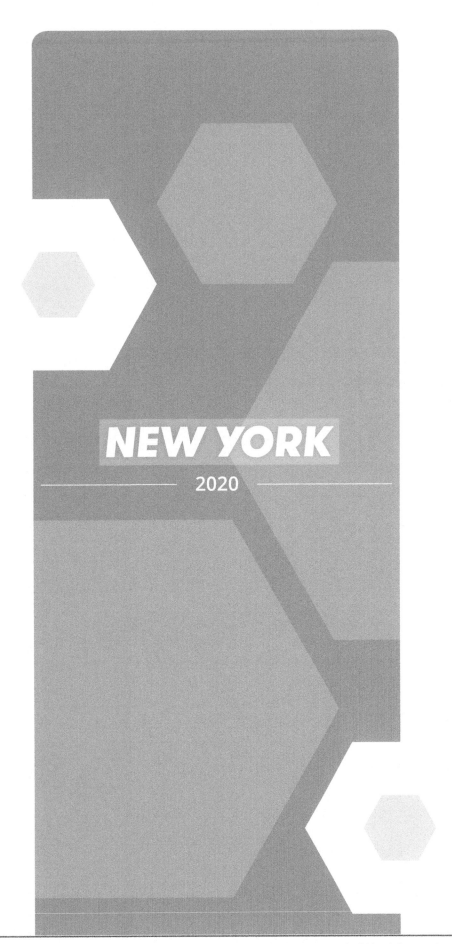

NEW YORK
2020

Albany Medical College

47 New Scotland Ave. MC 4
Albany, NY 12158
Phone: 518-262-5251
Email: paprogram@amc.edu

PROGRAM HIGHLIGHTS

Accreditation: Continuing

Degree Offered: Master (MSPAS)

Start Date: January annually

Program Length: 28 months

Class Capacity: 42 students

Tuition: $64,659

CASPA Participant: Yes

Supplemental Application: Yes ($60 fee)

Yellow Ribbon: No

Admissions: Rolling

Application Deadline: November 1

PREREQUISITE COURSEWORK

General Biology I and II with lab (8 credits), General Chemistry I and II with lab (8 credits), Biochemistry or Organic Chemistry or other advanced chemistry (3 credits), Anatomy and Physiology I and II with lab (8 credits), Microbiology with lab (4 credits), Psychology (3 credits), Statistics (3 credits), English Composition (3 credits). One Chemistry and one Biology course must be completed within the last 5 years. Prerequisites must be completed with a grade "C" or better. AP credits accepted.

GPA Requirement: No minimum

Healthcare Experience: 1,000 hours

PA Shadowing: Not required

Required Standardized Testing: GRE

Letters of Recommendation: Three required; no one specific

Seat Deposit: $500

ALBANY MEDICAL COLLEGE

MISSION:

The Center for Physician Assistant Studies, in support of Albany Medical Center's mission as an academic health sciences center, has a responsibility to educate Physician Assistant students from demographically diverse backgrounds to meet the future primary and specialty health care needs of the region and the country by providing highly skilled, cost-effective, patient-centered care in a variety of settings. This mission will be advanced through commitment to the values of Quality and Excellence, Collaboration, Confidentiality, Respect and Compassion, Integrity, Responsibility, Diversity, and Community Service.

CLASS OF 2021

Overall GPA: 3.64

Science GPA: 3.58

GRE Verbal: 62nd percentile

GRE Quantitative: 55th percentile

GRE Analytical: 61st percentile

Average Healthcare Experience: 2,977 hours

PANCE SCORES

5-year First Time Pass: 97%

Most Recent First Time Pass: 88%

CURRICULUM STRUCTURE

Didactic: 16 months

Clinical: 12 months

Rotations: 10 mandatory, 2 elective (variable duration)

Portfolio Project: Required for graduation

UNIQUE PROGRAM FEATURES

Reputation: Albany Medical College is among the oldest PA Programs in the nation (42 years) and has been continuously accredited since 1972.

Rotations: All students complete at least two rotations in underserved, rural, and culturally diverse settings. Students also complete a comprehensive interprofessional care rotation as well as a community practice preceptorship as their final rotation.

Clarkson University

1001 Clarkson Hall
Box 5882
Potsdam, NY 13699
Phone: 315-268-7942
Email: pa@clarkson.edu

PROGRAM HIGHLIGHTS

Accreditation: Continuing

Degree Offered: Master (MSPAS)

Start Date: January annually

Program Length: 28 months

Class Capacity: 30 students

Tuition: $108,087

CASPA Participant: Yes

Supplemental Application: Yes ($50 fee)

Yellow Ribbon: No

Admissions: Rolling

Application Deadline: March 1

PREREQUISITE COURSEWORK

Biology (3 credits), Anatomy and Physiology (6 credits), Microbiology (3 credits), Chemistry (6 credits), Social Sciences/Humanities (3 credits), Statistics (3 credits), Genetics (3 credits), Psychology (3 credits). Courses must be complete or in progress at the time of application. Prerequisites must be completed with a grade "C" or better. AP credits are not accepted.

GPA Requirement: Overall GPA 3.0; Science GPA 3.0; Prerequisite GPA 3.0

Healthcare Experience: 500 hours (100 hours must be complete at the time of application submission)

PA Shadowing: 8 hours

Required Standardized Testing: GRE (competitive score is >40th percentile and 4.0 on analytical)

Letters of Recommendation: Three required; one from an MD, PA or NP

Seat Deposit: $1,000

CLARKSON UNIVERSITY

MISSION:

The mission of the Clarkson University Department of Physician Assistant Studies is to educate Physician Assistants to become highly skilled and compassionate health care providers. The program will encourage an interdisciplinary approach with an emphasis on patient-centered care.

NO CLASS STATISTICS REPORTED

PANCE SCORES

5-year First Time Pass: 95%

Most Recent First Time Pass: 89%

CURRICULUM STRUCTURE

Didactic: 13 months

Clinical: 14 months (+ 1 summative month)

Rotations: 7 mandatory, 2 elective, 1 clinical research elective (each 5 weeks)

Master's Project: Required for graduation

UNIQUE PROGRAM FEATURES

Pre-PA: Up to 10 seats in each cohort are held for Clarkson pre-PA students and Clarkson students are given additional points in the admissions process.

Community Service: Students have volunteered for the local Hospice, Food Bank, Christmas Fund, Office of the Aging, blood pressure screenings, Relay for Life, and a Red Cross blood drive. Many students recently went on a mission trip to the Dominican Republic with plans in place to continue yearly missions.

Teaching Modalities: In addition to traditional lectures, the program utilizes problem-based learning as well as simulation medicine to teach students critical thinking and clinical skills.

Cornell University

570 Lexington Avenue, 9th floor
New York, NY 10022
Phone: 646-962-7277
Email: mshspa@med.cornell.edu

PROGRAM HIGHLIGHTS

Accreditation: Continuing

Degree Offered: Master (MSHS)

Start Date: March annually

Program Length: 26 months

Class Capacity: 42 students

Tuition: $91,260

CASPA Participant: Yes

Supplemental Application: Yes ($60 fee)

Yellow Ribbon: Yes

Admissions: Non-rolling

Application Deadline: September 1

PREREQUISITE COURSEWORK

Biology with lab (2 courses), Chemistry with lab (2 courses), Microbiology (1 course), Biochemistry (1 course), Anatomy and Physiology (2 courses), English Composition (1 course). Recommended courses: Statistics, Medical Terminology, Research Methods.

GPA Requirement: No minimum (but overall GPA of 3.0 is expected)

Healthcare Experience: 500 hours

PA Shadowing: Preferred, not required

Required Standardized Testing: GRE

Letters of Recommendation: Two required; one from a physician or PA and one academic letter (i.e., from a prior instructor)

Seat Deposit: $700

CORNELL UNIVERSITY

MISSION:

The principal mission of the Weill Cornell Graduate School MSHS Physician Assistant Program is to educate highly competent, compassionate, and culturally sensitive physician assistants drawn from diverse backgrounds and experiences, who will be capable of practicing and excelling in varied clinical and academic settings.

CLASS OF 2021

Overall GPA: 3.60

Science GPA: 3.60

PANCE SCORES

5-year First Time Pass: 98%

Most Recent First Time Pass: 97%

CURRICULUM STRUCTURE

Didactic: 10 months

Clinical: 16 months

Rotations: 10 mandatory, 5 selective (each 4 weeks)

Master's Thesis: Required for graduation

UNIQUE PROGRAM FEATURES

Surgical Focus: The Cornell PA program has a focus on surgery in didactic and clinical curricula, although all aspects of primary care are covered as well in order to properly prepare students for the PANCE. Students are allowed to focus on medicine in elective rotations as well.

239

CUNY School of Medicine

160 Convent Avenue
Harris Hall Suite 15
New York, NY 10031
Phone: 212-650-7745
Email:
paprogadmissions@med.cuny.edu

PROGRAM HIGHLIGHTS

Accreditation: Continuing

Degree Offered: Master (MSPAS)

Start Date: August annually

Program Length: 28 months

Class Capacity: 35 students

Tuition: $45,507 (in-state, including fees); $75,092 (out-of-state, including fees)

CASPA Participant: Yes

Supplemental Application: No

Yellow Ribbon: No

Admissions: Non-rolling

Application Deadline: January 15

PREREQUISITE COURSEWORK

Biology I and II with lab (8 credits), Chemistry I and II with lab (8 credits), Microbiology with lab (3 credits), Statistics (3 credits). Two of the following are also required: Cell and Molecular Biology (3 credits), Genetics (3 credits), Mammalian Physiology (3 credits), Anatomy and Physiology I and II with lab (8 credits), Biochemistry (3 credits). Two courses may be pending at the time of application. Microbiology, Statistics and the two-course option must be completed within 7 years of application. Prerequisites must be completed with a grade "C" or better. AP credits are reviewed on a case-by-case basis.

GPA Requirement: Overall GPA 3.0; Prerequisite GPA 3.0

Healthcare Experience: Preferred, not required

PA Shadowing: Not reported

Required Standardized Testing: None

Letters of Recommendation: Three required; one should be from a physician or physician assistant

Seat Deposit: $250

CUNY SCHOOL OF MEDICINE

MISSION:

The mission of the CUNY School of Medicine Physician Assistant Program is to improve the health of underserved communities and to eliminate healthcare disparity by providing increased access to physician assistant education to students from traditionally underrepresented populations. Through education and mentoring, we will create a workforce that will provide highly skilled health services to the communities of greatest need.

NO CLASS STATISTICS REPORTED

PANCE SCORES

5-year First Time Pass: 90%

Most Recent First Time Pass: 92%

CURRICULUM STRUCTURE

Didactic: 12 months

Clinical: 12 months

Research: 4 months

Rotations: 9 mandatory, 1 elective (each 5 weeks)

Research Methods Project: Required for graduation

UNIQUE PROGRAM FEATURES

Diversity: The Physician Assistant Program is committed to increasing the number of physician assistants of African-American, Latino, and other ethnic backgrounds, whose communities have historically been underserved.

Community Service: The PA student society is very active in community service activities and statewide and national PA conferences.

CUNY York College

94-20 Guy Brewer Boulevard
Jamaica, NY 11451
Phone: 718-262-2823
Email: paprogram@york.cuny.edu

PROGRAM HIGHLIGHTS

Accreditation: Continuing

Degree Offered: Master (MSPAS)

Start Date: August annually

Program Length: 28 months

Class Capacity: 30 students

Tuition: $43,581 (in-state, including fees);
$82,606 (out-of-state, including fees)

CASPA Participant: Yes

Supplemental Application: Yes ($125 fee)

Yellow Ribbon: No

Admissions: Non-rolling

Application Deadline: January 15

PREREQUISITE COURSEWORK

General Biology (2 semesters), General
Chemistry (2 semesters), Biochemistry (1
semester), Human Anatomy and Physiology
(2 semesters), Microbiology (1 semester),
Statistics (1 semester), Behavioral Science
(2 semesters). Anatomy and Physiology
must be completed within the last 5 years,
while Statistics and other sciences must
be completed within the last 10 years.
Recommended courses: Organic Chemistry.

GPA Requirement: Overall GPA 3.0

Healthcare Experience: 500 hours (400 hours
at the time of application submission)

PA Shadowing: Preferred, not required

Required Standardized Testing: GRE

Letters of Recommendation: Three required;
preferably from professors, health care
professionals and employers

Seat Deposit: $250

CUNY YORK COLLEGE

MISSION:

The York College Physician Assistant program seeks to recruit and educate students from the diverse surrounding communities to become highly competent, compassionate, and culturally aware providers of excellent medical care to underserved urban areas. Incorporated in our mission is a priority on increasing access to medical professional education for racial and ethnic minorities, financially disadvantaged students, and first-generation college graduates. Our program is committed to providing strong supports so that we may also expect high performance from our students.

NO CLASS STATISTICS REPORTED

PANCE SCORES

5-year First Time Pass: 90%

Most Recent First Time Pass: 79%

CURRICULUM STRUCTURE

Didactic: 16 months

Clinical: 12 months

Rotations: 9 mandatory (each 5 weeks)

UNIQUE PROGRAM FEATURES

Online Portfolio: Students complete the portfolio during clinical year which is designed to demonstrate integrative learning, professional development, and evidence based critical thinking.

241

PROGRAM HIGHLIGHTS

Accreditation: Continuing

Degree Offered: Combined BS/MS

Start Date: August annually

Program Length: 4.5 years

Class Capacity: 40 students

Tuition: $99,529 (including fees)

CASPA Participant: Yes (for transfers only)

Supplemental Application: Additional PA application required if applying as a high school senior

Yellow Ribbon: No

Admissions: Rolling

Application Deadline: October 1

PREREQUISITE COURSEWORK

Three years of math, one year of Chemistry and one year of Biology. Math and science subjects must have a minimum grade of at least 83 (B-).

GPA Requirement: Overall GPA 3.0 (also must rank in the top 25% of graduating high school class); Science GPA 3.0 (if transfer)

Healthcare Experience: 80 hours

PA Shadowing: Not required

Required Standardized Testing: Combined SAT score of at least 1170 (Math & Critical Reading sections) or a composite ACT score of 24 or higher

Letters of Recommendation: Three required; one should be from a healthcare provider or professional (e.g., a physician, RN, PA, etc.) who has observed the candidate in a healthcare setting (either volunteer or employment)

Seat Deposit: $250

D'YOUVILLE COLLEGE

MISSION:

The mission of the D'Youville Physician Assistant department is to prepare exemplary clinicians with the highest professional standards.

NO CLASS STATISTICS REPORTED

PANCE SCORES

5-year First Time Pass: 95%

Most Recent First Time Pass: 92%

CURRICULUM STRUCTURE

Pre-professional: 2 years

Didactic: 1 year

Clinical: 1.5 years

Rotations: 10 mandatory, 2 elective (each 2-8 weeks)

Research Project: Required for graduation

UNIQUE PROGRAM FEATURES

Combined Program: This is primarily an entry-level program for college freshmen. All other transfer students must apply through CASPA. See additional details on the program's website. Few students each year are accepted through CASPA.

Community Education Project: During your clinical phase, you'll have the opportunity to work with your preceptor to design and implement a community education project at a clinical site during your Primary Care core rotation. You'll research topics important to the lives of the patients you'll serve at the primary care site, develop patient education materials related to the promotion of good health and disease prevention, and present the results of your project at the end of your clinical phase.

Interdisciplinary Education Lab: Students from 8 health professions programs come together for IEL. The curriculum emulates real-life patient scenarios, in a controlled, simulated environment. The actors follow scripts with scenarios spanning the arc of care -- from recovery to after-care and ongoing or developing complications. Skilled instructors guide students every step of the way.

Daemen College

4380 Main Street
Amherst, NY 14226
Phone: 716-839-8563
Email: contactus@daemen.edu

PROGRAM HIGHLIGHTS

Accreditation: Continuing

Degree Offered: Master (MS); combined BS/MS available as well

Start Date: September annually

Program Length: 33 months

Class Capacity: 65 students (15-25 seats available for graduate applicants)

Tuition: $100,581

CASPA Participant: Yes

Supplemental Application: Yes (no fee)

Yellow Ribbon: Yes

Admissions: Non-rolling

Application Deadline: January 15

PREREQUISITE COURSEWORK

Biology with lab (8 credits), General Chemistry (8 credits), Calculus (3 credits), Psychology and/or Sociology (9 credits), Anatomy and Physiology with lab (8 credits), Microbiology with lab (4 credits), Organic Chemistry or Biochemistry with lab (4 credits). Must have a 3.0 GPA or better in Anatomy, Physiology, Microbiology and Organic/Biochem and these prerequisites must be completed within the last 5 years. At least 8 credits of higher science coursework must be completed within 12 months of entering the program. There may be no more than two grades below "C" in any college level course. There may be at most one outstanding course in progress at the time of application.

GPA Requirement: Overall GPA 3.0; Science GPA 3.0

Healthcare Experience: 120 hours

PA Shadowing: Preferred, not required

Required Standardized Testing: None

Letters of Recommendation: Three required; no one specific

Seat Deposit: $500

DAEMEN COLLEGE

MISSION:

The mission of the Daemen College Physician Assistant Program is to educate capable individuals to meet the challenges of providing quality health care services with the supervision of a licensed physician.

NO CLASS STATISTICS REPORTED

PANCE SCORES

5-year First Time Pass: 97%

Most Recent First Time Pass: 93%

CURRICULUM STRUCTURE

Didactic: 21 months

Clinical: 12 months

Rotations: 10 mandatory (each 4 weeks)

Research Project: Required for graduation

UNIQUE PROGRAM FEATURES

Community Service: The program founded Students Without Borders and makes an annual mission trip to the Dominican Republic. They are also active in providing free blood pressure and diabetes screenings to the local community.

Hofstra University

127 Hofstra University
Monroe Lecture Center, Room 113
Hempstead, NY 11549
Phone: 516-463-4074
Email: paprogram@hofstra.edu

PROGRAM HIGHLIGHTS

Accreditation: Continuing
Degree Offered: Master (MSPAS)
Start Date: September annually
Program Length: 28 months
Class Capacity: 57 students
Tuition: $110,442

CASPA Participant: Yes
Supplemental Application: No
Yellow Ribbon: Yes
Admissions: Rolling
Application Deadline: October 1

PREREQUISITE COURSEWORK

General Biology with lab (8 credits), General Chemistry with lab (8 credits), Human Physiology (4 credits), Human Anatomy (4 credits), Biochemistry or Organic Chemistry (3-4 credits), Microbiology (4 credits), Statistics (3 credits), Genetics or Cell Biology or other upper level Biology (3-4 credits). Physiology, Anatomy, Microbiology and Organic Chemistry or Biochemistry must be completed within the last 5 years.

GPA Requirement: Overall GPA 3.2; Science GPA 3.2

Healthcare Experience: 50 hours

PA Shadowing: Preferred, not required

Required Standardized Testing: None

Letters of Recommendation: Two required; no one specific

Seat Deposit: $1,500

HOFSTRA UNIVERSITY

MISSION:

The mission of the Hofstra University Department of Physician Assistant Studies is to educate physician assistant students to provide health care with clinical excellence, compassion, and dedication to the community.

NO CLASS STATISTICS REPORTED

PANCE SCORES

5-year First Time Pass: 98%

Most Recent First Time Pass: 96%

CURRICULUM STRUCTURE

Didactic: 12 months

Clinical: 12 months

Research: 4 months

Rotations: 7 mandatory, 1 elective (each 6 weeks)

Master's Research Project: Required for graduation

UNIQUE PROGRAM FEATURES

Freshman Entry Option: Option for a combined BS/MS program for students entering from high school.

Community Service: Students routinely participate in a variety of projects including a bone marrow drive and walks to raise money for cancer research. Some students even have used their summer vacation to complete mission trips in Nicaragua.

Simulation Training: Hofstra's PA program has integrated simulation experiences into the curriculum that emulate true to real life experiences as possible, further expanding student skills and knowledge. The program also uses innovative compilation of computer-assisted clinical educational program, provide a unique opportunity to enhance case-based learning.

Le Moyne College

Office of Graduate Admissions
1419 Salt Springs Road
Syracuse, NY 13214
Phone: 315-445-4745
Email: physassist@lemoyne.edu

PROGRAM HIGHLIGHTS

Accreditation: Continuing
Degree Offered: Master (MS)
Start Date: August annually
Program Length: 24 months
Class Capacity: 75 students
Tuition: $91,620

CASPA Participant: Yes
Supplemental Application: No
Yellow Ribbon: Yes
Admissions: Non-rolling
Application Deadline: October 1

PREREQUISITE COURSEWORK

Biology I and II with lab (2 semesters), Upper level Biology (4 courses, two of which must include lab), General Chemistry I and II with lab (2 semesters), Organic Chemistry or Biochemistry, Statistics or Calculus or Physics (2 semesters), Social Science (2 semesters), English Composition (1 semester). Prerequisites must be completed with a grade "C" or better.

GPA Requirement: Overall GPA 3.2; Science GPA 3.2; Prerequisite GPA 3.2

Healthcare Experience: 750 hours

PA Shadowing: Preferred, not required

Required Standardized Testing: None

Letters of Recommendation: Three required; at least one academic, if applicable, and/or from a professional in a health care field who can attest to your ability to be successful in a rigorous academic program as a health care provider

Seat Deposit: $750

LE MOYNE COLLEGE

MISSION:

The Le Moyne College Physician Assistant Program is dedicated to the education of students to become competent, caring, compassionate, and ethical providers of primary health care services with the supervision of a licensed physician. The program seeks to instill in each individual the desire to pursue a lifelong commitment to promote excellence in the delivery of patient care through continual self-assessment and advancement of one's medical skills and knowledge. This program prepares the student to work in a wide variety of settings under the supervision of licensed physicians, such as hospitals, private primary care facilities, nursing homes, and community centers.

NO CLASS STATISTICS REPORTED

PANCE SCORES

5-year First Time Pass: 96%

Most Recent First Time Pass: 93%

CURRICULUM STRUCTURE

Didactic: 12 months

Clinical: 12 months

Rotations: 7 mandatory, 1 elective (each 6 weeks)

Masters Project: Required for graduation

UNIQUE PROGRAM FEATURES

Humanities: Le Moyne is one of only a handful of PA programs that presents medical humanities courses as an integral part of training. The program focuses on a bio-psycho-social-spiritual approach in order to care for the whole person.

Community Service: Students complete many projects, including care packages for the homeless, blood drives, foot care clinics, and food/clothing collection for local organizations.

3+2 Track: Available for Le Moyne College biology majors, can earn a combined BS/MS in 5 years.

Veteran-Physician Assistant Bridge Path: The program has 3 paths for veteran admission including paths for those working on their undergraduate degree, those with an undergraduate degree but missing prerequisites, and those who have completed all application requirements.

Long Island University

1 University Plaza
Brooklyn, NY 11201
Phone: 718-488-1505
Email: robin.brizzi@liu.edu

PROGRAM HIGHLIGHTS

Accreditation: Continuing

Degree Offered: Master (MSPAS)

Start Date: August annually

Program Length: 28 months

Class Capacity: 42 students

Tuition: $107,414

CASPA Participant: Yes

Supplemental Application: No

Yellow Ribbon: Yes

Admissions: Non-rolling

Application Deadline: January 15

PREREQUISITE COURSEWORK

General Biology with lab (8 credits), General Chemistry with lab (8 credits), Human Anatomy with lab (4 credits), Human Physiology (3 credits), Microbiology (3 credits), Statistics (3 credits). Prerequisites must be completed within 10 years of matriculation. Prerequisites must be completed with a grade "C" or better. AP credits are not accepted.

GPA Requirement: Overall GPA 3.0; Science GPA 3.0

Healthcare Experience: 500 hours (400 hours must be complete at the time of application submission)

PA Shadowing: Preferred, not required

Required Standardized Testing: GRE

Letters of Recommendation: Three required; no one specific

Seat Deposit: $500

LONG ISLAND UNIVERSITY

MISSION:

The Division of Physician Assistant Studies supports Long Island University's mission through the education of men and women of all ethnic and socioeconomic backgrounds in the art and science of medicine in order that they may become competent, compassionate, high quality healthcare providers.

NO CLASS STATISTICS REPORTED

PANCE SCORES

5-year First Time Pass: 99%

Most Recent First Time Pass: 100%

CURRICULUM STRUCTURE

Didactic: 12 months

Clinical: 16 months

Rotations: 7 mandatory, 3 elective (each 5 weeks)

Capstone Project: Required for graduation

UNIQUE PROGRAM FEATURES

Community Service: Students have participated in the annual Breast Cancer Walk, Juvenile Diabetes Mellitus Walk, and HIV/AIDS walk, among other activities.

Interprofessional Education: Twice annually, over 500 students and 60 faculty members from LIU Pharmacy, the School of Health Professions (PA, PT, OT, RT, etc.) and the Harriet Rothkopf Heilbrunn School of Nursing at LIU Brooklyn participate in an Interprofessional Learning Experience, an interactive learning opportunity that is at the cutting edge of health care education.

Marist College

3399 North Road
Rotunda 381
Poughkeepsie, NY 12601
Phone: 845-575-3308
Email: pa-program@marist.edu

PROGRAM HIGHLIGHTS

Accreditation: Provisional

Degree Offered: Master (MSPAS)

Start Date: May annually

Program Length: 24 months

Class Capacity: 60 students

Tuition: $98,100

CASPA Participant: Yes

Supplemental Application: No

Yellow Ribbon: Yes

Admissions: Rolling

Application Deadline: January 15

PREREQUISITE COURSEWORK

Anatomy and Physiology I and II with lab (8 credits), General Biology I and II with lab (8 credits), General Chemistry I and II with lab (8 credits), Organic Chemistry I with lab (4 credits), Microbiology with lab (4 credits), Biochemistry I (3 credits) or Organic Chemistry II with lab (4 credits), Statistics (3 credits). Prerequisites must be completed with a grade "C" or better.

GPA Requirement: Overall GPA 3.0; Science GPA 3.0

Healthcare Experience: 500 hours

PA Shadowing: Not required

Required Standardized Testing: GRE or MCAT

Letters of Recommendation: Three required; one from a health care professional associated with the applicant's direct patient care experience

Seat Deposit: $750

MARIST COLLEGE

MISSION:

The Marist College Physician Assistant Program is committed to graduating entry-level, competent healthcare providers trained to practice ethically and culturally sensitive medicine in a team environment, and who will be life-long learners with a commitment to community service and the overall success of the profession.

CLASS OF 2021

Overall GPA: 3.47

Science GPA 3.35

Healthcare Experience: 2,061 hours

PANCE SCORES

5-year First Time Pass: 99% (based on two years of data)

Most Recent First Time Pass: 98%

CURRICULUM STRUCTURE

Didactic: 12 months

Clinical: 12 months

Rotations: 7 mandatory, 2 elective (each 5 weeks)

UNIQUE PROGRAM FEATURES

Facilities: The PA program is in a new state-of-the-art facility, which includes a gross anatomy laboratory, an 11-bed skills laboratory and a technologically advanced clinical simulation suite with a twin trauma bay and five traditional exam rooms.

Simulation: Students use both standardized patients and mannequins in the simulation lab for basic instruction and patient interaction, history taking and physical exam skills, diagnosis and documentation, clinical skills, and Objective Structured Clinical Examinations (OSCEs).

Mercy College

1200 Waters Place
Bronx, NY 10461
Phone: 718-678-8844
Email: PAProgram@mercy.edu

PROGRAM HIGHLIGHTS

Accreditation: Continuing

Degree Offered: Master (MSPAS)

Start Date: May annually

Program Length: 27 months

Class Capacity: 62 students

Tuition: $92,700

CASPA Participant: Yes

Supplemental Application: Yes ($40 fee)

Yellow Ribbon: No

Admissions: Non-rolling

Application Deadline: November 1

PREREQUISITE COURSEWORK

Biology I and II with lab, Chemistry I and II with lab, Microbiology with lab, Human Physiology, Upper level Biology (1 course), Biochemistry, Statistics. Biochemistry, Microbiology, and Human Physiology must be completed within the last 5 years and two of these must be completed at a 4-year institution. Upper level Biology also must be taken at a 4-year institution. Anatomy and Physiology I and II will not count as a substitute for Human Physiology. No more than 75 credits can be from a 2-year college. Recommended courses: Pathophysiology, Genetics, Neuroscience, Virology, Immunology, Human Anatomy.

GPA Requirement: Overall GPA 3.0; Science GPA 3.2

Healthcare Experience: 500 hours (250 of the hours must be completed in a primary care setting such as family medicine, outpatient internal medicine, pediatrics, or OB/GYN)

PA Shadowing: Not required

Required Standardized Testing: None

Letters of Recommendation: Three required; one must be from a PA, MD, or work supervisor

Seat Deposit: $800

MERCY COLLEGE

MISSION:

The mission of the Mercy College Graduate Program in Physician Assistant Studies is to educate physician assistants to provide quality, cost-effective, accessible health care, especially to underserved patients in the Tri-state area.

NO CLASS STATISTICS REPORTED

PANCE SCORES

5-year First Time Pass: 90%

Most Recent First Time Pass: 87%

CURRICULUM STRUCTURE

Didactic: 12 months

Clinical: 15 months

Rotations: 8 required, 1 elective (each 3-6 weeks)

Capstone Project: Required for graduation

UNIQUE PROGRAM FEATURES

Foreign Language: Medical Spanish is required as part of the curriculum.

Community Service: The program participates in international medical missions and students and faculty operate a mobile health vehicle that provides health screenings and education to members of the community twice a month.

Clinical Simulation Lab: The 12,000 square-foot space consists of several specialized labs designed to simulate different disciplines within a health care facility. The Labs also include control rooms, debriefing space and several large classrooms. Each are filled with state-of-the-art technology that give students real-world experience before they even begin their clinical experiences.

PROGRAM HIGHLIGHTS

Accreditation: Continuing
Degree Offered: Master (MSPAS)
Start Date: September annually
Program Length: 30 months
Class Capacity: 56 students
Tuition: $129,360

CASPA Participant: Yes
Supplemental Application: No
Yellow Ribbon: Yes
Admissions: Non-rolling
Application Deadline: October 1

PREREQUISITE COURSEWORK

Biology with lab (2 semesters),
General Chemistry I and II with lab
(2 semesters), Organic Chemistry
(1 semester), Biochemistry
(1 semester), Microbiology (1
semester), Psychology (1 semester),
Anatomy and Physiology I and
II (2 semesters), College Math
and Statistics (2 semesters).
Prerequisites must be completed
with a grade "B" or better and
within the last 5 years. At most
two prerequisites may be
outstanding by the application
deadline. AP credits are accepted.
Recommended courses: Genetics.

GPA Requirement: Overall GPA 3.0;
Science GPA 3.4

Healthcare Experience: 250 hours

PA Shadowing: Preferred, not
required

Required Standardized Testing:
None

Letters of Recommendation: Three
required; one from a PA, MD, or DO

Seat Deposit: $1,500

NEW YORK INSTITUTE OF TECHNOLOGY

MISSION:

The mission of the NYIT Department of Physician Assistant Studies is based on the belief that access for all persons to quality health care is a right. Thus, the mission of the program is to: educate qualified students to graduate as physician assistant students to provide high quality, compassionate, patient-centered health care as competent members of an interdisciplinary team to all populations seeking healthcare; educate physician assistant students to become life-long learners & critical thinkers who apply their medical knowledge and skills in practice with the highest levels of professionalism that governs the profession; and seek and encourage diversity in the recruitment of representatives of underserved populations within its faculty, staff, and student body, to serve a diverse population.

CLASS OF 2022

Male: 20%

Female: 80%

Overall GPA: 3.67

Science GPA: 3.65

Average Healthcare Experience (including shadowing): 2,263 hours

Average Age: 24

PANCE SCORES

5-year First Time Pass: 98%

Most Recent First Time Pass: 96%

CURRICULUM STRUCTURE

Didactic: 18 months

Clinical: 12 months

Rotations: 8 mandatory, 1 elective (each 4-8 weeks)

Research Project: Required for graduation

UNIQUE PROGRAM FEATURES

Admissions Preference: Priority for seats will be given to students from the 6-year BS/MS program who have met the requirements to transition into the graduate phase. The remaining seats will be open to external applicants. Typically 8-10 students enter annually from the 6-year pathway.

Global Health Certificate: The Center for Global Health offers a Certificate in Global Health and there are many opportunities to participate in service learning trips, both domestically and internationally.

Facilities: The department has a dedicated classroom/laboratory with audio-visual equipment, X-Ray Viewing Box, two electrocardiograph machines, and various human patient simulator models used for skills training. A state-of-the-art standardized patient laboratory has been developed for use by medical and physician assistant students to enhance skill acquisition. A cadaver lab provides a valuable hands-on approach to learning anatomy.

Interprofessional Education: An interprofessional educational initiative involving the School of Health Professions (nursing, physical therapy, occupational therapy, and PA programs) and the NYIT College of Osteopathic Medicine (D.O. program) is held annually. Students from these programs either participate in or observe a case-based scenario demonstrating a team-based approach to patient care. Students also work together to run simulated advanced patient codes.

Pace University

163 William Street, Fifth Floor
New York, NY 10038
Phone: 212-618-6050
Email: paprogram@pace.edu

PROGRAM HIGHLIGHTS

Accreditation: Continuing

Degree Offered: Master (MSPAS)

Start Date: July annually

Program Length: 26 months

Class Capacity: 80 students

Tuition: $105,000

CASPA Participant: Yes

Supplemental Application: Yes ($70 fee)

Yellow Ribbon: Yes

Admissions: Non-rolling

Application Deadline: September 1

PREREQUISITE COURSEWORK

Human Anatomy with lab (4 credits), Human Physiology (3 credits), General Biology with lab (8 credits), General Chemistry with lab (8 credits), Organic Chemistry or Biochemistry with lab (4 credits), Precalculus or Statistics (3 credits), Microbiology (3 credits), Genetics (3 credits). There may be no more than one grade less than a "B-" in a required prerequisite course. Prerequisites must be completed at the time of application e-submission to CASPA and within the last 10 years. AP credits are accepted.

GPA Requirement: Overall GPA 3.0; Science GPA 3.0

Healthcare Experience: 200 hours

PA Shadowing: Not required

Required Standardized Testing: None

Letters of Recommendation: Three required; one must be from a healthcare professional

Seat Deposit: $1,500

PACE UNIVERSITY - LENOX HILL

MISSION:

The mission of the Pace University-Lenox Hill Hospital Physician Assistant Program is to graduate physician assistants who demonstrate the competency necessary to function in diverse communities and settings. The program develops critical thinkers committed to professionalism, teamwork, and community engagement.

CLASS OF 2019

Male: 14%

Female: 86%

Overall GPA: 3.58

Science GPA: 3.50

Average Healthcare Experience: 1,719 hours

Average Age: 25

PANCE SCORES

5-year First Time Pass: 99%

Most Recent First Time Pass: 99%

CURRICULUM STRUCTURE

Didactic: 14 months

Clinical: 12 months

Rotations: 8 mandatory, 1 elective (each 5 weeks)

Research Method/Master Project: Required for graduation

UNIQUE PROGRAM FEATURES

Community Service: The Pace PA program is involved in a number of different volunteer projects throughout the year and raises funds for charitable organizations like the Susan G. Komen foundation and Leukemia and Lymphoma Society.

Rotations: The program boasts access to rotation sites in all five NYC boroughs as well as Connecticut and New Jersey. They also offer international rotation opportunities.

Pace University

861 Bedford Road
Pleasantville, NY 10570
Phone: 914-597-8319
Email: paplv@pace.edu

PROGRAM HIGHLIGHTS

Accreditation: Provisional

Degree Offered: Master (MSPAS)

Start Date: September annually

Program Length: 27 months

Class Capacity: 40 students

Tuition: $105,000

CASPA Participant: Yes

Supplemental Application: No

Yellow Ribbon: Yes

Admissions: Rolling

Application Deadline: January 15

PREREQUISITE COURSEWORK

Human Anatomy with lab (4 credits), Human Physiology (3 credits), General Biology with lab (8 credits), General Chemistry with lab (8 credits), Organic Chemistry or Biochemistry with lab (4 credits), Precalculus or Statistics (3 credits), Microbiology (3 credits). Prerequisites must be completed with a grade "B-" or better and within the last 7 years and by January 1st of the year of matriculation. AP credits are accepted.

GPA Requirement: Overall GPA 3.0; Science GPA 3.0

Healthcare Experience: 300 hours

PA Shadowing: 40 hours

Required Standardized Testing: None

Letters of Recommendation: Three required; one must be from a PA, MD, or DO

Seat Deposit: $1,500

PACE UNIVERSITY - PLEASANTVILLE

MISSION:

The mission of the Pace University, College of Health Professions, and Physician Assistant Studies Program - Pleasantville is to educate veterans and culturally diverse graduate students, providing an academically rigorous learning environment that promotes the intellectual, personal and professional growth of the students.

CLASS OF 2021

Male: 25%

Female: 75%

Overall GPA: 3.46

Science GPA: 3.38

Average Healthcare Experience: 3,312 hours

Average Age: 24

PANCE SCORES

5-year First Time Pass: N/A

Most Recent First Time Pass: N/A (have not graduated a class yet)

CURRICULUM STRUCTURE

Didactic: 15 months

Clinical: 12 months

Rotations: 8 mandatory, 1 elective (each 5 weeks)

Research Method/Master Project: Required for graduation

UNIQUE PROGRAM FEATURES

International Rotation: Students may choose to do their elective rotation abroad through Child Family Health International. The CFHI Global Health Education Program offers students a comprehensive clinical and cultural immersion experience in a developing country with local professionals working under vastly different circumstances from those found in the US, Canada or Europe.

Rochester Institute of Technology

Office of Admissions
- Bausch & Lomb Center
60 Lomb Memorial Drive
Rochester, NY 14623
Phone: 585-475-5151
Email: llwscl@rit.edu

PROGRAM HIGHLIGHTS

Accreditation: Continuing

Degree Offered: BS/MS

Start Date: September annually

Program Length: 30 months (graduate phase)

Class Capacity: 36 students

Tuition: $201,460 (for the total 5-year program)

CASPA Participant: No

Supplemental Application: Yes ($65 fee)

Yellow Ribbon: No

Admissions: Non-rolling; early decision available

Application Deadline: December 1

PREREQUISITE COURSEWORK

Not specifically mentioned; see program website for additional information. AP credits may be accepted.

GPA Requirement: Overall GPA 3.0

Healthcare Experience: Preferred, not required

PA Shadowing: Preferred, not required

Required Standardized Testing: None

Letters of Recommendation: Two required; no one specific

Seat Deposit: $300

ROCHESTER INSTITUTE OF TECHNOLOGY

MISSION:

Rochester Institute of Technology's Physician Assistant Program provides a foundation of science and liberal arts; and prepares students to provide compassionate, patient-centered healthcare. The Program is committed to developing the ethical values, medical knowledge, professionalism, and interpersonal communication skills essential for inter-professional, team-based, clinical practice.

NO CLASS STATISTICS REPORTED

PANCE SCORES

5-year First Time Pass: 94%

Most Recent First Time Pass: 100%

CURRICULUM STRUCTURE

Pre-professional: 2 years of undergraduate coursework

Didactic: 18 months

Clinical: 12 months

Rotations: 9 mandatory, 1 elective (each 5 weeks)

Capstone Project: Required for graduation

UNIQUE PROGRAM FEATURES

Dual Degree: RIT is a dual BS/MS program. Transfer students are accepted if space permits; however, students will typically enter as freshmen.

St. John's University

8000 Utopia Parkway
Queens, NT 11439
Phone: 718-990-8417
Email: medranor@stjohns.edu

PROGRAM HIGHLIGHTS

Accreditation: Continuing
Degree Offered: MSPA
Start Date: August annually
Program Length: 33 months
Class Capacity: 75 students
Tuition: $122,640

CASPA Participant: Yes
Supplemental Application: Yes
Yellow Ribbon: No
Admissions: Non-rolling
Application Deadline: January 15

PREREQUISITE COURSEWORK

General Biology I and II with lab (2 semesters), General Chemistry I and II with lab (2 semesters), Organic Chemistry I and II with lab or Organic Chemistry I with lab and Biochemistry (2 semesters), Human Anatomy and Physiology I and II with lab (2 semesters), Microbiology (1 semester), Behavioral Sciences (6 credits), English Composition, Calculus or higher math. Prerequisites or Bachelor's degree must be completed within the last 5 years.

GPA Requirement: Overall GPA 3.0; Science GPA 3.0

Healthcare Experience: Recommended, not required

PA Shadowing: Not required

Required Standardized Testing: None

Letters of Recommendation: Three required; no one specific

Seat Deposit: None

ST. JOHN'S UNIVERSITY

MISSION:

Conscious that culturally responsive healthcare is necessary to practice in diverse neighborhoods we strive to provide exceptional educational opportunities to men and women of varied races and socioeconomic backgrounds, so that our institution might continue its tradition of working as a partner with members of the local community. In this way, we will empower professionals to return to their own neighborhoods to promote preventive medicine and deliver affordable, high quality primary care.

NO CLASS STATISTICS REPORTED

PANCE SCORES

5-year First Time Pass: 93%

Most Recent First Time Pass: 84%

CURRICULUM STRUCTURE

Didactic: 20 months

Clinical: 13 months

Rotations: 9 mandatory, 1 elective (each 5 weeks)

Research Paper: Required for graduation

UNIQUE PROGRAM FEATURES

Facilities: Students benefit from high-tech classrooms, ultramodern science labs, and a 1.7 million volume library. The new D'Angelo Center is a five-story, 127,000-square-foot University and Student Center with classrooms, lecture halls, a Starbucks café and full-service food court.

Technology: State of the art technology is incorporated into the curriculum including a Simulation Lab, Anatomage Virtual Dissection Table for anatomy and other courses, and smart classrooms.

PROGRAM HIGHLIGHTS

Accreditation: Continuing

Degree Offered: Master (MS)

Start Date: June annually

Program Length: 24 months

Class Capacity: 70 students

Tuition: $59,512 (in-state, including fees); $97,346 (out-of-state, including fees)

CASPA Participant: Yes

Supplemental Application: Yes ($100 fee)

Yellow Ribbon: No

Admissions: Rolling

Application Deadline: October 1

PREREQUISITE COURSEWORK

General Biology (8 credits), Anatomy (3 credits), Physiology (3 credits), General Chemistry (8 credits), Biochemistry (3 credits), Organic Chemistry (3 credits), Microbiology (3 credits), Genetics (3 credits), Statistics or Biostatistics (3 credits), Arts/Humanities (6 credits), Social/Behavioral Science (9 credits), English Composition (3 credits). Science courses must be completed within 7 years of the application deadline. Prerequisites must be completed with a grade "C" or better.

GPA Requirement: Overall GPA 3.0; Science GPA 3.0

Healthcare Experience: 1,000 hours

PA Shadowing: Up to 200 hours may be counted toward healthcare experience

Required Standardized Testing: None

Letters of Recommendation: Three required; one academic letter, one health care letter, and one from a PA

Seat Deposit: $50

STONY BROOK UNIVERSITY

MISSION:

Mission: Our mission is to provide high quality graduate-level medical education in an interprofessional environment that fosters critical thinking and life-long learning. We seek to develop in our students the knowledge, attitudes, and skills necessary to be outstanding, compassionate health care providers. We promote professionalism, leadership, service and an appreciation of ethical values and diversity. Physician assistant education at Stony Brook emphasizes comprehensive patient-centered medical care across the lifespan and our curriculum focuses on the principles of evidence-based practice and the importance of scholarly activity.

PANCE SCORES

5-year First Time Pass: 97%

Most Recent First Time Pass: 98%

CURRICULUM STRUCTURE

Didactic: 12 months

Clinical: 12 months

Rotations: 9 mandatory, 1 elective (each 4-5 weeks)

Masters Project: Required for graduation

UNIQUE PROGRAM FEATURES

Admissions Preference: Preference is given to applicants who have demonstrated a commitment to working with underserved populations, demonstrated leadership activity and demonstrated a commitment to primary care.

Community Service: Students and faculty are involved in a number of events including fundraising for international relief, blood drives, book drives, and runs for cancer.

Underserved Focus: The majority of each of the last three entering classes participated in international medical missions to underserved areas on their own time. Additionally, almost all of the students in the last three entering classes had required clinical experiences in facilities designated as health professional shortage areas. These facilities serve some of the most diverse patient populations in the U.S.

Southampton Campus Expansion: The program will have a group of 25 students at the Stony Brook-Southampton campus for the majority of their pre-clinical education beginning with the Class of 2021. The remaining 45 students will be at the main campus.

SUNY Downstate Medical Center

450 Clarkson Avenue, MSC 60
Brooklyn, NY 11203
Phone: 718-270-2325
Email: PA.CHRP@downstate.edu

PROGRAM HIGHLIGHTS

Accreditation: Probation

Degree Offered: Master (MS)

Start Date: June annually

Program Length: 27 months

Class Capacity: 45 students

Tuition: $56,770 (in-state);
$104,930 (out-of-state)

CASPA Participant: No ($75 application fee)

Supplemental Application: No

Yellow Ribbon: No

Admissions: Early applications are encouraged

Application Deadline: January 3

PREREQUISITE COURSEWORK

Anatomy and Physiology I and II with lab (8 credits), General Biology I and II with lab (8 credits), General Chemistry I and II with lab (8 credits), Microbiology with lab (3 credits), Math (3 credits), General Psychology (3 credits), Abnormal or Life Span Psychology (3 credits), English (6 credits), Humanities/Social Science (6 credits), Upper level science (3-4 credits). Prerequisites should be completed within 8 years of the matriculation date and must be completed with a grade "C+" or better. Online coursework is not accepted. Recommended courses: Organic Chemistry, Genetics, Biochemistry, Embryology, Histology, Pathophysiology, Pharmacology, Statistics, other upper level sciences.

GPA Requirement: Overall GPA 3.0

Healthcare Experience: 500 hours (plus 250 hours of non-clinical volunteer work)

PA Shadowing: Preferred, not required

Required Standardized Testing: None

Letters of Recommendation: Three required; one should be from a PA, MD or NP and one from a current/former professor

Seat Deposit: $50

SUNY DOWNSTATE MEDICAL CENTER

MISSION:

The mission of the SUNY Downstate Medical Center Physician Assistant Program is to cultivate the development of professionally, competent and culturally diverse Physician Assistants to provide compassionate healthcare for an evolving urban population.

CLASS OF 2020

Overall GPA: 3.48

Science GPA: 3.59

PANCE SCORES

5-year First Time Pass: 90%

Most Recent First Time Pass: 86%

CURRICULUM STRUCTURE

Didactic: 15 months

Clinical: 12 months

Rotations: 9 mandatory, 1 elective (each 3-6 weeks)

Masters Project: Required for graduation

UNIQUE PROGRAM FEATURES

Brooklyn Free Clinic: Students volunteer during their didactic year providing care to community members under the guidance of faculty.

PROGRAM HIGHLIGHTS

Accreditation: Continuing

Degree Offered: Master (MSPAS)

Start Date: June annually

Program Length: 27 months

Class Capacity: 35 students

Tuition: $56,770 (in-state); $104,930 (out-of-state)

CASPA Participant: Yes

Supplemental Application: Yes ($65 fee)

Yellow Ribbon: No

Admissions: Rolling

Application Deadline: December 1

PREREQUISITE COURSEWORK

Anatomy and Physiology I and II with lab, General Biology I and II with lab, General Chemistry I and II with lab, Organic Chemistry or Biochemistry with lab, Microbiology with lab, Genetics, Statistics, English Composition, English elective, Medical Terminology (certificate or college credit), Behavioral/Social Science (2 semesters). One Biology and one Chemistry course need to be completed within 5 years of matriculation into the program. Prerequisites must be completed with a grade "C" or better.

GPA Requirement: Overall GPA 3.0

Healthcare Experience: 1,000 hours

PA Shadowing: Preferred, not required (up to 200 hours may count towards healthcare experience)

Required Standardized Testing: GRE

Letters of Recommendation: Three required; one from a college professor, one from a PA, and one from a physician or other healthcare professional

Seat Deposit: $150

SUNY UPSTATE MEDICAL CENTER

MISSION:

The mission of the Physician Assistant Program is to educate highly qualified physician assistants with patient centered values who practice medicine confidently and ethically by demonstrating academic excellence and clinical competence. Our emphasis is on serving the medically underserved populations in Upstate New York.

NO CLASS STATISTICS REPORTED

PANCE SCORES

5-year First Time Pass: 96%

Most Recent First Time Pass: 97%

CURRICULUM STRUCTURE

Didactic: 15 months

Clinical: 12 months

Rotations: 9 mandatory, 2 elective (each 4 weeks)

Master's Project: Required for graduation

UNIQUE PROGRAM FEATURES

Admissions: Preference is given to applicants with an expressed desire to work in rural and medically underserved communities.

Rotations: Students live in an assigned medically underserved community in Upstate New York for 12 months, completing all clinical rotations in that designated region.

PROGRAM HIGHLIGHTS

Accreditation: Continuing

Degree Offered: Bachelor (BS) and Master (MSPAS)

Start Date: August annually (Bay Shore); January annually (NUMC)

Program Length: 28 months

Class Capacity: 65 students (Bay Shore); 32 students (NUMC)

Tuition: $110,040

CASPA Participant: Yes

Supplemental Application: Yes ($25 fee)

Yellow Ribbon: Yes

Admissions: Rolling

Application Deadline: January 15 (Bay Shore); October 1 (NUMC)

PREREQUISITE COURSEWORK

General Biology I and II with lab (8 credits), General Chemistry I and II with lab (8 credits), Organic Chemistry or Biochemistry (4 credits), Anatomy and Physiology I and II (8 credits), Behavioral Science (6 credits), English (6 credits), Humanities (6 credits), Math (3 credits), Statistics (3 credits). Prerequisites must be completed with a grade "C" or better. Prerequisites may be planned or in progress at the time of application but all must be complete a full semester prior to the start of the program. AP credits are accepted for exam scores of 4 or 5.

GPA Requirement: Overall GPA 3.0; Science GPA 3.0

Healthcare Experience: 200 hours

PA Shadowing: 20 hours

Required Standardized Testing: None

Letters of Recommendation: Three required; one must be from a PA

Seat Deposit: $1,500

TOURO COLLEGE (BAY SHORE AND NASSAU UNIVERSITY MEDICAL CENTER)

MISSION:

The mission of the Bay Shore Campus/Nassau University Medical Center Physician Assistant Program is to educate capable students to meet the challenges of providing health care services under the supervision of a licensed physician. The program curriculum is designed both to educate its graduates to function as traditionally trained generalists, and to provide enrichment in hospital-based and private office settings.

CLASS OF 2019

Overall GPA: 3.58

Science GPA: 3.54

PANCE SCORES

5-year First Time Pass: 97%

Most Recent First Time Pass: 100% (Bay Shore), 93% (NUMC)

CURRICULUM STRUCTURE

Didactic: 12 months

Clinical: 16 months

Rotations: 8 mandatory, 2 elective (each 5 weeks)

Capstone Project: Required for graduation

UNIQUE PROGRAM FEATURES

Preferred Candidacy: Touro College students who have completed 34 or more undergraduate credits in the School of Health Sciences' Undergraduate Studies department may qualify for "preferred candidacy" status to the Bay Shore Campus or NUMC Physician Assistant programs. These students are guaranteed an interview if they meet admissions requirements.

Forensic Medicine: This elective rotation provides students with the opportunity to observe and perform the tasks associated with PAs who work as Forensic (medico-legal) Investigators. Working with Forensic Pathologists, students are exposed to and participate in the forensic autopsy, and also spend time in the forensic serology and toxicology labs. They are introduced to forensic anthropology, forensic odontology and forensic photography.

Touro College

232 West 40th Street
New York, NY 10018
Phone: 646-795-4510
Email: enrollhealth@touro.edu

PROGRAM HIGHLIGHTS

Accreditation: Continuing

Degree Offered: Bachelor (BS) and Master (MSPAS)

Start Date: August annually

Program Length: 32 months

Class Capacity: 45 students

Tuition: $144,160 (including fees)

CASPA Participant: Yes

Supplemental Application: Yes ($25 fee)

Yellow Ribbon: No

Admissions: Rolling

Application Deadline: January 15

PREREQUISITE COURSEWORK

General Biology I and II with lab (8 credits), General Chemistry I and II with lab (8 credits), Organic Chemistry or Biochemistry (4 credits), Anatomy and Physiology I and II (8 credits), Behavioral Science (6 credits), English (6 credits), Humanities (6 credits), Math (3 credits), Statistics (3 credits). Prerequisites must be completed with a grade "C" or better and within the last 10 years. AP credits are accepted for exam scores of 4 or 5.

GPA Requirement: Overall GPA 3.0; Science GPA 3.0

Healthcare Experience: 200 hours

PA Shadowing: 20 hours

Required Standardized Testing: None

Letters of Recommendation: Three required; one must be from a PA

Seat Deposit: $1,500

TOURO COLLEGE (MANHATTAN)

MISSION:

The mission of the Touro College Physician Assistant Programs is to educate capable students to meet the challenges of providing health care services under the supervision of a licensed physician. The program also strives to excel in the education and training of physician assistants who will serve the health care needs of the community with competence, compassion, and dedication.

CLASS OF 2020

Overall GPA: 3.58

Science GPA: 3.55

PANCE SCORES

5-year First Time Pass: 89%

Most Recent First Time Pass: 93%

CURRICULUM STRUCTURE

Didactic: 16 months

Clinical: 16 months

Rotations: 8 mandatory, 2 elective (each 5 weeks)

Capstone Project: Required for graduation

UNIQUE PROGRAM FEATURES

Timing: This program accommodates individuals who wish to embark on a career as a PA but may have other life circumstances that prevent them from being able to participate in the traditional didactic curriculum during the daytime, as courses are offered evenings from 4PM-9PM and Sundays from 9AM-5PM only.

Research Module: Students complete their final semester with a research module including courses in Applied Epidemiology & Biostatistics, Research Methods & Literature Review, and Evidence-Based Medicine to give the students the tools they need to evaluate medical literature and apply it to practice.

Wagner College

1 Campus Road
Staten Island, NY 10301
Phone: 718-420-4142
Email: paprogram@wagner.edu

PROGRAM HIGHLIGHTS

Accreditation: Continuing

Degree Offered: Bachelor (BS), Master (MS)

Start Date: June annually

Program Length: 36 months

Class Capacity: 40 students

Tuition: $157,248

CASPA Participant: Yes

Supplemental Application: Yes ($60 fee)

Yellow Ribbon: No

Admissions: Non-rolling

Application Deadline: December 1

PREREQUISITE COURSEWORK

Human Anatomy and Physiology I and II, General Chemistry I and II, Organic Chemistry, Medical Ethics or Medical Anthropology, Biostatistics or Statistics, two of the following (Microbiology, General Pathology or Genetics). Prerequisites must be completed with a grade "C+" or better.

GPA Requirement: Overall GPA 3.2; Science GPA 3.0

Healthcare Experience: Not required

PA Shadowing: Not required

Required Standardized Testing: None

Letters of Recommendation: Three required; no one specific

Seat Deposit: $300

WAGNER COLLEGE

MISSION:

To prepare professional academic clinicians committed to providing quality health care to all individuals.

NO CLASS STATISTICS REPORTED

PANCE SCORES

5-year First Time Pass: 94%

Most Recent First Time Pass: 94%

CURRICULUM STRUCTURE

Pre-professional: 2 years

Didactic: 15 months

Clinical: 21 months

Rotations: 14 mandatory, clerkship elective

Thesis Project: Required for graduation

UNIQUE PROGRAM FEATURES

Direct Entry: A direct entry track for college freshmen for the combined BS/MS degree is available. Most students are accepted via this pathway and the program accepts few if any graduate students each year.

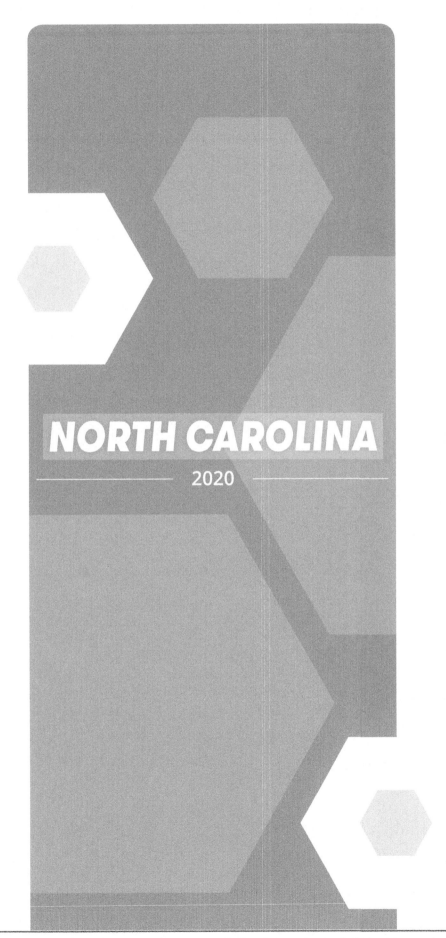

NORTH CAROLINA

2020

Campbell University

PO Box 1090
Buies Creek, NC 27506
Phone: 910-893-1690
Email: paga@campbell.edu

PROGRAM HIGHLIGHTS

Accreditation: Continuing

Degree Offered: Master (MPAP)

Start Date: August annually

Program Length: 24 months

Class Capacity: 54 students

Tuition: $85,500

CASPA Participant: Yes

Supplemental Application: Yes ($50 fee)

Yellow Ribbon: Yes

Admissions: Rolling

Application Deadline: September 1

PREREQUISITE COURSEWORK

Biology (1 semester), Human Anatomy and Physiology with lab (2 semesters), Microbiology with lab (1 semester), Chemistry with lab (1 semester), Organic Chemistry or Biochemistry (1 semester), Statistics or Biostatistics (1 semester), Psychology (1 semester). All prerequisites must be completed no later than December 31st of the year prior to matriculation and with a grade "C" or better. Recommended courses: Genetics.

GPA Requirement: Overall GPA or Last 60 Credit GPA 3.2; Prerequisite GPA 3.4 (recommended)

Healthcare Experience: 1,000 hours

PA Shadowing: 20 hours (recommended)

Required Standardized Testing: GRE (preference for those with score >300 and analytical >4.0)

Letters of Recommendation: Three required; preference is given to applicants with two out of three letters from physicians, PAs or clinical supervisors, and others familiar with your clinical experience

Seat Deposit: $1,000

CAMPBELL UNIVERSITY

MISSION:

Centered on the core values of faith, learning and service, Campbell's PA program prepares students to be compassionate, competent and professional health care providers.

CLASS OF 2018

Overall GPA: 3.41

GRE Verbal: 153

GRE Quantitative: 152

GRE Analytical: 4.2

Average Healthcare Experience: 5,268 hours

Average Age: 24.8

PANCE SCORES

5-year First Time Pass: 98%

Most Recent First Time Pass: 95%

CURRICULUM STRUCTURE

Didactic: 12 months

Clinical: 12 months

Rotations: 8 mandatory, 2 elective (each 4 weeks)

Evidence-Based Medicine Paper: Required for graduation

UNIQUE PROGRAM FEATURES

Dual Degree Program: Campbell University offers a dual degree PA/MS in Public Health and PA/MS in Clinical Research.

Facilities: The Hall of Medical Sciences is a 96,500 square foot facility that contains a simulation center for standardized patients, a physical assessment lab, 12 OSCE rooms, and an anatomy lab. It includes student group rooms, a resource library, a small café, and sophisticated technical equipment for hands-on, real-life application.

Community Service: The Wallace Student Society completes community service projects with a focus on prevention and health promotion in rural communities through patient education and charity fundraising.

263

Duke University

DUMC Box 104780
Durham, NC 27710
Phone: 919-681-3161
Email: paadmission@mc.duke.edu

PROGRAM HIGHLIGHTS

Accreditation: Continuing

Degree Offered: Master (MHS)

Start Date: August annually

Program Length: 24 months

Class Capacity: 90 students

Tuition: $87,036

CASPA Participant: Yes

Supplemental Application: Yes ($50 fee)

Yellow Ribbon: Yes

Admissions: Rolling

Application Deadline: October 1

PREREQUISITE COURSEWORK

Anatomy (3 credits), Physiology (3 credits), Microbiology (3 credits), Other Biology (6 credits), Chemistry with lab (8 credits), Statistics (2 credits). No more than two prerequisites may be pending at the time of application. Prerequisites must be completed by December 31st of the year prior to matriculation, within the last 10 years, and with a grade "C" or better. AP credits are not accepted. Recommended Courses: Genetics, Cell Biology, Molecular Biology, Embryology, Histology, Immunology.

GPA Requirement: No minimum

Healthcare Experience: 1,000 hours

PA Shadowing: Preferred, not required

Required Standardized Testing: GRE

Letters of Recommendation: Three required; at least one must be from a healthcare professional who can speak to your patient care qualifications

Seat Deposit: $1,125

DUKE UNIVERSITY MEDICAL CENTER

MISSION:

The Duke Physician Assistant Program's mission is to educate caring, competent primary care physician assistants who practice evidence-based medicine, are leaders in the profession, dedicated to their communities, culturally sensitive, and devoted to positive transformation of the health care system.

CLASS OF 2021

Overall GPA: 3.51-3.85

Science GPA: 3.39-3.87

GRE Verbal: 156-160

GRE Quantitative: 153-159

GRE Analytical: 4.5-5

Average Healthcare Experience: 3,270-7,854 hours

PANCE SCORES

5-year First Time Pass: 98%

Most Recent First Time Pass: 97%

CURRICULUM STRUCTURE

Didactic: 12 months

Clinical: 12 months

Rotations: 9 mandatory, 2 elective (each 4-8 weeks)

UNIQUE PROGRAM FEATURES

History: The PA profession originated at Duke in the mid-1960s with Dr. Eugene Stead and thus, Duke is the oldest PA program in the nation.

Community Service: Students in the Duke PA Program have a long tradition of taking time out of their busy academic schedules to participate in community service and fundraising. Specific opportunities are available to view on their website and have included involvement in diaper drives, food drives, trash collection, Habitat for Humanity, and others.

Research: Duke has established a research section to advance scholarship on the PA profession.

Medical Spanish: This elective is available to students during didactic year.

East Carolina University

4310 Health Sciences Building
600 Moye Boulevard/MS 668
Greenville, NC 27834
Phone: 252-744-1100
Email: PAAdmissions@ecu.edu

PROGRAM HIGHLIGHTS

Accreditation: Continuing
Degree Offered: Master (MSPA)
Start Date: August annually
Program Length: 27 months
Class Capacity: 36 students
Tuition: $39,076 (in-state, including fees); $85,098 (out-of-state, including fees)

CASPA Participant: Yes
Supplemental Application: Yes ($75 graduate school application fee)
Yellow Ribbon: No
Admissions: Rolling
Application Deadline: September 1

PREREQUISITE COURSEWORK

Human Anatomy and Physiology I and II with lab (8 credits), Genetics (3 credits), General Chemistry or higher with lab (8 credits), Microbiology (3 credits), Psychology (3 credits), Statistics (3 credits). It is preferred that all courses be completed within the last 5 years and applicants may have one pending prerequisite as long as it is completed by December 31st of the application year. It is recommended that prerequisites be completed with a grade "B" or better (no more than two grades of "C" will be accepted). AP credits are accepted for Psychology and Statistics prerequisites. Recommended Course: Biochemistry.

GPA Requirement: Overall GPA 3.0; Prerequisite GPA 3.0

Healthcare Experience: 1,000 hours (750 must be complete at the time of application)

PA Shadowing: Preferred, not required

Required Standardized Testing: GRE

Letters of Recommendation: Three required; should be from medical professionals, supervisors, and professors

Seat Deposit: $500

EAST CAROLINA UNIVERSITY

MISSION:

The mission of the Department of Physician Assistant Studies is to provide educational experiences which prepare physician assistant graduates to enhance access to primary medical care, with a hope to increase care for the citizens of rural and medically-underserved Eastern North Carolina and beyond. We seek to achieve this mission in an educational community where faculty, staff, clinical instructors, students, and other health care providers work together in an atmosphere of mutual respect, cooperation, compassion, and commitment.

CLASS OF 2021

Overall GPA: 3.70

Science GPA: 3.60

Prerequisite GPA: 3.70

GRE Total: 308

GRE Analytical: 4.5

PANCE SCORES

5-year First Time Pass: 100%

Most Recent First Time Pass: 100%

CURRICULUM STRUCTURE

Didactic: 15 months

Clinical: 12 months

Rotations: 8 mandatory, 2 elective (each 4-8 weeks)

UNIQUE PROGRAM FEATURES

Admissions Preference: Applicants must be residents of North Carolina, South Carolina, Virginia, Tennessee, Georgia, or Washington D.C. with preference given to those from North Carolina. Additionally, 35-50% of accepted students are typically from rural communities.

International Rotations: Students can complete an international rotation as one of their electives.

Rotation Sites: Most of the rotation sites are found in health care provider shortage areas, in line with the mission of the program to help relieve this shortage in North Carolina.

Medical Simulation: Students complete medical simulations with virtual reality simulators, high fidelity patient simulators, and simulated live patients while also learning procedure skills using models and task trainers.

Elon University

2750 Campus Box
Elon, NC 27244
Phone: 336-278-7600
Email: gradadm@elon.edu

PROGRAM HIGHLIGHTS

Accreditation: Continuing
Degree Offered: Master (MSPA)
Start Date: January annually
Program Length: 24 months
Class Capacity: 38 students
Tuition: $95,986

CASPA Participant: Yes
Supplemental Application: No
Yellow Ribbon: Yes
Admissions: Rolling
Application Deadline: November 1

PREREQUISITE COURSEWORK

Human Anatomy with lab and Physiology (7 credits), General Chemistry with lab (4 credits), Additional Chemistry with lab (4 credits), Microbiology (3 credits), Upper Level Science (3 credits), Psychology (3 credits). Science courses must be completed within 10 years of program matriculation and five of the six science courses must be completed at the time of application. Prerequisites must be completed with a grade "C" or better. AP credits are not accepted. Recommended courses: Biochemistry, Cell and Molecular Biology, Exercise Physiology, Genetics, Immunology, Organic Chemistry.

GPA Requirement: Overall GPA 3.2; Science GPA 3.0

Healthcare Experience: 250 hours

PA Shadowing: 20 hours

Required Standardized Testing: GRE (minimum score of 297 and 3.0 on analytical)

Letters of Recommendation: Three required; one must be from a PA or other healthcare provider

Seat Deposit: $1,000

ELON UNIVERSITY

MISSION:

The Elon University Department of Physician Assistant Studies embraces the overall mission of the University and seeks to fulfill the Departmental vision of "Learning. Caring. Serving. Leading."

CLASS OF 2021

Male: 18%

Female: 82%

Overall GPA: 3.75

Science GPA: 3.73

GRE Verbal: 155

GRE Quantitative: 153

GRE Analytical: 4.0

Average Healthcare Experience: 3,480 hours

Average Age: 25

PANCE SCORES

5-year First Time Pass: 98%

Most Recent First Time Pass: 100%

CURRICULUM STRUCTURE

Didactic: 12 months

Clinical: 12 months

Rotations: 7 mandatory, 1 elective (each 3-6 weeks)

Master's Project: Required for graduation

UNIQUE PROGRAM FEATURES

Facilities: The program's dedicated teaching space includes two classrooms, a clinical skills laboratory, five simulated exam rooms, a cardiopulmonary auscultation lab, wet dissection/clinical procedure lab and six small group study rooms. Shared space with the DPT program includes a human donor anatomy lab, locker rooms, and numerous student common spaces. Additional equipment will include a Harvey™ Cardiopulmonary simulator, high definition cameras for use with clinical skills examinations, and state-of-the-art classroom technology.

Global Learning Opportunity: Elon University School of Health Sciences has a program to develop global clinicians and informed leaders through clinical or service-learning experiences that take place in a culturally unique clinical setting with cultural immersion.

Gardner Webb University

PO Box 7252
College of Health Sciences
Boiling Springs, NC 28017
Phone: 704-406-2017
Email:
paprogram@gardner-webb.edu

PROGRAM HIGHLIGHTS

Accreditation: Probation

Degree Offered: Master (MPAS)

Start Date: January annually

Program Length: 28 months

Class Capacity: 36 students

Tuition: $88,200

CASPA Participant: Yes

Supplemental Application: Yes ($100 fee)

Yellow Ribbon: No

Admissions: Rolling

Application Deadline: September 1

PREREQUISITE COURSEWORK

Human Anatomy and Physiology I and II with lab (2 semesters), General Biology with lab (1 semester), Other Biology with lab (1 semester), Microbiology with lab (1 semester), General Chemistry with lab (1 semester), Other Chemistry with lab (1 semester), Organic Chemistry with lab (1 semester), Statistics (1 course), Psychology (1 course), Medical Terminology. Two prerequisites may be in progress at the time of application but must be completed before September 1st prior to matriculation. Prerequisites must be completed with a grade "B-" or better. AP credits are accepted for exam scores of 4 or 5.

GPA Requirement: Overall GPA 3.0; Prerequisite GPA 3.0

Healthcare Experience: 1,000 hours

PA Shadowing: Not required

Required Standardized Testing: None

Letters of Recommendation: Three required; one must be from a health care provider (PA, NP, MD, DO)

Seat Deposit: $1,500

GARDNER WEBB UNIVERSITY

MISSION:

To develop knowledgeable and caring Physician Assistants who practice competent patient-centered primary care in diverse environments.

CLASS OF 2021

Overall GPA: 3.47

Science GPA: 3.41

PANCE SCORES

5-year First Time Pass: 96% (based on four years of data)

Most Recent First Time Pass: 97%

CURRICULUM STRUCTURE

Didactic: 16 months

Clinical: 12 months

Rotations: 8 mandatory, 1 elective (each 3-6 weeks)

UNIQUE PROGRAM FEATURES

Underserved Focus: All students will complete a 3-week clinical rotation with an underserved population, in line with the program's service values. The program is also developing international mission opportunities for students.

Virtual Cadaver Lab: The program has built a $300,000 virtual cadaver lab to enhance the anatomy course and for use in the medical and surgical curriculum. They also have a robotics lab component.

High Point University

Graduate Admissions - Norcross Hall
One University Parkway
High Point, NC 27268
Phone: 336-841-9504
Email: PAprogram@highpoint.edu

PROGRAM HIGHLIGHTS

Accreditation: Continuing

Degree Offered: Master (MPAS)

Start Date: June annually

Program Length: 27 months

Class Capacity: 35 students

Tuition: $94,500 (including fees)

CASPA Participant: Yes

Supplemental Application: No

Yellow Ribbon: Yes

Admissions: Rolling

Application Deadline: October 1

PREREQUISITE COURSEWORK

Human or Vertebrate Anatomy with lab (4 credits), Human or Vertebrate Physiology (3 credits), Biological Science with lab (8 credits), Upper Level Human Biological Science (3 credits), Microbiology with lab (3 credits), General/Inorganic Chemistry with lab (4 credits), Additional Chemistry with lab (4 credits), Statistics (3 credits), Psychology (3 credits), Humanities and Social Sciences (9 credits, at least one upper level course), Medical Terminology (course credit or certificate). Only one prerequisite course may be in progress during the fall semester of the year of application, and science courses must be completed within 10 years of program matriculation. Prerequisites must be completed with a grade "C" or better. AP credits are accepted for exam scores of 4 or 5 provided that the course appears on your college transcript.

GPA Requirement: Overall GPA 3.2; Science GPA 3.2

Healthcare Experience: 200 hours

PA Shadowing: 15 hours

Required Standardized Testing: GRE

Letters of Recommendation: Three required; one should be from a professor and one from a supervisor

Seat Deposit: $1,000

HIGH POINT UNIVERSITY

MISSION:

The mission of the High Point University Physician Assistant Studies program is to deliver a student-centered, experiential curriculum grounded in high academic and ethical standards. The program strives to develop compassionate physician assistants who are self-directed lifelong learners prepared to provide evidence-based, patient-centered care as members of an interprofessional health care team.

CLASS OF 2020

Overall GPA: 3.74

Science GPA: 3.69

GRE Verbal: 154

GRE Quantitative: 153

Average Healthcare Experience: 1,835 hours

PANCE SCORES

5-year First Time Pass: 98% (based on two years of data)

Most Recent First Time Pass: 100%

CURRICULUM STRUCTURE

Didactic: 15 months

Clinical: 12 months

Rotations: 7 mandatory, 2 elective (each 5 weeks)

Master's Project: Required for graduation

UNIQUE PROGRAM FEATURES

Students First: The faculty is committed to maximizing the student educational experience through innovative and stimulating learning experiences, mentoring relationships with students, small student to faculty ratios, and feedback and support for professional development.

Experiential Learning: The program provides opportunities for medical simulation, standardized patients, task trainers, problem-based learning, case-based learning, team-based learning and other emerging technologies. They have a state of the art Center for Medical Simulation.

Staying Ahead of the Curve: The program is committed to preparing healthcare professionals for the world as it is going to be in the future through maximizing the use of health information technology.

Lenoir-Rhyne University

625 7th Avenue NE
Box 7475
Hickory, NC 28603
Phone: 828-328-7129
Email: kelly.powell@lr.edu

PROGRAM HIGHLIGHTS

Accreditation: Provisional

Degree Offered: Master (MSPAS)

Start Date: January annually

Program Length: 27 months

Class Capacity: 48 students

Tuition: $88,885

CASPA Participant: Yes

Supplemental Application: No

Yellow Ribbon: No

Admissions: Rolling

Application Deadline: March 1

PREREQUISITE COURSEWORK

Biology I and II with Lab, Microbiology with lab, Chemistry I and II with lab, Organic Chemistry I and II, Anatomy and Physiology I and II with lab, Biochemistry with lab, Medical Terminology, Genetics, Psychology, Sociology or Social Science, Statistics, Upper level Math, Physics. At most two prerequisites may be pending at the time of application. Prerequisites must be completed with a grade "C" or better and within the last 10 years. AP credits are not accepted. BLS certification is required prior to matriculation.

GPA Requirement: Overall GPA 3.0; Science GPA 3.0; Prerequisite GPA 3.0

Healthcare Experience: Preferred, not required

PA Shadowing: Preferred, not required

Required Standardized Testing: GRE (>301 total)

Letters of Recommendation: Three required; one from a medical provider (MD, DO, PA, or NP), one from a professor and one from an employer or coach

Seat Deposit: $1,000

LENOIR-RHYNE UNIVERSITY

MISSION:

The Mission of the Master of Science in Physician Assistant Studies Program is to educate highly qualified physician assistants from diverse faith, geographic, socioeconomic and cultural backgrounds; preparing them to become competent and compassionate health care professionals, providing quality healthcare to diverse populations in medically underserved areas locally, nationally and internationally.

CLASS OF 2019

Overall GPA: 3.32

Science GPA: 3.22

GRE Total: 307

Average Healthcare Experience: 2,567 hours

PANCE SCORES

5-year First Time Pass: 98% (based on two years of data)

Most Recent First Time Pass: 97%

CURRICULUM STRUCTURE

Didactic: 15 months

Clinical: 12 months

Rotations: 7 mandatory, 1 elective (each 6 weeks)

Capstone Project: Required for graduation

UNIQUE PROGRAM FEATURES

Preference: Veterans, especially those with medical experience will be given favorable consideration.

3+2 Track: Available for competitive undergraduate Lenoir-Rhyne students.

269

Methodist University

5107 College Center Drive
Fayetteville, NC 28312
Phone: 910-630-7615
Email: paprogram@methodist.edu

PROGRAM HIGHLIGHTS

Accreditation: Continuing

Degree Offered: Master (MMS)

Start Date: August annually

Program Length: 27 months

Class Capacity: 40 students

Tuition: $92,743

CASPA Participant: Yes

Supplemental Application: No

Yellow Ribbon: Yes

Admissions: Rolling

Application Deadline: January 15

PREREQUISITE COURSEWORK

Microbiology with lab (4 credits), Anatomy and Physiology with lab (4 credits), Additional Animal/Human Biology courses (8 credits), General Chemistry I and II with lab (8 credits), Organic Chemistry I and II with lab (8 credits), Biochemistry (3 credits), Statistics (3 credits), Psychology (6 credits), Medical Terminology (1 semester). Prerequisites must be completed with a grade "C" or better. Applicants can apply with courses in progress but they must then be completed with a grade "B+" or higher. AP credits are accepted.

GPA Requirement: No minimum (but overall GPA 3.0 and prerequisite GPA 3.2 are recommended)

Healthcare Experience: 500 hours

PA Shadowing: Not required

Required Standardized Testing: GRE (score >297 recommended or 50th percentile in each section)

Letters of Recommendation: Three required; one from a professor or advisor, one from a medical professional with whom you have worked clinically, and one from an employer or other professor or medical co-worker/supervisor

Seat Deposit: $1,000

METHODIST UNIVERSITY

MISSION:

To develop competent clinicians within a supportive, engaging, culturally diverse environment which fosters spiritual, academic and social growth. Our graduates will become integrated into communities striving for excellence in healthcare through compassion, professionalism, and lifelong learning.

CLASS OF 2021

Male: 25%

Female: 75%

Overall GPA: 3.34

Prerequisite GPA: 3.50

GRE Verbal: 154

GRE Quantitative: 153

GRE Analytical: 4.0

Average Healthcare Experience: 4,743 hours

Average Age: 27

PANCE SCORES

5-year First Time Pass: 98%

Most Recent First Time Pass: 92%

CURRICULUM STRUCTURE

Didactic: 13.5 months

Clinical: 13.5 months

Rotations: 9 mandatory, 2 elective (each 5 weeks)

Clinical Research Project: Required for graduation

UNIQUE PROGRAM FEATURES

Facilities: The program has a dedicated 8,000 square foot facility with two classrooms, nine offices, locker rooms, a kitchen, library, lounge, and clinical exam laboratory. Students also have a 7,200 square foot lecture hall and gross anatomy lab.

Interprofessional Education: At numerous times throughout didactic and clinical year students interact with Athletic Training, Health Care Administration, Kinesiology, Nursing, and Physical Therapy students.

Pfeiffer University

48380 US Hwy 52
Misenheimer, NC 28109
Phone: 704-463-3167
Email: pfeifferpa@pfeiffer.edu

PROGRAM HIGHLIGHTS

Accreditation: Provisional

Degree Offered: Master (MSPAS)

Start Date: January annually

Program Length: 27 months

Class Capacity: 36 students

Tuition: $99,094 (including fees)

CASPA Participant: Yes

Supplemental Application: No

Yellow Ribbon: No

Admissions: Rolling

Application Deadline: September 1

PREREQUISITE COURSEWORK

Anatomy and Physiology I and II (2 semesters), Microbiology with lab (1 semester), Organic Chemistry with lab (1 semester), Genetics (1 semester), Biochemistry (1 semester), Psychology (1 semester), Statistics (1 semester), Medical Terminology (1 semester or CE credit). Prerequisites must be completed within the last 7 years. AP credits are not accepted.

GPA Requirement: Overall GPA 3.0; Prerequisite GPA 3.2 (both recommended)

Healthcare Experience: 500 hours

PA Shadowing: 24 hours

Required Standardized Testing: PA-CAT, CASPer

Letters of Recommendation: Three required; letters should be from physicians, PAs, NPs, research mentors, professors or volunteer coordinators/supervisors who had direct interaction with the applicant and can attest to his/her qualities, strengths and suitability for a career as a PA

Seat Deposit: $500

PFEIFFER UNIVERSITY

MISSION:

The mission of the Pfeiffer University Master of Science in Physician Assistant Studies program is to educate servant leaders from diverse backgrounds as physician assistants who will provide exceptional healthcare in an inter-professional setting--serving rural medically underserved populations through community involvement, public health policy and advocacy.

NO CLASS STATISTICS REPORTED

PANCE SCORES

5-year First Time Pass: N/A

Most Recent First Time Pass: N/A (have not graduated a class yet)

CURRICULUM STRUCTURE

Didactic: 15 months

Clinical: 12 months

Rotations: 8 mandatory, 1 elective (each 5 weeks)

Graduate Research Project: Required for graduation

UNIQUE PROGRAM FEATURES

Facilities: The Pfeiffer University Center for Health Sciences will feature the Center for Advanced Clinical Simulation Education (CACSE). The CACSE will include four simulated ICU rooms, one Surgical Suite and one Emergency Department Trauma Bay; each of these rooms is equipped with a high fidelity, computerized human simulator. Additionally, the CACSE will feature a fully functional clinic with six exam rooms, where physician assistant students alongside board certified and licensed physician assistant faculty, will provide much-needed community health services.

Scholarly Concentrations: In response to the critical need of health care providers in the areas of Behavioral and Mental Health and Rural Medicine, the Pfeiffer University MS-PAS program is offering Scholarly Concentrations in Behavioral and Mental Health and Rural Medicine. The Scholarly Concentrations are offered during the clinical phase of the program

271

University of North Carolina

Bondurant Hall, CB 7121
Chapel Hill, NC 27599
Phone: 919-962-8008
Email: paprogram@unc.edu

PROGRAM HIGHLIGHTS

Accreditation: Provisional

Degree Offered: Master (MHS)

Start Date: January annually

Program Length: 24 months

Class Capacity: 20 students

Tuition: $56,718 (in-state);
$101,748 (out-of-state)

CASPA Participant: Yes

Supplemental Application: Yes ($85 fee)

Yellow Ribbon: Yes

Admissions: Rolling

Application Deadline: September 1

PREREQUISITE COURSEWORK

Human Anatomy and Physiology (or Special Operations Combat Medics Course), Biochemistry or Organic Chemistry (3 credits), Microbiology (3 credits), Sociology or Psychology (3 credits), Statistics or Biostatistics (3 credits), Medical Terminology. It is strongly recommended that prerequisites be completed within the last 7 years. Prerequisites must be completed with a grade "C" or better. Two courses may be in progress at the time of application but must be completed by August 31st. AP credits are not accepted.

GPA Requirement: Overall (or Last 60 Credit) GPA 3.0; Prerequisite GPA >3.2

Healthcare Experience: 1,000 hours

PA Shadowing: Not required

Required Standardized Testing: GRE (scores >150 in each section and 3.5 in analytical preferred)

Letters of Recommendation: Three required; preference given to applicants with at least two of the three letters from experienced health care professionals who have observed or supervised you in a clinical setting

Seat Deposit: $1,000

UNIVERSITY OF NORTH CAROLINA

MISSION:

The mission of the University of North Carolina at Chapel Hill Physician Assistant program is to promote high-quality, accessible, patient-centered health care for the people of North Carolina and the nation through excellence in education, scholarship, and clinical service. The UNC PA program is committed to the health care and workforce needs of North Carolinians and will use an inter-professional approach to prepare skilled and compassionate health care practitioners across the continuum of life.

CLASS OF 2022

Overall GPA: 3.32

Prerequisite GPA: 3.71

GRE Total: 306

Average Healthcare Experience: 4,000 hours

PANCE SCORES

5-year First Time Pass: 90% (based on two years of data)

Most Recent First Time Pass: 94%

CURRICULUM STRUCTURE

Didactic: 12 months

Clinical: 12 months

Rotations: 7 mandatory, 2 elective (each 4-6 weeks)

Capstone Project: Required for graduation

UNIQUE PROGRAM FEATURES

Non-Traditional and Veteran Focus: The program strives to provide education to non-traditional students, with attention to all veterans, especially those who have served in medical military settings such as the special forces medics, for careers in medically underserved areas. In the past 4 years, 37% of students were veterans.

Underserved Focus: The program prepares generalist PAs to practice in rural or urban medically underserved areas through emphasis on health promotion, disease prevention, cultural competency, and primary care.

Interprofessional Education: Students collaborate in curricular components designed to foster inter-professionalism with physical therapy, occupational therapy and audiology students.

Wake Forest University

Medical Center Boulevard
Winston Salem, NC 27157
Phone: 336-716-4356
Email: paadmit@wakehealth.edu

PROGRAM HIGHLIGHTS

Accreditation: Continuing

Degree Offered: Master (MMS)

Start Date: June annually

Program Length: 24 months

Class Capacity: 88 students

Tuition: $82,914

CASPA Participant: Yes

Supplemental Application: Yes ($100 fee)

Yellow Ribbon: Yes

Admissions: Rolling

Application Deadline: September 1

PREREQUISITE COURSEWORK

Genetics (3 credits), General Chemistry or Organic Chemistry (3 credits), Biochemistry (3 credits), Anatomy and Physiology (6 credits), Microbiology (3 credits), Statistics (2 credits), Medical Terminology (1 course). Prerequisites must be completed by December 31st of the year of application and with a grade "C" or better. It is strongly recommended that any prerequisite coursework older than 5 years be repeated. Science prerequisites should also be completed with a lab component when applicable.

GPA Requirement: No minimum

Healthcare Experience: 1,000 hours

PA Shadowing: Preferred, not required

Required Standardized Testing: GRE, CASPer

Letters of Recommendation: Three required; one must be from a healthcare professional

Seat Deposit: $1,000

WAKE FOREST UNIVERSITY (BOWMAN GRAY)

MISSION:

The mission of the Wake Forest School of Medicine Physician Assistant (PA) Program is to produce highly capable, compassionate PAs who deliver patient-centered care, make significant contributions to the health care community and continually advance the PA profession.

NO CLASS STATISTICS REPORTED

PANCE SCORES

5-year First Time Pass: 99%

Most Recent First Time Pass: 99%

CURRICULUM STRUCTURE

Didactic: 12 months

Clinical: 12 months

Rotations: 7 mandatory, 1 selective, 2 elective (each 4 weeks)

Graduate Project: Required for graduation

UNIQUE PROGRAM FEATURES

Inquiry-Based Learning: The curriculum is centered around inquiry-based, small-group, self-directed learning based on real patient medical problems. In inquiry-based learning (IBL), learners are progressively given more and more responsibility for their own education and become increasingly independent of the teacher for their education.

Dual Degree: The MMS-PhD is a 5- to 7-year program that combines a Master of Medical Science in Physician Assistant Studies with a PhD in Molecular Medicine and Translational Science (MMTS). The program targets students interested in clinical research, community research, and the translation of knowledge into improved human health.

Emerging Leaders Program: The Emerging Leaders Program is a sequential degree program in which students can earn an MA in Management and then earn an MMS in Physician Assistant Studies in 34 months, or a Master of Studies in Law followed by MMS in Physician Assistant Studies in 36 months.

One Program, Two Locations: The Wake Forest PA Program is accredited for up to 64 students for the Winston-Salem campus and up to 24 students at the Boone campus.

Wingate University

220 N Camden St
Wingate, NC 28174
Phone: 704-233-8051
Email: pa@wingate.edu

PROGRAM HIGHLIGHTS

Accreditation: Continuing

Degree Offered: Master (MPAS)

Start Date: August annually

Program Length: 27 months

Class Capacity: 55 students
(between two campuses)

Tuition: $91,000

CASPA Participant: Yes

Supplemental Application: No

Yellow Ribbon: No

Admissions: Rolling

Application Deadline: January 15

PREREQUISITE COURSEWORK

Human Anatomy and Physiology I
and II with lab (8 credits), Genetics
(3 credits), Microbiology with lab (4
credits), Organic Chemistry with lab
(4 credits), Biochemistry (3 credits),
General Psychology (3 credits),
Statistics (3 credits), Medical
Terminology. Prerequisites must
be completed with a grade "C-" or
better. AP credits are accepted for
the Psychology prerequisite.

GPA Requirement: Science GPA 3.2

Healthcare Experience: 500 hours

PA Shadowing: Not required

Required Standardized Testing: GRE

Letters of Recommendation: Two
required; one must be from a
healthcare provider (MD, DO, PA or
NP)

Seat Deposit: $1,500

WINGATE UNIVERSITY

MISSION:

The Wingate University Physician Assistant Program is dedicated to developing educated, productive and ethical physician assistants to serve the healthcare needs of the community in which they practice.

CLASS OF 2020

Male: 27%

Female: 73%

Minority: 16%

Science GPA: >3.2 for 80% of students

GRE Total: >300 for 100% of students

Average Healthcare Experience: >1,000 hours for 79% of students

PANCE SCORES

5-year First Time Pass: 99%

Most Recent First Time Pass: 98%

CURRICULUM STRUCTURE

Didactic: 12 months

Clinical: 15 months

Rotations: 8 mandatory, 2 elective (each 5 weeks)

Capstone Project: Required for graduation

UNIQUE PROGRAM FEATURES

One Program, Two Locations: The Wingate Program is accredited for up to 55 students, 40 of which are placed at the Wingate campus and 15 of which are placed at the Hendersonville campus. Each campus follows the same curriculum, utilizing synchronous distance learning.

PA Advantage Program: Approximately 10% of students are accepted through this pathway, which guarantees high school seniors an interview into the PA program if they meet certain criteria throughout their tenure at Wingate.

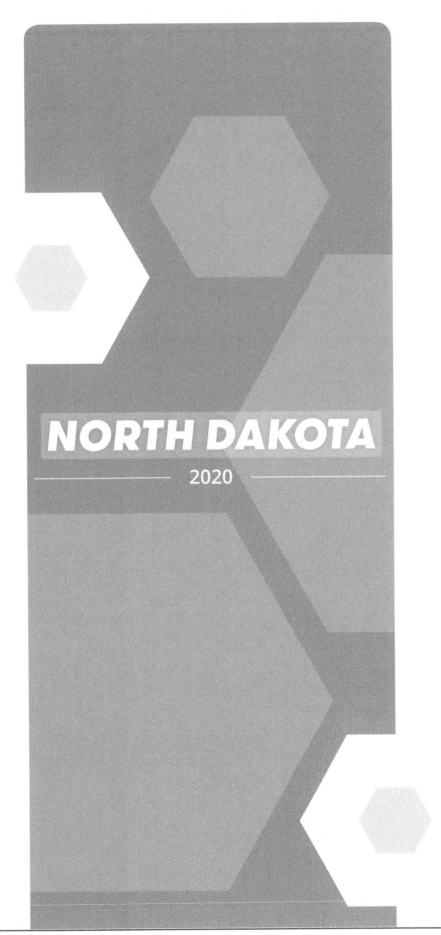

NORTH DAKOTA

2020

PROGRAM HIGHLIGHTS

Accreditation: Continuing

Degree Offered: Master (MPAS)

Start Date: May annually

Program Length: 24 months

Class Capacity: 35 students

Tuition: $40,808 (in-state); $51,826 (contiguous states); $61,212 (out-of-state)

CASPA Participant: Yes

Supplemental Application: Yes ($35 fee)

Yellow Ribbon: Yes

Admissions: Non-rolling

Application Deadline: September 1

PREREQUISITE COURSEWORK

Track 1: Human Anatomy (3 credits), Human Physiology (3 credits), Microbiology, Medical Terminology, Statistics. Track 2: Track 1 courses plus Psychology (3 credits) and two of Organic Chemistry, Biochemistry, Cellular Biology or Molecular Biology (6 credits). Prerequisites must be completed with a grade "B" or better, except Organic Chemistry and Biochemistry, which require a "C" or better. Recommended courses: Pharmacology, Genetics.

GPA Requirement: Overall GPA 3.0; Prerequisite GPA 3.0

Healthcare Experience: Track 1: Licensed/Certified Health Care Professional with minimum of 3 years experience. Track 2: Science-based educational background and minimum of 500 (1,000 preferred) hours of direct patient care.

PA Shadowing: Not required

Required Standardized Testing: None

Letters of Recommendation: Three required; one educational, one clinical, and one personal letter

Seat Deposit: $500

UNIVERSITY OF NORTH DAKOTA

MISSION:

The primary mission of the University of North Dakota Department of Physician Assistant Studies is to prepare selected students to become competent physician assistants working collaboratively with physicians, emphasizing primary care in rural and/or underserved communities.

NO CLASS STATISTICS REPORTED

PANCE SCORES

5-year First Time Pass: 93%

Most Recent First Time Pass: 97%

CURRICULUM STRUCTURE

Students begin with 2 semesters of online basic science coursework. They then return to campus over the next year and a half for several 2-6 week sessions of didactic primary care instruction. Between didactic sessions students complete primary care clerkships and specialty clerkships. During clerkships students are responsible for additional online coursework as well.

Thesis/Dissertation: Required for graduation

UNIQUE PROGRAM FEATURES

Track 1 Admissions: In this track, licensed or certified healthcare providers apply as a pair with a preceptor who has agreed to precept the student on their primary care clerkships throughout the program. Preference is given to pairs that have the clinical site in rural (<25,000 population) areas and/or are working with underserved populations.

Track 2 Admissions: In this track, students complete additional prerequisites and 500 hours of lower-level healthcare experience to be eligible for admissions. Students are placed by the program into their primary care clerkships and specialty clerkships. They apply as individuals.

Unique Curriculum: UND's PA Program is a unique hybrid of online coursework with alternating classroom and clinical experiences. The didactic primary care sessions are immediately followed by a clinical practice experience, providing quick application of concepts, resulting in greater development and retention of clinical competencies.

Admissions Preference: Residents from North Dakota, Montana, Minnesota and South Dakota are given admissions preference, although qualified out-of-state applicants are also readily accepted. Applicants from rural or underserved communities are also awarded preference.

277

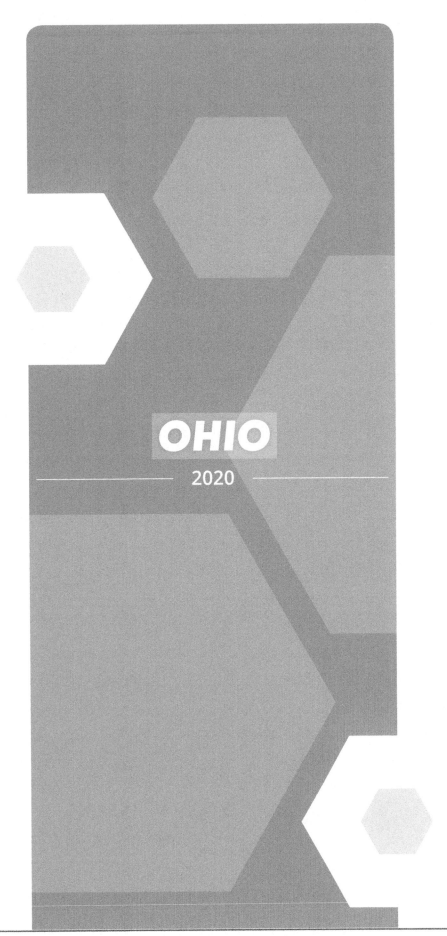

OHIO

2020

Baldwin Wallace University

275 Eastland Road
Berea, OH 44017
Phone: 440-826-8012
Email: paprogram@bw.edu

PROGRAM HIGHLIGHTS

Accreditation: Continuing
Degree Offered: Master (MMS)
Start Date: May annually
Program Length: 24 months
Class Capacity: 32 students
Tuition: $85,000 (including fees)

CASPA Participant: Yes
Supplemental Application: Yes (no fee)
Yellow Ribbon: No
Admissions: Rolling
Application Deadline: November 1

PREREQUISITE COURSEWORK

Biology I and II with lab, Anatomy and Physiology I and II with lab, Microbiology with lab, General Chemistry I and II with lab, Organic Chemistry I with lab, Introductory Psychology, English Composition, Statistics or Biostatistics, Medical Terminology. Prerequisites must be completed with a grade "C" or better and within the last 7 years. Some prerequisites may be in progress at the time of application. AP credits may be accepted. Recommended courses: Biochemistry, Genetics, Immunology, Histology, Embryology, Endocrinology, Epidemiology, Neuroscience, Pathophysiology, Virology, Medical/Bioethics, Public Health, Developmental/Abnormal Psychology, Algebra.

GPA Requirement: Overall GPA 3.0; Science GPA 3.0

Healthcare Experience: Preferred, not required

PA Shadowing: 40 hours

Required Standardized Testing: GRE

Letters of Recommendation: Three required; one from a physician or PA, one from a college professor or advisor, and one from a work manager or supervisor

Seat Deposit: $1,500

BALDWIN WALLACE UNIVERSITY

MISSION:

To educate talented physician assistants who strive to promote the PA profession, understand the primary care workforce needs of the future, and act competently when providing excellent patient care utilizing an evidence-based and dynamic team approach.

CLASS OF 2021

Overall GPA: 3.83

Science GPA: 3.89

PANCE SCORES

5-year First Time Pass: 100%

Most Recent First Time Pass: 100%

CURRICULUM STRUCTURE

Didactic: 12 months

Clinical: 12 months

Rotations: 8 mandatory, 3 elective (each 4 weeks)

Research Project: Required for graduation

UNIQUE PROGRAM FEATURES

Admission Preferences: Preference is given to previous graduates of Baldwin Wallace University, Ohio residents and those with previous direct patient care experience.

Leadership and Public Health Curriculum: Students take courses in healthcare leadership and public health and policy, which are designed to give students the foundation to become effective leaders and understand how healthcare reform and public health policy impact PA practice.

PROGRAM HIGHLIGHTS

Accreditation: Provisional

Degree Offered: Master (MSPAS)

Start Date: May annually

Program Length: 27 months

Class Capacity: 36 students

Tuition: $92,372

CASPA Participant: Yes

Supplemental Application: No

Yellow Ribbon: No

Admissions: Rolling

Application Deadline: November 1

PREREQUISITE COURSEWORK

Biology with lab (4 credits), Human Anatomy with lab (4 credits), Human Physiology with lab (4 credits), Microbiology with lab (3 credits), Organic Chemistry with lab (8 credits), Biochemistry (3 credits), Psychology (3 credits), Statistics (3 credits), Medical Terminology (1 credit). Applicants may have up to two prerequisites in progress at the time of application but they must be completed no later than the fall semester of the year of application. Prerequisites must be completed within the last 10 years. AP credits may be accepted.

GPA Requirement: Overall GPA 3.0; Science GPA 3.0 (or for the last 40 credit hours for both)

Healthcare Experience: 1,000 hours

PA Shadowing: Preferred, not required

Required Standardized Testing: GRE

Letters of Recommendation: Three required; one from a healthcare professional who has known the applicant for at least 6 months

Seat Deposit: $500

CASE WESTERN RESERVE UNIVERSITY

MISSION:

The CWRU Physician Assistant Program strives to improve access to health care through the education and development of compassionate, highly competent physician assistants who are prepared to provide quality, patient-centered care in a collaborative environment and who are dedicated to clinical competence, medical professionalism, leadership, community outreach, cultural humility, and innovation.

CLASS OF 2021

Male: 36%

Female: 64%

Minority: 41%

Overall GPA: 3.50

Science GPA: 3.50

Prerequisite GPA: 3.40

GRE Quantitative: 50th percentile

GRE Verbal: 56th percentile

GRE Analytical: 65th percentile

Average Healthcare Experience: 3,450 hours

PANCE SCORES

5-year First Time Pass: 100% (based on two years of data)

Most Recent First Time Pass: 100%

CURRICULUM STRUCTURE

Didactic: 15 months

Clinical: 12 months

Rotations: 8 mandatory, 1 primary care elective, 1 inpatient elective, 2 other elective (each 4 weeks)

Capstone Project: Required for graduation

UNIQUE PROGRAM FEATURES

Clinical Experience: As one of the top 25 medical schools in the nation, students will have the chance to practice in both the clinical environment of the program's top-notch affiliated hospitals and in the school's Mt. Sinai Skills and Simulation Center. Students also complete a longitudinal pre-clinical experience in the first year of study.

Elective Coursework: Students can electively study medical Spanish and research methods in addition to the regular PA curriculum.

Non-traditional Learning: Learning experiences that take place in non-traditional settings is one of the unique features of the Case PA program. Based on the program's goal to prepare students to address community health issues and health disparities in the context of societal and economic systems, they have created experiential learning and community outreach activities that are built into the curriculum.

Health Education Campus: In summer 2019, Case Western Reserve University and Cleveland Clinic opened the Health Education Campus to bring medical, nursing, dental medicine and physician assistant students together to learn with—and from—each other. Through the interprofessional education model, students come together for some of their traditional health courses, as well as new offerings focused specifically on elements of successful teams.

PROGRAM HIGHLIGHTS

Accreditation: Continuing

Degree Offered: Master (MPAS)

Start Date: May annually

Program Length: 27 months

Class Capacity: 60 students

Tuition: $89,446

CASPA Participant: Yes

Supplemental Application: No

Yellow Ribbon: No

Admissions: Rolling

Application Deadline: October 1

PREREQUISITE COURSEWORK

Organic Chemistry I and II with lab (8 credits), Biochemistry (4 credits), Human Anatomy and Physiology with lab (8 credits), Microbiology with lab (4 credits), General Biology with lab (4 credits), General Psychology (3 credits), Developmental or Abnormal Psychology (3 credits), Statistics (3 credits). Prerequisites may be in progress at the time of application but all must be completed within the last 10 years. Prerequisites must be completed with a grade "C" or better.

GPA Requirement: Prerequisite GPA 3.0

Healthcare Experience: Preferred, not required (250 hours recommended)

PA Shadowing: Preferred, not required

Required Standardized Testing: GRE, CASPer

Letters of Recommendation: Three required; no more than one may be from a professor

Seat Deposit: $500

KETTERING COLLEGE

MISSION:

The mission of the Kettering College physician assistant studies program is to provide, in a Christian environment, the academic and clinical experience necessary to develop competent empathetic professional health care providers who are dedicated to lifelong learning.

CLASS OF 2021

Male: 22%

Female: 78%

Overall GPA: 3.62

Prerequisite GPA: 3.57

Average Age: 23

PANCE SCORES

5-year First Time Pass: 99%

Most Recent First Time Pass: 100%

CURRICULUM STRUCTURE

Didactic: 15 months

Clinical: 12 months

Rotations: 7 mandatory, 1 elective (each 5 weeks)

Capstone Project: Required for graduation

UNIQUE PROGRAM FEATURES

Adventist Tradition: Students can complete courses in spirituality in healing and healthcare as well as two semesters of clinical ethics in line with the college's founding principles.

Admissions Preference: Bonus consideration is awarded to students who have completed at least 7 credit hours at Kettering College.

Service Learning: Students often complete community service including patient education and screenings at the free medical/dental clinic for the underserved in Dayton, Ohio.

PROGRAM HIGHLIGHTS

Accreditation: Continuing

Degree Offered: Master (MSPAS)

Start Date: May annually

Program Length: 27 months

Class Capacity: 26 students

Tuition: $86,800

CASPA Participant: Yes

Supplemental Application: No

Yellow Ribbon: No

Admissions: Rolling

Application Deadline: December 1

PREREQUISITE COURSEWORK

General Chemistry I and II with lab (2 courses), Organic Chemistry with lab (1 course), Biology I and II with lab (2 courses), Human Anatomy and Physiology I and II with lab (2 courses), Microbiology with lab (1 course), Genetics (1 course), Statistics (1 course), Psychology (1 course), English (2 courses), College Algebra (1 course), Medical Terminology (tested during interviews). Prerequisites must be completed with a grade "B" or better, except Organic Chemistry, which requires a "C" or better. Prerequisites should be completed within the last 7 years.

GPA Requirement: Overall GPA 3.2

Healthcare Experience: 250 hours

PA Shadowing: 50 hours (counts towards healthcare experience)

Required Standardized Testing: GRE

Letters of Recommendation: Three required; one from a physician or PA, one from a college professor, and one choice reference

Seat Deposit: $1,500

LAKE ERIE COLLEGE

MISSION:

To recruit exemplary individuals from diverse backgrounds while creating an environment of academic excellence, leadership, and scholarly activity that produces culturally competent, compassionate Physician Assistants who practice evidence-based medicine and who are dedicated to serving the healthcare needs of the community.

CLASS OF 2020

Overall GPA: 3.55

Average Healthcare Experience: 2,799 hours

PANCE SCORES

5-year First Time Pass: 100% (based on four years of data)

Most Recent First Time Pass: 100%

CURRICULUM STRUCTURE

Didactic: 15 months

Clinical: 12 months

Rotations:
7 mandatory,
3 elective
(each 4 weeks)

UNIQUE PROGRAM FEATURES

Admissions Preference: All Lake Erie College students and graduates who meet the minimum requirements will be granted an interview. Lake Erie College students and graduates will be given some preference in admission.

Early Clinical Experiences: These start within the first few weeks of the program and can include interprofessional tumor board, coroner's office, nursing homes, emergency departments, operating rooms and genetics laboratory.

Community Service: All students perform community-based projects and service. All have participated in a community service learning project and have continued with community projects including Fresh Air Camp, Geauga Faith Rescue Mission, Hospice of Western Reserve, Kids Kicking Cancer, Lake County Free Clinic, Medwish, oral health at local elementary schools, Relay for Life, and Victory Gallop.

Dual Degree: Students can apply 12 credits from the PA program to an MBA degree at Lake Erie and are automatically accepted into the MBA program if desired.

Student Bios: Available on the program's website to learn more about the typical student the program accepts.

Marietta College

215 Fifth Street
Marietta, OH 45750
Phone: 740-376-4458
Email: paprogram@marietta.edu

PROGRAM HIGHLIGHTS

Accreditation: Continuing

Degree Offered: Master (MSPAS)

Start Date: June annually

Program Length: 26 months

Class Capacity: 36 students

Tuition: $77,534

CASPA Participant: Yes

Supplemental Application: No

Yellow Ribbon Program: Yes

Admissions: Rolling

Application Deadline: November 1

PREREQUISITE COURSEWORK

Human or Mammalian Upper Level Biology (3 credits), General Chemistry I and II with lab (8 credits), Organic Chemistry with lab (4 credits), Microbiology with lab (3 credits), Human Anatomy with lab (3 credits), Human Physiology (3 credits), General Psychology (3 credits), Upper Level Psychology (3 credits), Statistics (3 credits). Prerequisites must be completed with a grade "C" or better, within the last 10 years, and should be completed by December prior to beginning the program. AP credits for up to two prerequisites will be accepted. Recommended courses: Genetics, Immunology, Virology, Biochemistry, Histology, Pathophysiology, Toxicology.

GPA Requirement: Prerequisite GPA 3.0

Healthcare Experience: Preferred, not required

PA Shadowing: Not required

Required Standardized Testing: GRE or MCAT

Letters of Recommendation: Three required; one should be from a healthcare professional who has known you for at least six months

Seat Deposit: $1,000

MARIETTA COLLEGE

MISSION:

The Marietta College Physician Assistant Program is dedicated to educating future physician assistants to provide quality health care to meet the needs of patients in Ohio and throughout the Appalachian region. The program accomplishes this mission by educating individuals who have the academic, clinical and interpersonal proficiencies necessary to practice as physician assistants.

CLASS STATISTICS (LAST 4 COHORTS)

Overall GPA: 3.66

Prerequisite GPA: 3.70

GRE Verbal: 152

GRE Quantitative: 151

Average Healthcare Experience: 2,500 hours

Average Age: 23

PANCE SCORES

5-year First Time Pass: 98%

Most Recent First Time Pass: 92%

CURRICULUM STRUCTURE

Didactic: 12 months

Clinical: 14 months

Rotations: 9 mandatory (each 5 weeks), 2 elective (each 4 weeks)

Capstone Project: Required for graduation

UNIQUE PROGRAM FEATURES

Admissions: Applicants who would like to be considered for "early" interviews must have their CASPA application completed by August 1 of the year of application. Marietta college students and alumni will be given special consideration. There is also a direct admissions pathway for a limited number of high school students.

Scholarship: Two students per class will be chosen to receive the Paul Spear Appalachia Scholarship, which is based on the applicant's desire to provide healthcare in the Southeastern Ohio and/or Appalachia area and financial need. The award covers half of the tuition for both the didactic and clinical phases of the Program as long as the student maintains a 3.0 GPA throughout the program. In repayment of the scholarship, the student commits to a one-for-one service agreement to practice in the Southeastern Ohio and/or Appalachia area for each year of the scholarship award.

285

Mount St. Joseph University

Graduate Admissions
5701 Delhi Road
Cincinnati, OH 45233
Phone: 513-244-4375
Email: PAprogram@msj.edu

PROGRAM HIGHLIGHTS

Accreditation: Provisional

Degree Offered: Master (MPAS)

Start Date: January annually

Program Length: 27 months

Class Capacity: 32 students

Tuition: $85,400 (including fees)

CASPA Participant: Yes

Supplemental Application: No

Yellow Ribbon: Yes

Admissions: Not reported

Application Deadline: December 1

PREREQUISITE COURSEWORK

General Chemistry with lab (2 semesters), Organic Chemistry with lab, Biochemistry, General Biology with lab (2 semesters), Microbiology, Anatomy and Physiology with lab (2 semesters), Developmental Psychology, Statistics. Prerequisites must be completed within the last 5 years and with a grade "C" or better.

GPA Requirement: Overall GPA 3.0; Science GPA 3.0

Healthcare Experience: 500 hours

PA Shadowing: 40 hours

Required Standardized Testing: GRE

Letters of Recommendation: Three required; one from a professor/supervisor, one from a PA, and one from a professional/social colleague

Seat Deposit: $1,000

MOUNT ST. JOSEPH UNIVERSITY

MISSION:

The specific mission of the Mount St. Joseph University Physician Assistant program is to educate outstanding, compassionate clinicians, fully prepared to deliver high quality, accessible health care, demonstrating commitment to life-long learning and ethical practice.

NO CLASS STATISTICS REPORTED

PANCE SCORES

5-year First Time Pass: N/A

Most Recent First Time Pass: N/A (have not graduated a class yet)

CURRICULUM STRUCTURE

Didactic: 12 months

Clinical: 15 months

Rotations: 9 mandatory, 2 elective (each 5 weeks)

UNIQUE PROGRAM FEATURES

Admissions Preference: Preference will be given to those applicants who are graduates of Mount St. Joseph University, veterans of the Armed Forces, residents of Greater Cincinnati, and applicants with significant prior health-care experience, shadowing, higher GPA and higher GRE.

Facilities: There is an on campus Simulation Lab featuring Simulation IQ with audiovisual recording capability and embedded electronic health record, as well as an Advanced Anatomy Lab including the AnatomageTM virtual anatomy program to supplement cadaver specimens.

Ohio Dominican University

Physician Assistant Studies
St. Albert Hall, Room 215
1216 Sunbury Road
Columbus, OH 43219
Phone: 614-251-4320
Email:
paprogram@ohiodominican.edu

PROGRAM HIGHLIGHTS

Accreditation: Continuing

Degree Offered: Master (MSPAS)

Start Date: August annually

Program Length: 27 months

Class Capacity: 50 students

Tuition: $77,362

CASPA Participant: Yes

Supplemental Application: No

Yellow Ribbon: No

Admissions: Non-rolling

Application Deadline: October 1

PREREQUISITE COURSEWORK

Inorganic/General Chemistry with lab (4 credits), Organic Chemistry with lab (4 credits), Biochemistry (3 credits), Human Anatomy and Physiology (6 credits), Microbiology with lab (4 credits), General Biology I and II (6 credits), Intro to Psychology (3 credits), Additional Upper Level Psychology (3 credits), College Algebra or Higher Math (3 credits), Statistics (3 credits), 4 Humanities courses (12 credits). Prerequisites must be completed with a grade "C" or better and ideally within the last 8 years. Preference is given to applicants with the majority of academic work completed prior to application.

GPA Requirement: Overall GPA 3.0; Science GPA 3.0

Healthcare Experience: 250 hours

PA Shadowing: Preferred, not required

Required Standardized Testing: GRE or MCAT

Letters of Recommendation: Two required; at least one should be from a clinician working in healthcare

Seat Deposit: $1,500

OHIO DOMINICAN UNIVERSITY

MISSION:

Ohio Dominican's Physician Assistant Studies Program will educate students to become well-qualified, competent physician assistants practicing in physician supervised primary care and specialty patient focused teams. The ODU PA Program embraces a holistic approach to the pursuit of excellence in academics, research, clinical practice and community service.

NO CLASS STATISTICS REPORTED

PANCE SCORES

5-year First Time Pass: 98%

Most Recent First Time Pass: 98%

CURRICULUM STRUCTURE

Didactic: 15 months

Clinical: 12 months

Rotations: 7 mandatory, 4 elective (each 4 weeks)

UNIQUE PROGRAM FEATURES

Admissions Preference: Preference will be given to current Ohio residents, graduates of Ohio Dominican University, past or present members of the armed forces, and those with significant health care experience.

Facilities: The state-of-the-art PA program building located in St. Albert Hall includes cadaver labs, simulation labs, wet labs, science classrooms, collaboration rooms, and a student lounge.

Mission Trips: There are medical mission trips available to students in places like Haiti and Dominican Republic.

Commitment to Service: ODU's PA Program is developing partnerships with organizations in Central Ohio to engage in service opportunities throughout the community. Further, all students will perform a service-component during the didactic phase for the course "Diverse & Vulnerable Patient Populations."

Ohio University

Division of Physician Assistant Practice
6805 Bobcat Way, Suite 112
Dublin, OH 43016
Phone: 614-793-5619
Email: painfo@ohio.edu;
paadmissions@ohio.edu

PROGRAM HIGHLIGHTS

Accreditation: Continuing

Degree Offered: Master (MPAP)

Start Date: May annually

Program Length: 27 months

Class Capacity: 45 students

Tuition: $58,300 (in-state);
$60,238 (out-of-state)

CASPA Participant: Yes

Supplemental Application: Yes ($50 fee)

Yellow Ribbon: No

Admissions: Non-rolling

Application Deadline: August 1

PREREQUISITE COURSEWORK

Human Anatomy with lab (4 credits), Human Physiology (3-4 credits), Biology with lab (8 credits), Microbiology with lab (3-4 credits), General Chemistry with lab (8 credits), Organic Chemistry with lab (4 credits), Biochemistry (3 credits), Statistics (3 credits), College Algebra or higher (3 credits), General Psychology (3 credits), Abnormal/Developmental/Physiological Psychology (3 credits), Medical Terminology (2 credits or completion of an online course). Prerequisites must be completed with a grade "C" or better. At most two prerequisites may be outstanding at the time of application. Anatomy and Physiology must be completed within the last 5 years. AP credits may be accepted.

GPA Requirement: Overall GPA 3.0; Science/Math GPA 3.0

Healthcare Experience: Required (no specific number of hours)

PA Shadowing: Not required

Required Standardized Testing: GRE

Letters of Recommendation: Two required; one from a physician or PA

Seat Deposit: $1,000

OHIO UNIVERSITY

MISSION:

The mission of the Ohio University Master of Physician Assistant Practice program is to prepare students to be leaders in PA practice in any clinical setting, with a particular emphasis on primary care in urban and rural underserved communities in the State of Ohio and throughout Appalachia, using an interprofessional team approach.

CLASS OF 2021

Overall GPA: 3.60

Science/Math GPA: 3.52

GRE Verbal: 153

GRE Quantitative: 151

GRE Analytical: 4.0

PANCE SCORES

5-year First Time Pass: 98% (based on three years of data)

Most Recent First Time Pass: 100%

CURRICULUM STRUCTURE

Didactic: 15 months

Clinical: 12 months

Rotations: 8 mandatory, 3 selective (each 4 weeks)

Graduate Research Project: Required for graduation

UNIQUE PROGRAM FEATURES

Admissions Preference: The OU PA Program is actively seeking candidates who are residents of Appalachia regions of Ohio and the US Military. The program defines U.S. Military as active duty, reserves or veteran status from the Army, Marine Corps, Navy, Air Force, Coast Guard and National Guard.

Underserved Focus: In keeping with the mission of Ohio University, students enrolled in the OUPA Program will complete a portion of their clinical training in medically underserved areas of Ohio.

University of Dayton

300 College Park
Fitz Hall 510
Dayton, OH 45469
Phone: 937-299-2900
Email: akidwell1@udayton.edu

PROGRAM HIGHLIGHTS

Accreditation: Probation

Degree Offered: Master (MPAP)

Start Date: August annually

Program Length: 27 months

Class Capacity: 40 students

Tuition: $78,988 (including some fees)

CASPA Participant: Yes

Supplemental Application: No

Yellow Ribbon: No

Admissions: Non-rolling

Application Deadline: November 1

PREREQUISITE COURSEWORK

Human Anatomy and Physiology with lab (8 credits), Microbiology with lab (3-4 credits), Organic Chemistry I and II with lab (8 credits), Biochemistry (3-4 credits), General Psychology (3 credits), second Psychology course (3 credits), Statistics (3-4 credits), Medical Terminology (2-3 credits). Up to two prerequisites may be in progress at the time of application. Prerequisites must be completed with a grade "C" or better. All science courses must be completed within the last 10 years. AP credits are accepted for up to two prerequisites.

GPA Requirement: Overall GPA 3.0; Science GPA 3.0; Prerequisite GPA 3.0

Healthcare Experience: 250 hours (+20 hours of community service required)

PA Shadowing: 20 hours

Required Standardized Testing: None

Letters of Recommendation: Three required; one from a recent college professor, one from a health care professional who has known the applicant for at least 6 months, and one of the applicant's choice

Seat Deposit: $1,000

UNIVERSITY OF DAYTON

MISSION:

The mission of the Department of Physician Assistant Education is to produce physician assistants who are committed to the service of the human person through the skillful, compassionate, and ethical provision of health care within the context of the Catholic Marianist tradition. We emphasize excellent generalist care for the whole person, particularly upholding dignity for society's most vulnerable, in a learning environment which emphasizes leadership, life-long learning, and service.

NO CLASS STATISTICS REPORTED

PANCE SCORES

5-year First Time Pass: 95% (based on three years of data)

Most Recent First Time Pass: 100%

CURRICULUM STRUCTURE

Didactic: 15 months

Clinical: 12 months

Rotations: 8 mandatory, 1 elective (each 4-10 weeks)

Capstone Project: Required for graduation

UNIQUE PROGRAM FEATURES

Facilities: State-of-the-art facilities include a student resource room and lounge, small group classrooms, mock examination rooms, and several simulation rooms. Rooms are equipped with the latest technology to maximize the use of devices, including tablets.

Admissions Preference: Special consideration is given to current University of Dayton students and graduates of other Marianist Universities.

289

The University of Findlay

Physician Assistant Program
1000 North Main Street
Findlay, OH 45840
Phone: 419-434-4529
Email: paprogram@findlay.edu

PROGRAM HIGHLIGHTS

Accreditation: Continuing

Degree Offered: Master (MPA)

Start Date: August annually

Program Length: 28 months

Class Capacity: 18 students

Tuition: $86,117

CASPA Participant: Yes

Supplemental Application: Yes ($50 fee)

Yellow Ribbon: Yes

Admissions: Non-rolling

Application Deadline: October 1

PREREQUISITE COURSEWORK

Human Anatomy and Physiology I and II with lab, Microbiology with lab, Human Genetics, General Chemistry I and II with lab, Basic Organic and Biochemistry with lab or Organic Chemistry I with lab, General Physics I with lab, Medical Terminology, Statistics or higher math, General Psychology. Prerequisites must be completed with a grade "C" or better, and there must be no more than two courses with a grade of "C". Prerequisites should be completed within the last 10 years but ideally within the last 5 years. AP credits are not accepted.

GPA Requirement: Overall GPA 3.0; Science GPA 3.0; Prerequisite GPA 3.0; Non-Science GPA 3.0

Healthcare Experience: Preferred, not required

PA Shadowing: Preferred, not required

Required Standardized Testing: None

Letters of Recommendation: Three required; ideally, one from a professor, one from an employer, and one from a clinician (PA, MD, NP)

Seat Deposit: $1,000

UNIVERSITY OF FINDLAY

MISSION:

The mission of the Physician Assistant program at The University of Findlay is to provide our students with the medical knowledge, technical skills, and experience in a variety of didactic and clinical settings necessary for them to become ethical, competent, and compassionate health care providers as part of the health care team. This mission complements the University of Findlay's mission, which is to equip students for meaningful lives and productive careers.

NO CLASS STATISTICS REPORTED

PANCE SCORES

5-year First Time Pass: 99%

Most Recent First Time Pass: 94%

CURRICULUM STRUCTURE

Didactic: 16 months

Clinical: 12 months

Rotations: 7 mandatory, 1 elective (each 6 weeks)

Capstone Project: Required for graduation

UNIQUE PROGRAM FEATURES

Small Class Size: The 18 student class allows for one-on-one mentoring of students by faculty and fosters a tight knit community for academic activities, social activities, and community service/engagement.

Admissions Preference: The program offers a small number of additional admission points to: applicants who have more extensive or more highly skilled healthcare experience, honorably discharged veterans, and to individuals who have taken at least 30 semester hours of coursework at The University of Findlay.

University of Mount Union

Physician Assistant Studies Program
1972 Clark Avenue
Alliance, OH 44601
Phone: 330-823-2419
Email: scarpill@mountunion.edu

PROGRAM HIGHLIGHTS

Accreditation: Continuing

Degree Offered: Master (MSPAS)

Start Date: May annually

Program Length: 27 months

Class Capacity: 40 students

Tuition: $80,500

CASPA Participant: Yes

Supplemental Application: No

Yellow Ribbon: No

Admissions: Non-rolling

Application Deadline: October 1

PREREQUISITE COURSEWORK

English Composition (3-4 credits), General Psychology (3-4 credits), General Biology I and II with lab or upper level Biology coursework (8 credits), Anatomy and Physiology I and II with lab (8 credits), Genetics (2-4 credits), Inorganic/General Chemistry with lab (3-4 credits), Organic Chemistry I with lab (3-4 credits), Elementary Statistics or Biostatistics (3-4 credits), Microbiology with lab (4 credits), Medical Terminology (assessed by a proficiency exam during orientation). Prerequisites must be completed with a grade "C" or better and within the last 10 years. Up to two prerequisites may be pending at the time of application.

GPA Requirement: Overall GPA 3.0; Science GPA 3.0; Prerequisite GPA 3.0

Healthcare Experience: Preferred, not required

PA Shadowing: 40 hours

Required Standardized Testing: GRE

Letters of Recommendation: Three required; one must be from a physician or PA

Seat Deposit: $1,500

UNIVERSITY OF MOUNT UNION

MISSION:

The mission of the Mount Union Physician Assistant Studies Program is to educate knowledgeable, competent, and compassionate physician assistants who, under physician supervision, provide patient care with professionalism and integrity.

NO CLASS STATISTICS REPORTED

PANCE SCORES

5-year First Time Pass: 99%

Most Recent First Time Pass: 100%

CURRICULUM STRUCTURE

Didactic: 15 months

Clinical: 12 months

Rotations: 8 mandatory, 2 elective (each 4 weeks)

Capstone Project: Required for graduation

UNIQUE PROGRAM FEATURES

Admissions Preference: Preference in the selection of students for the interview process will be given to University of Mount Union graduates who meet all other admissions prerequisites.

University of Toledo

3000 Arlington Avenue, Mail Stop 1027
Toledo, OH 43614
Phone: 419-383-5408
Email: physicianassistant@utoledo.edu

PROGRAM HIGHLIGHTS

Accreditation: Continuing

Degree Offered: Master (MSBS)

Start Date: August annually

Program Length: 27 months

Class Capacity: 30 students

Tuition: $63,102 (in-state, including fees); $102,302 (out-of-state, including fees)

CASPA Participant: Yes

Supplemental Application: Yes ($45 fee)

Yellow Ribbon: No

Admissions: Rolling

Application Deadline: October 1

PREREQUISITE COURSEWORK

Human Anatomy and Physiology I and II (6 credits), Inorganic/General Chemistry with lab (4 credits), Organic Chemistry or Biochemistry with lab (4 credits), Microbiology with lab (4 credits), Psychology (6 credits), Genetics (3 credits), College Algebra or Statistics or higher Math (3 credits), Medical Terminology (1 credit). Prerequisites must be completed within the last 8 years and with a grade "B-" or better. At most three prerequisites may be in progress at the time of interviews. AP credits are not accepted. Recommended courses: Introductory Psychology, Lifespan Psychology.

GPA Requirement: Overall GPA 3.4; Science GPA 3.4

Healthcare Experience: Not required

PA Shadowing: Not required

Required Standardized Testing: GRE

Letters of Recommendation: Three required; no one specific

Seat Deposit: $300

UNIVERSITY OF TOLEDO

MISSION:

The mission of the UT Physician Assistant Program is to provide a comprehensive and student-centered academic and clinical education to develop competent, compassionate, and primary care oriented PAs who are capable of providing high-quality, cost effective, patient centered health care in diverse settings.

CLASS OF 2018

Male: 33%

Female: 67%

Minority: 30%

PANCE SCORES

5-year First Time Pass: 89%

Most Recent First Time Pass: 93%

CURRICULUM STRUCTURE

Didactic: 17 months

Clinical: 10 months

Rotations: 7 mandatory, 1 elective (each 4 weeks), Primary Care preceptorship (8 weeks)

Scholarly Project: Required for graduation

UNIQUE PROGRAM FEATURES

Facilities: The UTPA Program and the College of Nursing share the fine facilities of the Collier Building on the Health Science Campus. The Physician Assistant Program classrooms and laboratories are state-of-the-art and include modern educational technology such as the Interprofessional Immersion Skill Center, The Center for Creative Instruction and The Ruth M. Hillebrand Clinical Skills Center.

Admissions Preference: The University of Toledo College of Medicine and Life Sciences value added groups (current Ohio residents, graduates of The University of Toledo, non-traditional, underrepresented in medicine and veterans) are given some degree of preference.

Underserved Focus: The UT PA Program students have multiple opportunities to provide care to the underserved populations in the community. Students may participate in the student-led Community Care Clinics (CCC), a free clinic established to provide primary care, women's health care, diabetes management, chiropractic services, and respiratory therapy to the underserved in the community. PA students also have an opportunity to volunteer with community physicians, PAs, and NPs at That Neighborhood Free Health Clinic. The College of Medicine and Life Sciences participates in medical mission teams with the Global Health Program. PA students have an opportunity annually to serve on the Honduras mission trip and the Nicaragua Medical Mission Trip.

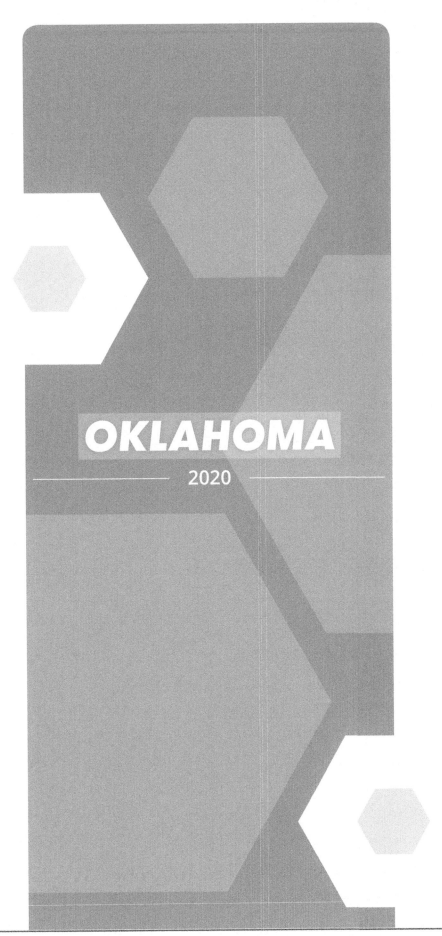

OKLAHOMA

2020

Oklahoma City University

2501 N. Blackwelder Ave
Oklahoma City, OK 73106
Phone: 405-208-6260
Email: paprogram@okcu.edu

PROGRAM HIGHLIGHTS

Accreditation: Provisional

Degree Offered: Master (MPAS)

Start Date: January annually

Program Length: 28 months

Class Capacity: 36 students

Tuition: $90,300

CASPA Participant: Yes

Supplemental Application: Yes ($60 fee)

Yellow Ribbon: No

Admissions: Non-rolling

Application Deadline: August 1

PREREQUISITE COURSEWORK

Biological Sciences (at least 5 courses totaling 15 credits), Chemistry (at least 3 courses, one of which must be Biochemistry), Psychology (2 courses). Prerequisites must be completed with a grade "C" or better and by August 15th of the year of application. Having a strong GPA in the last 60 credits makes you a more competitive applicant. Recommended courses: Anatomy, Physiology, Cell Biology, Molecular Biology, Embryology, Immunology, Microbiology.

GPA Requirement: Overall GPA 3.0

Healthcare Experience: Preferred, not required

PA Shadowing: Preferred, not required

Required Standardized Testing: None

Letters of Recommendation: Three required; preferably from individuals who can provide an objective evaluation of your work ethic, character, empathy, and academic performance

Seat Deposit: $150

OKLAHOMA CITY UNIVERSITY

MISSION:

To prepare physician assistants who are competent in the art and science of medicine so that they may improve lives in the communities they serve.

NO CLASS STATISTICS REPORTED

PANCE SCORES

5-year First Time Pass: 93% (based on two years of data)

Most Recent First Time Pass: 86%

CURRICULUM STRUCTURE

Didactic: 12 months

Clinical: 16 months

Rotations: 7 mandatory (each 4-8 weeks), 6 medicine/electives (each 4 weeks), 1 preceptorship (4 weeks)

UNIQUE PROGRAM FEATURES

Business Focus: The program has several courses to familiarize students with the business of medicine, including Operationalizing a Medical Practice; Health Care Financial Strategies; Accessing the Community; Reimbursement, Documentation of Care, Coding and Billing; and Contracts and Medical Law.

Clinical: Each student completes a 4-week rotation in one of the charity clinics in the Oklahoma City area as part of their clinical year.

University of Oklahoma, Oklahoma City

Physician Associate Program
College of Medicine
940 Stanton L. Young, Ste. 357
Oklahoma City, OK 73104
Phone: 405-271-2058
Email: infookc-pa@ouhsc.edu

PROGRAM HIGHLIGHTS

Accreditation: Continuing

Degree Offered: Master (MHS)

Start Date: June annually

Program Length: 27 months

Class Capacity: 50 students

Tuition: $46,886 (in-state, including fees); $87,516 (out-of-state, including fees)

CASPA Participant: Yes

Supplemental Application: Yes ($75 fee)

Yellow Ribbon: No

Admissions: Non-rolling

Application Deadline: October 1

PREREQUISITE COURSEWORK

College Algebra or higher, Introduction to Psychology, Psychology elective, General Chemistry I and II, Human Anatomy, Human Physiology, Microbiology, Pathogenic Microbiology or Immunology or Virology or Genetics. Prerequisites must be completed with a grade "C" or better. At most one science and one non-science prerequisite may be in progress after December 31st of the year prior to matriculation.

GPA Requirement: Overall GPA 3.0; Science GPA 3.0

Healthcare Experience: Preferred, not required

PA Shadowing: Preferred, not required (students encouraged to shadow at least 3 different PAs in different specialties)

Required Standardized Testing: GRE (waived if you already hold a Master's degree), CASPer

Letters of Recommendation: Three required; no one specific

Seat Deposit: $150

UNIVERSITY OF OKLAHOMA, OKLAHOMA CITY

MISSION:

Our mission is to attract the best talent in the region from diverse backgrounds and equip them with the capability to provide excellent patient care.

CLASS OF 2020

Male: 30%

Female: 70%

Minority: 36%

Overall GPA: 3.70

Science GPA: 3.70

GRE Total: 302

Average Age: 25

PANCE SCORES

5-year First Time Pass: 95%

Most Recent First Time Pass: 98%

CURRICULUM STRUCTURE

Didactic: 15 months

Clinical: 12 months

Rotations: 8 mandatory, 2 elective (each 4-8 weeks)

Research Project: Required for graduation

UNIQUE PROGRAM FEATURES

Original Programs: This program is one of the original six accredited programs in the United States and has maintained continuous accreditation since 1972.

PROGRAM HIGHLIGHTS

Accreditation: Continuing

Degree Offered: Master (MHS)

Start Date: June annually

Program Length: 30 months

Class Capacity: 24 students

Tuition: $45,690 (in-state);
$87,297 (out-of-state)

CASPA Participant: Yes

Supplemental Application: Yes ($75 fee)

Yellow Ribbon: Yes

Admissions: Non-rolling

Application Deadline: October 1

PREREQUISITE COURSEWORK

English Composition I and II (6 credits), College Algebra (3 credits), Psychology (6 credits), Chemistry (12 credits, at least 3 of which must be Organic Chemistry or Biochemistry with lab), Microbiology with lab (4 credits), Upper Division Science (6 credits), Human Anatomy with lab (4 credits), Human Physiology with lab (4 credits). Anatomy, Physiology, and Upper Division Sciences must be completed within the last 7 years. Prerequisites must be completed with a grade "C" or better. AP credit is accepted provided it was accepted by your college institution and appears on your official transcript. At most one science and one non-science prerequisite may be in progress after December 31st of the year prior to matriculation.

GPA Requirement: Overall GPA 3.0; Science GPA 3.0

Healthcare Experience: Preferred, not required

PA Shadowing: Not required

Required Standardized Testing: GRE, CASPer

Letters of Recommendation: Three required; no one specific

Seat Deposit: $150

UNIVERSITY OF OKLAHOMA, TULSA

MISSION:

The mission of the Physician Assistant Program at the OU-TU School of Community Medicine is to train physician assistants to provide quality health care to the citizens of Oklahoma with an emphasis on serving diverse and underserved communities.

NO CLASS STATISTICS REPORTED

PANCE SCORES

5-year First Time Pass: 100%

Most Recent First Time Pass: 100%

CURRICULUM STRUCTURE

Didactic: 15 months

Clinical: 15 months

Rotations: 9 mandatory, 1 elective, 1 selective, 1 preceptorship (each 2-8 weeks)

Capstone Project: Required for graduation

UNIQUE PROGRAM FEATURES

Clinics: Bedlam Evening Clinic and Physician Assistant Longitudinal (PAL) Student Clinics are unique educational features of the program, which afford students the opportunity to treat their own panel of patients from the community.

Summer Institute: This week-long immersive experience engages participants in a curriculum of reflective, experiential service learning. Participants interact with community members including patients, healthcare providers and community agencies to gain an understanding of the intricacies of the healthcare community within the Tulsa area. Participants also experience a poverty simulation designed to create an understanding of the challenges facing many members of the community.

Student Academy: Each month medical students and PA students learn to apply their knowledge in a topic-focused Student Academy. The students join together to discuss an important topic and work together in a collaborative environment. This collaborative session allows the students to work together across disciplines and prepares them to work together after completion of their respective programs.

297

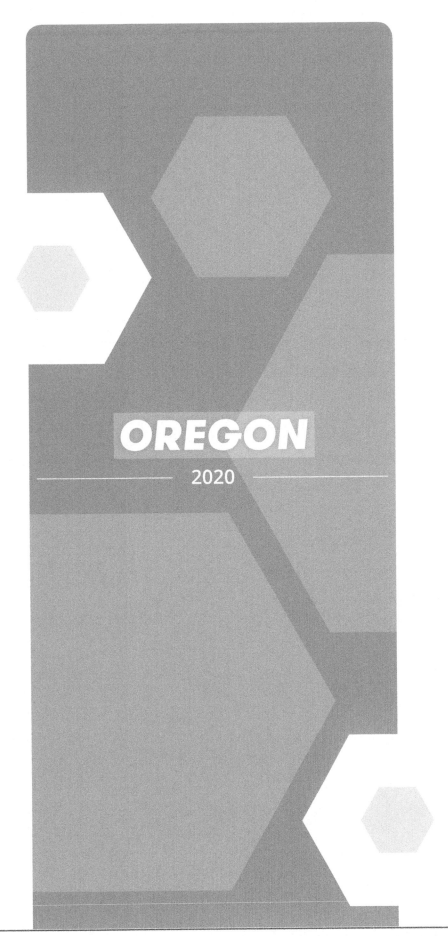

OREGON

2020

Oregon Health & Science University

Division of Physician Assistant Education
2730 SW Moody Avenue, Mail Code: CL5PA
Portland, OR 97201
Phone: 503-494-3633
Email: paprgm@ohsu.edu

PROGRAM HIGHLIGHTS

Accreditation: Continuing
Degree Offered: Master (MPAS)
Start Date: June annually
Program Length: 26 months
Class Capacity: 42 students
Tuition: $90,072

CASPA Participant: Yes
Supplemental Application: No
Yellow Ribbon: Yes
Admissions: Rolling
Application Deadline: August 1

PREREQUISITE COURSEWORK

Human Anatomy and Physiology with lab (2 semesters), Microbiology with lab (1 semester), Biology (6 credits), Chemistry (6 credits), General or Developmental Psychology (3 credits), Biostatistics or Statistics (3 credits). Prerequisites must be completed with a grade "C" or better and by December 31st prior to the year of matriculation. Overall, students must have completed 30 credit hours of Biology, Chemistry and Physics and also must have completed Anatomy and Physiology within 5 years of program matriculation. AP credits are accepted if they appear on your official college transcript. Recommended courses: Genetics, Biochemistry, Pharmacology, Pathophysiology, Immunology, Spanish.

GPA Requirement: Overall GPA 3.0; Science GPA 3.0 (preferred)

Healthcare Experience: 2,000 hours

PA Shadowing: Preferred, not required

Required Standardized Testing: None

Letters of Recommendation: Three required; preferably one from a PA, MD, or DO, one from a current or former work supervisor, and one from an academic source such as a professor or advisor

Seat Deposit: $700

OREGON HEALTH & SCIENCE UNIVERSITY

MISSION:

The Mission of the OHSU Physician Assistant Program is to: Prepare physician assistants for the practice of medicine and the delivery of primary care services to diverse populations, including the medically underserved; contribute to meeting the health workforce needs of Oregon; provide a model of excellence in physician assistant education; and advance the physician assistant profession in the state.

CLASS OF 2021

Overall GPA: 3.42

Average Healthcare Experience: 3 years

Average Age: 28.8

PANCE SCORES

5-year First Time Pass: 98%

Most Recent First Time Pass: 98%

CURRICULUM STRUCTURE

Didactic: 12 months

Clinical: 14 months

Rotations: 9 mandatory, 2 elective (each 4 weeks)

Community Outreach Project: Required for graduation

UNIQUE PROGRAM FEATURES

Admissions Preference: The program gives preference to residents of Oregon, Veterans, non-resident applications with Oregon Heritage, and resident and non-resident applications with superior achievements or interest/experience in rural health, underserved populations and/or primary care.

Rural Track: The Oregon Rural Scholars PA Program (ORSPAP) is an elective rural track program specifically designed to prepare students who wish to practice medicine in rural areas with the skills needed to practice in such a setting.

PROGRAM HIGHLIGHTS

Accreditation: Continuing
Degree Offered: Master (MSPAS)
Start Date: May annually
Program Length: 27 months
Class Capacity: 59 students
Tuition: $102,240

CASPA Participant: Yes
Supplemental Application: Yes ($55 fee)
Yellow Ribbon: No
Admissions: Non-rolling
Application Deadline: September 1

PREREQUISITE COURSEWORK

Human Anatomy and Physiology I and II with lab (2 semesters), Microbiology or Bacteriology (1 semester), General Chemistry I and II with lab (2 semesters), Organic Chemistry or Biochemistry (1 semester), Statistics (3 credits), Psychology or Sociology (3 credits). All prerequisites must be completed by December 31st of the year prior to entering the program. AP credits are accepted for the Statistics and Psychology/Sociology prerequisites. Recommended courses: Pharmacology, Medical Terminology, Spanish, Abnormal Psychology, Development Psychology, Aging and Disabilities, Public Health, Technical Writing, Communications.

GPA Requirement: Science GPA 3.0; GPA (Last 45 Credits) 3.0

Healthcare Experience: 1,000 hours

PA Shadowing: Not required (counts towards healthcare experience)

Required Standardized Testing: None

Letters of Recommendation: Two required; at least one should be from a physician, PA or NP with whom you have worked or shadowed

Seat Deposit: $1,000

PACIFIC UNIVERSITY

MISSION:

The School of Physician Assistant Studies prepares and mentors students within an innovative curriculum to provide quality care for a diverse global community focusing on primary care for underserved and rural populations.

CLASS OF 2021

Male: 37%

Female: 63%

Science GPA: 3.74

Last 45 Credits GPA: 3.88

Average Healthcare Experience: 4,150 hours

Average Age: 28

PANCE SCORES

5-year First Time Pass: 99%

Most Recent First Time Pass: 96%

CURRICULUM STRUCTURE

Didactic: 14 months

Clinical: 13 months

Rotations: 7 mandatory (each 6-12 weeks)

Graduate Project: Required for graduation

UNIQUE PROGRAM FEATURES

Curriculum Design: The curriculum uses system-based modules. In the morning students attend traditional lectures, while in the afternoon they focus on case-based small group learning and simulation exercises.

Unique Tracks: The program offers several different tracks depending on applicant interest including a rural health care track and global health care track.

Community Service: Students participate in community service projects that include staffing of a low-cost clinic and healthcare screening for the homeless.

Outreach Initiatives: The program has a Hawaii Outreach Initiative and a Veterans Outreach initiative aimed at garnering more student interest from these groups and giving some admissions preference to students in either category.

Student Perspectives: Available on the program website to learn more about why students chose Pacific.

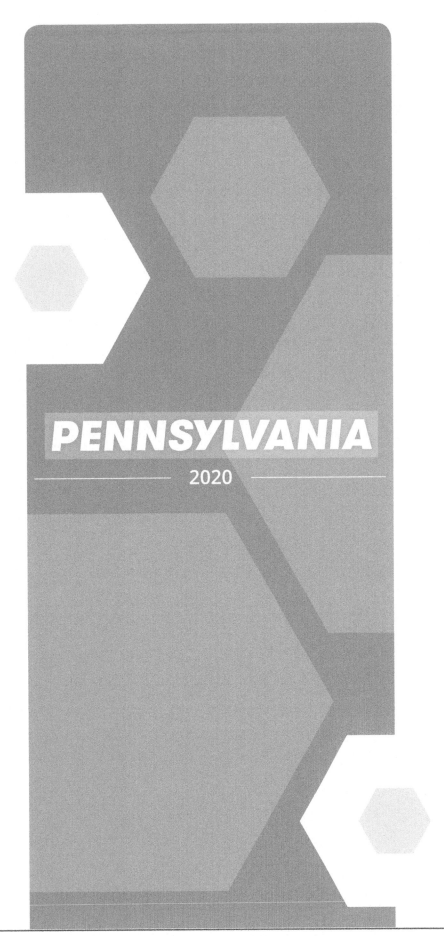

PENNSYLVANIA
2020

Arcadia University

450 South Easton Road
Glenside, PA 19038
Phone: 215-572-2888
Email: admiss@arcadia.edu

PROGRAM HIGHLIGHTS

Accreditation: Continuing

Degree Offered: Master (MMS)

Start Date: May annually

Program Length: 24 months

Class Capacity: 56 students

Tuition: $93,042

CASPA Participant: Yes

Supplemental Application: No

Yellow Ribbon: No

Admissions: Rolling

Application Deadline: October 1

PREREQUISITE COURSEWORK

Biological Sciences (5 courses, to include Anatomy, Physiology, and Microbiology; Biochemistry is recommended), Chemistry (3 courses, to include at least one semester of Organic Chemistry), Psychology (1 semester), Statistics (1 semester). Prerequisites must be completed within the last 10 years. AP credits are accepted provided they are listed on your college transcript.

GPA Requirement: None (overall GPA 3.0 recommended)

Healthcare Experience: 200 hours

PA Shadowing: Preferred, not required

Required Standardized Testing: GRE or MCAT

Letters of Recommendation: Three required; ideally, one should be from a professor and one from a practicing licensed physician or PA

Seat Deposit: $500

ARCADIA UNIVERSITY

MISSION:

Arcadia University's Physician Assistant Program is dedicated to training highly competent, globally aware physician assistants who are prepared to be life-long learners. The Program is committed to fostering excellence in patient care and promoting professionalism, leadership, cultural competency, scholarship, and service.

CLASS OF 2021

Overall GPA: 3.65

Science GPA: 3.56

GRE Total: 312

GRE Analytical: 4.30

Average Healthcare Experience: 2,724 hours

PANCE SCORES

5-year First Time Pass: 100%

Most Recent First Time Pass: 99%

CURRICULUM STRUCTURE

Didactic: 12 months

Clinical: 12 months

Rotations: 7 mandatory, 3 elective (each 4 weeks)

UNIQUE PROGRAM FEATURES

Dual Degree: There is an option to get a dual MPH. The MPH program focuses on population health and includes the disciplines of epidemiology and biostatistics with an in-depth fieldwork thesis project oriented toward a student's primary area of research interest. Students complete the coursework for the MPH in the year prior to entering the Physician Assistant program.

Pre-PA Track: There is a 4+2 track available for incoming undergraduates.

Rotations: International rotations are available. To date, Arcadia PA students have studied in over twenty countries around the world, including South Africa, Bolivia, Costa Rica, Guatemala, India, Scotland, England and Belize.

Community Service: The program typically organizes a one-week medical service trip in late spring to bring PA students, alumni and faculty to communities in need. Past service trips have traveled to places including Appalachia, Belize, Panama, Nicaragua and Guatemala.

Articulation Agreement: Arcadia University has an articulation agreement with West Chester University.

PROGRAM HIGHLIGHTS

Accreditation: Continuing

Degree Offered: Master (MPAS)

Start Date: August annually

Program Length: 24 months

Class Capacity: 80 students

Tuition: $111,356 (including fees)

CASPA Participant: Yes

Supplemental Application: No

Yellow Ribbon: No

Admissions: Non-rolling

Application Deadline: October 1

PREREQUISITE COURSEWORK

General Biology I and II with lab (2 semesters), General Chemistry I and II with lab (2 semesters), Organic Chemistry with lab (1 semester), Anatomy with lab (1 semester), Physiology (1 semester), Microbiology (1 semester), General Psychology (1 semester), English (1 semester), Medical Terminology (1 semester). Prerequisites must be completed with a grade "B-" or better. All prerequisites must be completed by June 1st prior to the August matriculation and within the last 10 years. Recommended courses: Genetics, Statistics, Nutrition, Developmental Psychology, Advanced Anatomy and Physiology, Pathophysiology, Cadaver Lab Dissection.

GPA Requirement: Overall GPA 3.25; Science GPA 3.25

Healthcare Experience: Preferred, not required

PA Shadowing: 32 hours

Required Standardized Testing: GRE

Letters of Recommendation: Three required; one academic letter, one from a volunteer or work supervisor, and one of the applicant's choice

Seat Deposit: $800

CHATHAM UNIVERSITY

MISSION:

To strive for excellence in physician assistant education whose graduates are known as outstanding clinicians in the community and leaders in the profession trained by faculty who are recognized for developing and researching innovative curricular methods. The Chatham University MPAS Program is dedicated to producing knowledgeable, compassionate, ethical, and clinically skillful graduates that are ready to provide health care services to all persons without exclusion and who are willing to become the future leaders and educators of the profession.

CLASS OF 2021

Male: 15%

Female: 85%

Overall GPA: 3.71

Science GPA: 3.66

GRE Total: 304

GRE Analytical: 4.5

Average Age: 24

PANCE SCORES

5-year First Time Pass: 99%

Most Recent First Time Pass: 99%

CURRICULUM STRUCTURE

Didactic: 12 months

Clinical: 12 months

Rotations: 7 mandatory, 2 elective (duration not specified)

UNIQUE PROGRAM FEATURES

Curriculum: Chatham University utilizes a hybrid model of problem-based learning, lecture, and online activity that challenges students to be self-directed and prepares students for the evidence-based, problem-oriented world of clinical medicine.

Articulation Agreements: Chatham University's PA program has articulation agreements with the following colleges: Allegheny College, Grove City College, Saint Vincent College, Washington and Jefferson College, and Waynesburg University.

Student Perspective: Visit the program's website for video testimonials from current students.

Desales University

Physician Assistant Program
2755 Station Avenue
Center Valley, PA 18034
Phone: 610-282-1100 x1415
Email: mspas@desales.edu

PROGRAM HIGHLIGHTS

Accreditation: Continuing

Degree Offered: Master (MSPAS)

Start Date: August annually

Program Length: 24 months

Class Capacity: 80 students

Tuition: $81,000

CASPA Participant: Yes

Supplemental Application: No

Yellow Ribbon: No

Admissions: Rolling

Application Deadline: December 1

PREREQUISITE COURSEWORK

Human Anatomy and Physiology I and II (6 credits), English Composition I and II (6 credits), General Biology (3 credits), General Chemistry (3 credits), Microbiology (3 credits), Organic Chemistry (3 credits), Psychology (3 credits), Statistics (3 credits). Anatomy, Physiology and Microbiology must be completed within the last 5 years; exceptions may be considered for applicants who have been active in the medical field since taking the course. At most three prerequisites may be planned or in progress at the time of application.

GPA Requirement: Overall GPA 3.0; Science GPA 3.0

Healthcare Experience: 500 hours

PA Shadowing: Preferred, not required (counts towards healthcare experience)

Required Standardized Testing: GRE or MCAT

Letters of Recommendation: Three required; no one specific

Seat Deposit: $1,000

DESALES UNIVERSITY

MISSION:

The mission of the Physician Assistant Program is consistent with the enduring Christian Humanistic traditions of DeSales University and seeks to graduate physician assistants who dedicate themselves to the total well-being of the patient. Graduates of the Program will deliver competent and compassionate health care including preventative services and wellness education to patients of diverse populations in a variety of settings. They will consider the patient holistically in the context of family, community, and society, and incorporate ethical principles into a patient-focused practice. They will serve their patients by using evidence-based medicine and promoting life-long learning in the profession.

NO CLASS STATISTICS REPORTED

PANCE SCORES

5-year First Time Pass: 99%

Most Recent First Time Pass: 100%

CURRICULUM STRUCTURE

Didactic: 12 months

Clinical: 12 months

Rotations: 8 mandatory, 1 elective (each 5 weeks)

UNIQUE PROGRAM FEATURES

Pre-PA Track: In addition to the traditional master's program pathway for new graduate students, DeSales also provides program planning at the undergraduate level with 3+2 and 4+2 options that can culminate with an MSPAS.

Community Service: The students run a free clinic at a local homeless shelter. The DeSales Free Clinic allows PA students to deliver competent and compassionate medical care to one of the area's most vulnerable populations. The clinic is open two evenings per week to the men seeking shelter or enrolled in a recovery program at the Allentown Rescue Mission.

Facilities: The Gambet center is a new 77,000 sq. ft., $27 million facility that includes state-of-the-science simulation laboratories to replicate clinical scenarios specific to adult, pediatric and birthing care for undergraduate and graduate health care degree programs, as well as gross anatomy lab and a standardized patient lab.

Rotations: The DeSales program is proud to offer international rotations; five-week rotations are offered in Peru and Tanzania, one-week rotations are offered in Honduras.

307

Drexel University

1601 Cherry Street, 6th Floor,
MS#6504
Philadelphia, PA 19102
Phone: 267-359-5741
Email: paadmissions@drexel.edu

PROGRAM HIGHLIGHTS

Accreditation: Continuing

Degree Offered: Master (MHS)

Start Date: September annually

Program Length: 27 months

Class Capacity: 80 students

Tuition: $91,962

CASPA Participant: Yes

Supplemental Application: No

Yellow Ribbon: Yes

Admissions: Rolling

Application Deadline: September 1

PREREQUISITE COURSEWORK

Human Anatomy and Physiology I and II with lab (8 credits), General Biology I and II with lab (8 credits), General Chemistry with lab (4 credits), Microbiology (3 credits), Psychology (3 credits), Genetics (3 credits), Medical Terminology (1 credit). It is strongly recommended that A&P be completed within 3-5 years of application. Prerequisites must be completed with a grade "B-" or better and by the end of the fall semester prior to matriculation. AP credits are accepted. Recommended courses: Abnormal and Developmental Psychology, Biochemistry, Critical Thinking, Death & Dying, Embryology, Ethics, Foreign Language, Intro to Pharmacology, Logic, Nutrition, Organic Chemistry, Pathophysiology, Advanced Anatomy, Philosophy, Public Speaking, Research Design, Sociology, Statistics.

GPA Requirement: Overall GPA 3.0; Science GPA 3.0

Healthcare Experience: 500 hours (additionally, preference is given to applicants with at least 100 hours of community service/volunteer work)

PA Shadowing: Preferred, not required

Required Standardized Testing: None

Letters of Recommendation: Two required (up to five accepted/encouraged); preferably from individuals who have been in a supervisory capacity over the applicant or academic instructors who have personal knowledge of the applicant

Seat Deposit: $500

DREXEL UNIVERSITY

MISSION:

The mission of the program is to: educate qualified primary care physician assistants; improve health care delivery in rural and urban medically underserved areas; and promote the physician assistant profession.

CLASS OF 2021

Overall GPA: 3.63

Science GPA: 3.60

Average Healthcare Experience: 2,996 hours

PANCE SCORES

5-year First Time Pass: 97%

Most Recent First Time Pass: 90%

CURRICULUM STRUCTURE

Didactic: 12 months

Clinical: 15 months

Rotations: 6 mandatory (each 5 weeks), plus Primary Care practicum

Graduate Project: Required for graduation

UNIQUE PROGRAM FEATURES

3+2 Track: This program has an accelerated dual-degree BS/MHS option for highly qualified students whereby they can complete the curriculum in 5 ¼ years as opposed to the traditional 6 ¼ years.

Post-Master's Certificate in Geriatrics: The program offers a post-master's certificate in Geriatrics which consists of three didactic courses and one clinical practicum. The certificate program is offered part-time for working professionals and is one year in length; the program begins in the Winter Term of each year (January), and runs through the Fall term of the following year (December).

Duquesne University

John G Rangos School of Health Sciences
600 Forbes Avenue
Pittsburgh, PA 15282
Phone: 412-396-5914
Email: rshs@duq.edu

PROGRAM HIGHLIGHTS

Accreditation: Probation

Degree Offered: BS/Master (MPAS)

Start Date: August annually

Program Length: Pre-professional + 27 months

Class Capacity: 40 students

Tuition: $261,427 (entire undergraduate and masters program)

CASPA Participant: No

Supplemental Application: No

Yellow Ribbon: No

Admissions: Rolling; option for early action

Application Deadline: December 1

PREREQUISITE COURSEWORK

Since students apply in high school, the only prerequisites for applying are advanced science and math coursework (minimum of 7 units), demonstration of leadership skills, involvement in extracurricular activities, and demonstration of knowledge of the PA profession. AP credits are not accepted.

GPA Requirement: Overall GPA 3.0 (high school)

Healthcare Experience: Not required

PA Shadowing: Preferred, not required

Required Standardized Testing: SAT or ACT (a composite math and verbal SAT score of at least 1,170 or a composite ACT score of at least 24)

Letters of Recommendation: One required; from an academic source such as a teacher or counselor

Seat Deposit: $500

DUQUESNE UNIVERSITY

MISSION:

The mission of the Duquesne University Department of Physician Assistant Studies is five-fold: to prepare trainees with the necessary knowledge and skills to reliably perform the role of a physician assistant; to promote a lifelong responsibility for ongoing learning and active participation in a changing health care environment; to instill a professional identity in each student based on the education for the mind, heart and spirit that is achieved at Duquesne; to prepare graduates to provide quality primary health care among rural, urban and minority populations; and to expand knowledge beyond primary care.

NO CLASS STATISTICS REPORTED

PANCE SCORES

5-year First Time Pass: 93%

Most Recent First Time Pass: 77%

CURRICULUM STRUCTURE

Pre-Professional: 3 years

Didactic: 14 months

Clinical: 12 months

Rotations: 7 mandatory, 1 elective (each 6 weeks)

Master's Project: Required for graduation

UNIQUE PROGRAM FEATURES

Program: This is the first five-year entry-level Master's degree program in the nation. "Entry level" students come into Duquesne University as freshmen, complete the five year curriculum, and earn both a Bachelor of Science in Health Sciences degree and a Master of Physician Assistant Studies degree.

Articulation Agreements: Articulation agreements currently exist with Athlone Institute of Technology, LaRoche College, St. Vincent College, and Westminster College. In the past, these agreements have allowed for a limited number of students to complete the first few years at one of these institutions and then transfer into the third year of the Physician Assistant curriculum if and when seats are available.

Gannon University

Morosky Academic Center
150 W. 10th St.
Erie, PA 16541
Phone: 814-871-5643
Email: schlick001@gannon.edu

PROGRAM HIGHLIGHTS

Accreditation: Continuing

Degree Offered: BS/Master (MPAS)

Start Date: August annually

Program Length: 44 months

Class Capacity: 58 students

Tuition: $203,705 (for the 5-year program)

CASPA Participant: No

Supplemental Application: No

Yellow Ribbon: No

Admissions: Ten early admission seats are offered to high school students, and admissions is very competitive so early application is advised; admissions for graduate applicants is based on available space

Application Deadline: December 1

PREREQUISITE COURSEWORK

Biology (8 credits), Chemistry (8 credits), Psychology (3 credits), Statistics (3 credits), Medical Terminology (3 credits or demonstrated competency), Human Anatomy with lab (4 credits), Human Physiology with lab (4 credits), Microbiology with lab (4 credits), Genetics (3 credits), Research (3 credits). Prerequisites must be completed within the last 7 years.

GPA Requirement: Overall GPA 3.0

Healthcare Experience: 30 hours

PA Shadowing: Not required (counts towards healthcare experience)

Required Standardized Testing: None

Letters of Recommendation: Three required; letters should be from individuals who are familiar with the student's academic and professional background

Seat Deposit: $300

GANNON UNIVERSITY

MISSION:

The Gannon University Physician Assistant Program strives to provide a stimulating learning environment, highly qualified and motivated faculty, as well as modern facilities that offer Physician Assistant students the opportunity to become well-prepared primary care providers who are leaders in their field and community.

NO CLASS STATISTICS REPORTED

PANCE SCORES

5-year First Time Pass: 95%

Most Recent First Time Pass: 91%

CURRICULUM STRUCTURE

Pre-Professional: 3 years

Didactic: 12 months

Clinical: 12 months

Rotations: 6 mandatory, 2 elective (each 5 weeks)

Capstone/Research Project: Required for graduation

UNIQUE PROGRAM FEATURES

Program: This program is primarily a 5-year program starting at the undergraduate level. Requirements listed above are for when seats are available for post-baccalaureate candidates.

Curriculum Focus: This program places heavy emphasis on family medicine/primary care, with four of the core rotations focusing on this area of medicine.

King's College

133 North River Street
Wilkes-Barre, PA 18711
Phone: 570-208-5853
Email: PAadmissions@kings.edu

PROGRAM HIGHLIGHTS

Accreditation: Continuing

Degree Offered: Master (MSPAS)

Start Date: August annually

Program Length: 24 months

Class Capacity: 75 students

Tuition: $87,792

CASPA Participant: Yes

Supplemental Application: No

Yellow Ribbon: No

Admissions: Rolling

Application Deadline: October 1

PREREQUISITE COURSEWORK

Anatomy and Physiology I and II (8 credits), General Biology (8 credits), General Chemistry (8 credits), Microbiology (4 credits), Organic Chemistry (4 credits), Genetics (3 credits). Prerequisites should be completed with labs and must be completed with a grade "C-" or better. Prerequisites cannot be taken online. Candidates cannot have more than two outstanding prerequisite courses in the spring prior to the start of the program in August.

GPA Requirement: Overall GPA 3.2; Science GPA 3.2

Healthcare Experience: 500 hours (300 of these must be direct patient care)

PA Shadowing: Required (no specific number of hours; counts towards healthcare experience)

Required Standardized Testing: None

Letters of Recommendation: Two required; recommended that one be from a professional that the applicant has worked with clinically and one from someone academic

Seat Deposit: $820

KING'S COLLEGE

MISSION:

The Department of Physician Assistant Studies educates students in a primary care-based curriculum that emphasizes the mastery of knowledge, technical skills, critical thinking, and moral reasoning. King's Department of PA Studies fosters excellence in teaching and faculty scholarship, and forms highly competent professional healthcare providers committed to patient-centered, compassionate care, and the inherent dignity of every person.

NO CLASS STATISTICS REPORTED

PANCE SCORES

5-year First Time Pass: 97%

Most Recent First Time Pass: 91%

CURRICULUM STRUCTURE

Didactic: 10.5 months

Clinical: 13.5 months

Rotations: 8 mandatory, 1 elective (each 6 weeks)

Capstone Project: Required for graduation

UNIQUE PROGRAM FEATURES

Pre-PA Track: A combined 5-year BS/MS program is offered.

Admissions: Seats were not available for graduate applicants for the class beginning in fall of 2020. Availability of seats for graduate applicants can be found on the program's website.

Lock Haven University

Physician Assistant Program
432 Railroad Street
Lock Haven, PA 17745
Phone: 570-484-2929
Email: lbeers@lockhaven.edu

PROGRAM HIGHLIGHTS

Accreditation: Continuing

Degree Offered: Master (MHS)

Start Date: May annually

Program Length: 24 months

Class Capacity: 72 students

Tuition: $61,792 (in-state); $84,463 (out-of-state)

CASPA Participant: Yes

Supplemental Application: No

Yellow Ribbon: No

Admissions: Not reported

Application Deadline: October 1

PREREQUISITE COURSEWORK

General Chemistry I and II (2 semesters), Biology or Zoology (2 semesters), Human Anatomy and Physiology (2 semesters), Microbiology (1 semester), Human Genetics (1 semester), Statistics (1 semester). Prerequisites must be completed with a grade "B" or better. Anatomy and Physiology must be completed within the last 5 years, all others within 10 years. Science courses with labs are preferred. AP credits are not accepted. Recommended courses: Organic Chemistry, Biochemistry, Physics, Developmental Psychology, Behavioral Sciences.

GPA Requirement: Overall GPA 3.0

Healthcare Experience: Preferred, not required

PA Shadowing: Preferred, not required

Required Standardized Testing: GRE (minimum 50th percentile and 3.5 analytical)

Letters of Recommendation: Three required; no one specific

Seat Deposit: $1,000

LOCK HAVEN UNIVERSITY

MISSION:

The mission of the program is to educate highly-skilled Physician Assistants who: are capable of providing quality health care; have expertise in the health care needs of the medically underserved; are prepared to critically evaluate, and become leaders in bringing about improvement in the medical and social systems that affect the health of underserved populations; and will seek and retain employment as primary care Physician Assistants in medically underserved areas of the Commonwealth of Pennsylvania.

CLASS OF 2014

Male: 28%

Female: 72%

Overall GPA: 3.55

Science GPA: 3.43

GRE Verbal: 153

GRE Quantitative: 154

GRE Analytical: 4.1

Average Age: 24

PANCE SCORES

5-year First Time Pass: 97%

Most Recent First Time Pass: 94%

CURRICULUM STRUCTURE

Didactic: 12 months

Clinical: 12 months

Rotations: 7 mandatory, 1 elective (each 6 weeks)

UNIQUE PROGRAM FEATURES

Multiple Campuses: The Lock Haven program has expanded and now offers PA education at its Clearfield, Coudersport, and Harrisburg campuses. Lectures are delivered simultaneously to all campuses via fully interactive video conferencing.

Pre-PA Track: A 3+2 combined BS/MHS program is offered for incoming undergraduates. A minimum of five students enrolled in the 3+2 track, following a successful interview, are admitted each year.

Scholarship: Some scholarships are available through numerous benefactors of the Lock Haven University Physician Assistant Program.

Marywood University

2300 Adams Avenue
Scranton, PA 18509
Phone: 570-348-6298
Email: paprogram@marywood.edu

PROGRAM HIGHLIGHTS

Accreditation: Continuing

Degree Offered: Master (MPAS)

Start Date: May annually

Program Length: 24 months

Class Capacity: 60 students

Tuition: $81,370

CASPA Participant: Yes

Supplemental Application: No

Yellow Ribbon: Yes

Admissions: Rolling

Application Deadline: October 1

PREREQUISITE COURSEWORK

General Biology I and II with lab (2 semesters), General Chemistry I and II with lab (2 semesters), Anatomy and Physiology I and II with lab (2 semesters), Organic Chemistry I and II with lab (2 semesters), Microbiology with lab (1 semester), Immunology with lab (or other upper level science course such as Molecular Biology, Cell Biology, Virology), Medical Terminology (within the last 2 years). Applicants may apply with courses planned or in progress. Prerequisites should be completed within the last 7 years and with a grade "C" or better. AP credits are not accepted.

GPA Requirement: Overall GPA 3.0; Prerequisite GPA 3.0

Healthcare Experience: 500 hours

PA Shadowing: 50 hours (counts towards healthcare experience)

Required Standardized Testing: GRE

Letters of Recommendation: Three required; one must be from a PA with whom you have shadowed/worked during actual patient-care activities

Seat Deposit: $500

MARYWOOD UNIVERSITY

MISSION:

The Physician Assistant Program at Marywood University is committed to providing students with an exceptional education in a supportive and nurturing environment. This professional education will include the biomedical and clinical knowledge necessary to diagnose, treat, educate, and empower patients in a variety of settings across the lifespan.

CLASS OF 2021

Overall GPA: 3.58

Prerequisite GPA: 3.43

GRE Total: 296

Average Healthcare Experience: 1,942 hours

PANCE SCORES

5-year First Time Pass: 96%

Most Recent First Time Pass: 96%

CURRICULUM STRUCTURE

Didactic: 12 months

Clinical: 12 months

Rotations: 9 mandatory, 1 elective (each 5 weeks)

UNIQUE PROGRAM FEATURES

Pre-PA Track: Students in the pre-professional phase are required to maintain an overall GPA of 3.00, as well as a 3.00 average in all prerequisite science courses and/or labs to be considered for admission to the professional phase. Students who have successfully met all required liberal arts core requirements and science prerequisites may apply for admission to the professional program, following their second year as pre-PA.

Clinical Tracks: Unique to Marywood's PA Program, students may choose to focus their studies and clinical experience by applying for acceptance to one the following Clinical Tracks during the clinical phase of the program: Emergency Medicine, Orthopedics/Sports Medicine, Hospitalist, General Surgery.

Student Society: M.U.P.A.S.S. is an organization comprised of PA students. This organization is committed to increasing awareness of the PA profession and promoting health and wellness on campus, in the community and on a national level. Members of this society will participate in health related awareness activities, conferences as well as encourage service and scholarship by its members.

Facilities: The program's Physical Assessment Lab includes 22 exam tables and 5 private exam rooms for practical education and individual testing of history taking and physical examination techniques. In addition, there are X-ray view boxes, operating room scrub sinks and a variety of teaching models.

Student Perspectives: Available on the program website for you to learn what current students love about the Marywood program.

Mercyhurst University

501 East 38th Street
Erie, PA 16546
Phone: 814-824-2598
Email: paprogram@mercyhurst.edu

PROGRAM HIGHLIGHTS

Accreditation: Continuing

Degree Offered: Master (MPAS)

Start Date: May/June annually

Program Length: 24 months

Class Capacity: 30 students

Tuition: $89,822

CASPA Participant: Yes

Supplemental Application: No

Yellow Ribbon: No

Admissions: Not reported

Application Deadline: December 1

PREREQUISITE COURSEWORK

Biology with lab (8 credits), General and Organic Chemistry with lab (12 credits), Biochemistry (3 credits), Anatomy with lab (4 credits), Physiology (3 credits), Microbiology with lab (4 credits), Genetics (3 credits), Statistics (3 credits), Psychology (3 credits), Medical Terminology (1 credit). A minimum of 12 credits of the prerequisite courses including Physiology and Microbiology must be completed within the last 5 years. Prerequisites must be completed with a grade "C" or better. AP credits are not accepted.

GPA Requirement: Overall GPA 3.2; Prerequisite GPA 3.2

Healthcare Experience: 200 hours

PA Shadowing: Not required

Required Standardized Testing: GRE

Letters of Recommendation: Three required; no one specific

Seat Deposit: $1,090

MERCYHURST UNIVERSITY

MISSION:

The mission of the Department of Physician Assistant Studies (DPAS) is to prepare students with the highest quality academic and clinical training. The program will prepare physician assistants to be leaders in the profession, proficient in meeting the challenges of healthcare, while providing compassionate, quality care to the diverse communities in which they serve.

NO CLASS STATISTICS REPORTED

PANCE SCORES

5-year First Time Pass: 97% (based on three years of data)

Most Recent First Time Pass: 93%

CURRICULUM STRUCTURE

Didactic: 12 months

Clinical: 12 months

Rotations: 7 mandatory, 2 elective (each 4-5 weeks)

Thesis Project: Required for graduation

UNIQUE PROGRAM FEATURES

Community Service: All Physician Assistant Students must earn 20 hours of service while in the program. In 2017, six students completed a medical mission trip in Honduras.

Admissions Preference: Preference will be given to qualified Mercyhurst graduates.

Misericordia University

301 Lake Street
Dallas, PA 18612
Phone: 570-674-6716
Email:
MUPAInquiry@misericordia.edu

PROGRAM HIGHLIGHTS

Accreditation: Provisional

Degree Offered: Master (MSPAS)

Start Date: July annually

Program Length: 25 months

Class Capacity: 20 students

Tuition: $99,743 (including fees)

CASPA Participant: Yes

Supplemental Application: No

Yellow Ribbon: No

Admissions: Rolling

Application Deadline: March 1

PREREQUISITE COURSEWORK

Anatomy and Physiology I and II
with lab (8 credits), Microbiology
with lab (3 credits), Biochemistry
(3 credits), Genetics (3 credits),
Statistics (3 credits), Medical
Terminology (1 credit). Prerequisites
must be completed with a grade
"B" or better and within the last 10
years. At most two prerequisites
may be planned or in progress at
the time of application.

GPA Requirement: Overall GPA 3.2;
Science GPA 3.2

Healthcare Experience: 500 hours

PA Shadowing: Not required

Required Standardized Testing:
None

Letters of Recommendation: Two
required; having one from a PA,
physician, NP or other healthcare
provider will be scored at a higher
value

Seat Deposit: $500

MISERICORDIA UNIVERSITY

MISSION:

The Misericordia University Physician Assistant Program strives
to attract intellectually talented and caring students who will be
educationally transformed and mentored to become competent
and compassionate Physician Assistants.

NO CLASS STATISTICS REPORTED

PANCE SCORES

5-year First Time
Pass: N/A

Most Recent First
Time Pass: N/A (have
not graduated a class
yet)

CURRICULUM STRUCTURE

Didactic: 12 months

Clinical: 13 months

Rotations: 7
mandatory,
1 elective (each 6
weeks)

Research Project:
Required for
graduation

UNIQUE PROGRAM FEATURES

Facilities: Misericordia University
has a 7,575 square foot, custom
designed PA educational facility
within the Trocaire Building on
its main campus. Key features of
this space include a dedicated
PA didactic year classroom with
state of the art 'smart-technology',
an open-floor-plan physical
assessment and procedural skills
lab with 11 examination areas, 4
private physical examination rooms
which may be used for refining
examination skills or objective
structured clinical examinations
(OSCEs), a PA student study area,
and private offices for all PA
program faculty and staff. Also,
a high level, state-of-the-art, new
cadaver lab will open Fall 2020.

Admissions Preference:
Applicants who have completed
their undergraduate degree at
Misericordia University or whose
home residence is in one of the
eleven northeastern Pennsylvania
counties receive special
consideration in the admission
process of the Misericordia
University Physician Assistant
Program. Applicants who are
active duty military or who are U.S.
military veterans also receive special
consideration.

Penn State College of Medicine

500 University Drive
Mail Code H152
Hershey, PA 17033
Phone: 717-531-0003 (ext. 285595)
Email:
psupaprogram@pennstatehealth.psu.edu

PROGRAM HIGHLIGHTS

Accreditation: Continuing

Degree Offered: Master (MPAS)

Start Date: May annually

Program Length: 24 months

Class Capacity: 30 students

Tuition: $75,104

CASPA Participant: Yes

Supplemental Application: Yes (no fee)

Yellow Ribbon: No

Admissions: Non-rolling (through early application is encouraged)

Application Deadline: January 15

PREREQUISITE COURSEWORK

General Biology (1 semester), Anatomy and Physiology (2 semesters), Microbiology (1 semester), General or Principles of Chemistry (1 semester), Biochemistry or Organic Chemistry (1 semester), General Psychology (1 semester), Statistics or Biostatistics (1 semester), English Composition (2 semesters). Labs are highly recommended with any science course. Anatomy, Physiology and Microbiology must be completed within the last 5 years unless you have been working full time and continuously in healthcare since completion of this coursework. Courses may be planned or in progress at the time of application. AP credits are accepted.

GPA Requirement: Overall GPA 3.0; Science GPA 3.0

Healthcare Experience: 500 hours

PA Shadowing: Not required

Required Standardized Testing: GRE or MCAT or PCAT or DAT

Letters of Recommendation: Three required; no one specific

Seat Deposit: $1,000

PENN STATE UNIVERSITY

MISSION:

The Physician Assistant Program's mission is to prepare graduates to be academically, clinically, professionally and culturally competent in the delivery of health care services, to develop critical thinking and application skills, and to provide compassionate and comprehensive care to the patients they will serve. Our graduates will improve the health of their patients and the populations they serve in an efficient and cost-conscious manner.

CLASS OF 2021

Male: 40%

Female: 60%

Minority: 47%

Overall GPA: 3.70

Science GPA: 3.70

GRE Verbal: 160

GRE Quantitative: 158

GRE Analytical: 4.5

Average Healthcare Experience: 3,561 hours

Average Age: 26

PANCE SCORES

5-year First Time Pass: 100% (based on four years of data)

Most Recent First Time Pass: 100%

CURRICULUM STRUCTURE

Didactic: 12 months

Clinical: 12 months

Rotations: 8 mandatory, 1 elective (each 5 weeks)

UNIQUE PROGRAM FEATURES

Admissions Preference: In accordance with the PA Program's mission and goals, special consideration for admission is given to applicants who are veterans, who are from underrepresented populations or who are from economically or educationally disadvantaged backgrounds. Special consideration is also given to those applicants who have graduated from or will be graduating from Penn State University.

Acceptance: The Penn State PA Program has early assurance programs with the following institutions: Franklin and Marshall College and Lebanon Valley College.

Financial Assistance: For clinical sites for mandatory rotations located more than one hour from campus, housing or financial support is given to these students.

Pennsylvania College of Technology

Physician Assistant Program
Dif 22, One College Avenue
Williamsport, PA 17701
Phone: 570-327-4519
Email: pa@pct.edu

PROGRAM HIGHLIGHTS

Accreditation: Continuing

Degree Offered: BS/MS

Start Date: August annually

Program Length: 24 months

Class Capacity: 30 students

Tuition: $39,621 (in-state);
$61,028 (out-of-state)

CASPA Participant: No (but plans to be in 2021 or 2022)

Supplemental Application: No

Yellow Ribbon: No

Admissions: Rolling

Application Deadline: March 1

PREREQUISITE COURSEWORK

For post-grads with a Bachelor's Degree: General Chemistry I and II with lab (2 semesters), General Biology I and II with lab (2 semesters), Anatomy and Physiology I and II with lab (2 semesters), Biochemistry (1 semester), Organic Chemistry with lab (1 semester), Microbiology with lab (1 semester), Physics (1 semester), Genetics (1 semester). Prerequisites must be completed with a grade "B" or better.

GPA Requirement: Prerequisite GPA 3.0

Healthcare Experience: 300 hours

PA Shadowing: 16 hours

Required Standardized Testing: CASPer

Letters of Recommendation: No

Seat Deposit: $150

PENNSYLVANIA COLLEGE OF TECHNOLOGY

MISSION:

The School of Nursing & Health Sciences at Pennsylvania College of Technology is committed to preparing professional and competent practitioners. Our programs are structured to support and develop essential qualities of caring, accountability, a credible work ethic, critical judgment, information literacy, and effective interpersonal skills to address social demands. Graduates will be prepared to enter or advance within the health professions workforce and be eligible for initial or continuing licensure, certification, and advanced education.

NO CLASS STATISTICS REPORTED

PANCE SCORES

5-year First Time Pass: 87%

Most Recent First Time Pass: 93%

CURRICULUM STRUCTURE

Didactic: 12 months (PA didactic coursework begins in the fourth year of undergrad)

Clinical: 12 months (the fifth year of the sequence)

Rotations: 7 mandatory, 2 elective (duration not specified)

Capstone Project: Required for graduation

UNIQUE PROGRAM FEATURES

Admissions: Starting Fall 2018, the Physician Assistant Studies (PA) degree at Penn College became a combined Bachelor/Master of Science degree. In this 3+2 program, students will complete the pre-professional phase over the course of the first three years, and the professional phase the last two years. After five years, successful students will graduate with a combined BS/MS Physician Assistant Studies degree.

Extracurricular: In 2018, PA students participated in the medical care of players and coaches in the Little League World Series.

Rotations: International rotations may be available during the clinical year.

317

Philadelphia College of Osteopathic Medicine

Office of Admissions
4170 City Avenue
Philadelphia, PA 19131
Phone: 215-871-6772
Email: PAadmissions@pcom.edu

PROGRAM HIGHLIGHTS

Accreditation: Continuing

Degree Offered: Master (MS)

Start Date: June annually

Program Length: 26 months

Class Capacity: 87 students (between two campuses)

Tuition: $97,603

CASPA Participant: Yes

Supplemental Application: No (but $75 fee)

Yellow Ribbon: No

Admissions: Rolling

Application Deadline: December 1

PREREQUISITE COURSEWORK

General Biology I and II with lab (8 credits), Other Biology (3 credits), Anatomy and Physiology I and II with lab (8 credits), General Chemistry I and II with lab (8 credits), Other Chemistry (3 credits), Health-related Science course (Nutrition, Immunology, Virology, Microbiology, Genetics, Cell Biology) or Physics (3 credits), Social Sciences (9 credits), Math (6 credits). Prerequisites must be completed with a grade "C" or better and within the last 10 years. At most two science/math prerequisites may be planned or in progress at the time of application. AP credits are accepted provided the course and credits appear on your college transcript.

GPA Requirement: Overall GPA 3.0; Science GPA 3.0

Healthcare Experience: 200 hours

PA Shadowing: Preferred, not required

Required Standardized Testing: None

Letters of Recommendation: Three required; one from a physician, PA, or NP

Seat Deposit: $500

PHILADELPHIA COLLEGE OF OSTEOPATHIC MEDICINE

MISSION:

The mission of the PCOM Physician Assistant Program is to educate highly qualified physician assistants, preparing them to become competent and compassionate health care providers, supported through scholarly activity and a broad range of clinical practice experiences.

CLASS OF 2021
PHILADELPHIA (P) AND GEORGIA (G) CAMPUSES

Male: 20% (P), 12.5% (G)

Female: 80% (P), 87.5% (G)

Minority: 35% (P), 25% (G)

Overall GPA: 3.68 (P & G)

Science GPA: 3.65 (P), 3.61 (G)

Average Age: 24 (P), 25 (G)

PANCE SCORES

5-year First Time Pass: 99%

Most Recent First Time Pass: 96%

CURRICULUM STRUCTURE

Didactic: 14 months

Clinical: 12 months

Rotations: 7 mandatory (each 6 weeks), 1 elective (4 weeks)

Research Practicum: Required for graduation

UNIQUE PROGRAM FEATURES

Distant Campus: The PCOM PA program has an affiliated distant campus in Suwanee, Georgia as noted above.

Saint Francis University

Department of PA Sciences
117 Evergreen Drive, PO Box 600
Loretto, PA 15940
Phone: 814-472-3130
Email: pa@francis.edu

PROGRAM HIGHLIGHTS

Accreditation: Continuing
Degree Offered: Master (MPAS)
Start Date: May annually
Program Length: 24 months
Class Capacity: 55 students
Tuition: $104,704

CASPA Participant: Yes
Supplemental Application: No
Yellow Ribbon: Yes
Admissions: Rolling
Application Deadline: August 1

PREREQUISITE COURSEWORK

Chemistry with lab (2 semesters), Human Anatomy and Physiology with lab (2 semesters), Microbiology with lab (1 semester), Psychology (1 semester), Statistics or upper level Math (1 semester). Prerequisites not completed prior to interview must be subsequently completed with a grade "B" or better.

GPA Requirement: Overall GPA 3.0; Science GPA 3.0 (competitive applicants have a 3.4 overall and prerequisite GPA)

Healthcare Experience: 100 hours

PA Shadowing: 40 hours (counts towards healthcare experience)

Required Standardized Testing: None

Letters of Recommendation: Three required; no one specific

Seat Deposit: $800

SAINT FRANCIS UNIVERSITY

MISSION:

To educate individuals as physician assistants to provide competent, compassionate and comprehensive health care to people and communities in need, as expressed through the Franciscan tradition.

NO CLASS STATISTICS REPORTED

PANCE SCORES

5-year First Time Pass: 98%

Most Recent First Time Pass: 100%

CURRICULUM STRUCTURE

Didactic: 12 months

Clinical: 12 months

Rotations: 8 mandatory, 1 elective (each 5 weeks)

UNIQUE PROGRAM FEATURES

Direct Entry: The program offers a 3+2 pre-PA track available for entering undergraduates and the number of seats available for graduate student applicants is limited.

Facilities: Currently there are plans for a new Health Science building, which will include state-of-the-art facilities, including a simulation lab.

Curriculum: During the didactic year, students participate in multiple clinical experiences, in such settings as the operating room, emergency department and a family practice office. This allows students to begin applying their medical knowledge and skills early on in their training. The didactic curriculum also blends lecture format with small-group critical-thinking sessions and simulated patient encounters.

Community Service: Numerous community service activities are available through on and off-campus events, such as free clinics, health fairs and medical mission trips. As an example, the Hugs United Spring Break Mission Trip is comprised of a dedicated group of volunteers of students, faculty, and alumni that heads to the Dominican Republic to work closely with an orphanage and provide much needed love and support.

Rotations: International clinical rotation opportunities are available.

PROGRAM HIGHLIGHTS

Accreditation: Continuing

Degree Offered: Master (MMS)

Start Date: August annually

Program Length: 25 months

Class Capacity: 50 students

Tuition: $86,100

CASPA Participant: Yes

Supplemental Application: No

Yellow Ribbon: No

Admissions: Rolling

Application Deadline: December 1

PREREQUISITE COURSEWORK

Anatomy and Physiology I and II with lab (8 credits), Biology I and II with lab (8 credits), Chemistry I and II with lab (8 credits), Microbiology (3 credits), Organic Chemistry (3 credits), Psychology (3 credits), Statistics or Biostatistics (3 credits), English Composition (3 credits). Prerequisites must be completed with a grade "C" or better and within the last 10 years. Prerequisites may be in progress at the time of application. Recommended courses: Medical Terminology, Physics, Genetics, Immunology, Embryology, Histology, Biochemistry, Cell Biology, Public Speaking, Ethics, Developmental or Abnormal Psychology.

GPA Requirement: Overall GPA 3.0; Science GPA 3.0

Healthcare Experience: 300 hours

PA Shadowing: 20 hours

Required Standardized Testing: GRE

Letters of Recommendation: Three required; one must be from a PA

Seat Deposit: $1,000

SALUS UNIVERSITY

MISSION:

To graduate collaborative clinicians who will serve the healthcare needs of a global community with intelligence, compassion, and integrity.

CLASS OF 2021

Male: 14%

Female: 86%

Minority: 20%

Overall GPA: 3.70

Science GPA: 3.66

Prerequisite GPA: 3.70

GRE Verbal: 155

GRE Quantitative: 155

GRE Analytical: 4.0

Average Age: 23

PANCE SCORES

5-year First Time Pass: 96%

Most Recent First Time Pass: 98%

CURRICULUM STRUCTURE

Didactic: 12 months

Clinical: 13 months

Rotations: 8 mandatory, 2 elective (each 5 weeks)

Capstone Project: Required for graduation

UNIQUE PROGRAM FEATURES

Partnership Agreement: Salus University has teamed with other universities to acknowledge their commitment to the training of future practitioners of primary healthcare by joining in an articulation agreement. Salus has a 3+2 program in conjunction with Western New England University and a 4+2 program with Messiah College, Cedar Crest College, Indiana University of Pennsylvania, Rosemont College and University of the Sciences.

Curriculum: Students' clinical exposure begins in the new, state of the art clinical assessment lab and patient care begins in the first year. There are also numerous service learning opportunities.

Seton Hill University

1 Seton Hill Drive
Greensburg, PA 15601
Phone: 724-838-4208
Email: gadmit@setonhill.edu

PROGRAM HIGHLIGHTS

Accreditation: Continuing

Degree Offered: Master (MSPA)

Start Date: January annually

Program Length: 27 months

Class Capacity: 50 students

Tuition: $100,298

CASPA Participant: Yes

Supplemental Application: No

Yellow Ribbon: Yes

Admissions: Non-rolling

Application Deadline: January 15

PREREQUISITE COURSEWORK

Human Anatomy and Physiology I and II with lab (2 semesters), Chemistry I and II with lab (2 semesters), Organic Chemistry I and II with lab (2 semesters), Microbiology with lab (1 semester), Biochemistry (1 semester), Abnormal Psychology or Lifespan Development (1 semester), Statistics (1 semester), Medical Terminology (1 course). Prerequisites must be completed within the last 7 years. AP credits are not accepted.

GPA Requirement: Overall GPA 3.2; Prerequisite GPA 3.2

Healthcare Experience: 300 hours

PA Shadowing: 12 hours (at least 4 hours in three different medical or surgical specialties)

Required Standardized Testing: None

Letters of Recommendation: Three required; no one specific

Seat Deposit: $1,000

SETON HILL UNIVERSITY

MISSION:

The Physician Assistant Program at Seton Hill University is dedicated to the use of mobile technology to provide students with a quality academic and clinical education. All students will be trained as effective team members. Program emphasis is on delivering optimal care in an efficient, effective and professional manner.

NO CLASS STATISTICS REPORTED

PANCE SCORES

5-year First Time Pass: 93%

Most Recent First Time Pass: 84%

CURRICULUM STRUCTURE

Didactic: 15 months

Clinical: 12 months

Rotations: 8 mandatory, 2 elective (duration not specified)

Grand Rounds Presentations: Required for graduation

UNIQUE PROGRAM FEATURES

Direct Entry: There is a combined 5-year BS/MS option available.

Facilities: The JoAnne Woodyard Boyle Health Sciences Center provides new clinical and research labs, classrooms, study areas and a "vibe" fresh market for students taking courses in the natural and health sciences.

Slippery Rock University

Physician Assistant Program
220 West Prairie Street
Harrisville, PA 16038
Phone: 724-738-2425
Email: pa.program@sru.edu

PROGRAM HIGHLIGHTS

Accreditation: Provisional

Degree Offered: Master (MSPAS)

Start Date: June annually

Program Length: 24 months

Class Capacity: 52 students

Tuition: $77,493 (in-state, including fees); 110,362 (out-of-state, including fees)

CASPA Participant: Yes

Supplemental Application: No

Yellow Ribbon: No

Admissions: Rolling

Application Deadline: December 1

PREREQUISITE COURSEWORK

General Biology with lab (3-4 credits), Anatomy and Physiology I and II with lab (6-8 credits), Microbiology with lab (3-4 credits), Genetics (3-4 credits), General Chemistry I and II with lab (6-8 credits), Organic Chemistry (3-4 credits), Statistics (3 credits), Psychology (3 credits), English (6 credits), Medical Terminology (1 credit). Biology and Chemistry prerequisites must be completed with a grade "C" or better. Prerequisites may be outstanding at the time of application. AP credits are accepted for the English prerequisite only. Recommended courses: Upper level Biology or Biochemistry.

GPA Requirement: Overall GPA 3.25; Science GPA 3.25; Prerequisite GPA 3.25

Healthcare Experience: Preferred, not required

PA Shadowing: 50 hours (at least 25 of these hours must be with more than one PA in more than one area of medicine)

Volunteer Experience: 100 hours

Required Standardized Testing: None

Letters of Recommendation: Two required; one from a PA highly recommended

Seat Deposit: $500

SLIPPERY ROCK UNIVERSITY

MISSION:

The overarching objective of the PA Program is to prepare future physician assistants; who demonstrate competencies or ability to acquire competencies in effective and appropriate application of medical knowledge, interpersonal and communication skills, patient care, professionalism, practice-based learning and improvement, and systems-based practice; to practice patient-centered care in a team environment, while advancing the profession and helping to meet the medical needs of the region, state, nation, and world.

CLASS OF 2019

Male: 22%

Female: 78%

Prerequisite GPA: 3.68

Average Age: 23.8

PANCE SCORES

5-year First Time Pass: 95% (based on two years of data)

Most Recent First Time Pass: 93%

CURRICULUM STRUCTURE

Didactic: 12 months

Clinical: 12 months

Rotations: 9 mandatory (two completed in special needs populations), 1 elective (each 3-4.5 weeks)

UNIQUE PROGRAM FEATURES

Curriculum: SRU's unique curriculum will expose students to clinical practice in the first year and train students to be competent in helping individuals with special needs.

Travel: Opportunities will arise for students to participate in medical mission trips abroad or within the U.S. Trips will be organized and led by PA faculty and will focus on teambuilding, leadership, and life experience while providing care to those in medically underserved regions.

Affordability: SRU's PA program claims to be the most affordable in western Pennsylvania. Graduates' starting salaries can be more than the cost of their educational investment.

Temple University

Medicine Education
& Research Bldg
3500 North Broad Street, Suite 124
Philadelphia, PA 19140
Phone: 215-707-3656
Email: pa-admissions@temple.edu

PROGRAM HIGHLIGHTS

Accreditation: Provisional

Degree Offered: Master (MMS)

Start Date: June annually

Program Length: 26 months

Class Capacity: 30 students

Tuition: $86,229 (in-state); $90,441 (out-of-state)

CASPA Participant: Yes

Supplemental Application: Yes ($60 fee)

Yellow Ribbon: No

Admissions: Rolling

Application Deadline: January 15

PREREQUISITE COURSEWORK

General Biology I and II with lab (8 credits), General Chemistry I and II with lab (8 credits), Organic Chemistry with lab (4 credits), Biochemistry (3 credits), Human Anatomy (4 credits), Human Physiology (3 credits), Statistics (2 credits), Psychology (3 credits), Medical Terminology (2 credits), two of the following: Genetics, Molecular Biology, Immunology, Microbiology, Cell Biology. Prerequisites must be completed with a grade "C" or better and within the last 10 years.

GPA Requirement: Overall GPA 3.0

Healthcare Experience: 400 hours (plus 50 hours volunteer experience recommended)

PA Shadowing: 100 hours (strongly preferred)

Required Standardized Testing: GRE or MCAT

Letters of Recommendation: Three required; one from a PA, MD or NP, one from a professor with whom you completed prerequisite science course work, and one of your choice

Seat Deposit: $500

TEMPLE UNIVERSITY LEWIS KATZ SCHOOL OF MEDICINE

MISSION:

Temple University Physician Assistant Program will develop physician assistants who are recognized as leaders, educators and innovators in the delivery of high-quality healthcare that is accessible, affordable, compassionate and respectful of cultural diversity in the delivery of healthcare to all patients, especially those within our communities.

FIRST TWO COHORT STATISTICS

Overall GPA: 3.50

Science GPA: 3.25

PANCE SCORES

5-year First Time Pass: 100% (based on one year of data)

Most Recent First Time Pass: 100%

CURRICULUM STRUCTURE

Didactic: 14 months

Clinical: 12 months

Rotations: 7 mandatory, 2 elective (each 5 weeks)

Capstone Clinical Research Project: Required for graduation

UNIQUE PROGRAM FEATURES

Interdisciplinary Study: The Physician Assistant program is part of interprofessional education at the Lewis Katz School of Medicine. Interprofessional education is a collaborative exercise that involves students from the School of Medicine as well as from Temple University's College of Public Health, Maurice H. Kornberg School of Dentistry, School of Pharmacy, and School of Podiatric Medicine.

Facilities: The William Maul Measey Institute for Clinical Simulation and Patient Safety allows students to learn basic clinical skills and teamwork in a safe learning environment throughout the curriculum under the teaching and guidance of the PA program faculty.

Thomas Jefferson University

130 S. 9th Street, 6th floor
Philadelphia, PA 19107
Phone: 215-503-8890
Email: TJU.Admissions@jefferson.edu

PROGRAM HIGHLIGHTS

Accreditation: Continuing

Degree Offered: Master (MSPAS)

Start Date: May annually

Program Length: 27 months

Class Capacity: 48 students

Tuition: $83,168

CASPA Participant: Yes

Supplemental Application: No

Yellow Ribbon: No

Admissions: Rolling

Application Deadline: November 1

PREREQUISITE COURSEWORK

General Biology I and II with lab (8 credits), General Chemistry I and II with lab (8 credits), Anatomy with lab (4 credits), Physiology with lab (4 credits), Microbiology with lab (4 credits), Statistics (3 credits), Psychology (3 credits), Medical Terminology (1 credit), English/College Writing (3 credits). Prerequisites must be completed with a grade "B" or better and within the last 10 years. At most two prerequisites may be outstanding at the time of application. AP credits are not accepted. Recommended courses: Biochemistry, Genetics, Organic Chemistry, Physics, Intro to Pharmacology.

GPA Requirement: Overall GPA 3.25; Science GPA 3.25

Healthcare Experience: 200 hours

PA Shadowing: Required (no specific number of hours)

Required Standardized Testing: None

Letters of Recommendation: Three required; preferably one academic, one patient care and one additional academic or patient care

Seat Deposit: $1,000

THOMAS JEFFERSON UNIVERSITY CENTER CITY CAMPUS

MISSION:

The mission of the Center City Physician Assistant Studies Program is to use our model of interprofessional education to educate skilled, compassionate physician assistants prepared to provide leadership through our evolving healthcare system, dedicated to lifelong learning and service to the community.

NO CLASS STATISTICS REPORTED

PANCE SCORES

5-year First Time Pass: 100% (based on three years of data)

Most Recent First Time Pass: 100%

CURRICULUM STRUCTURE

Didactic: 15 months

Clinical: 12 months

Rotations: 7 mandatory, 1 elective (each 5 weeks)

Graduate Project: Required for graduation

UNIQUE PROGRAM FEATURES

Facilities: A 66-seat, 1,605 square foot, state-of-the-art classroom and an additional 2,935 square foot laboratory space within the Dorrance Hamilton Building is dedicated for primary use by the PA program. PA students also have access to the Dr. Robert & Dorothy Rector Clinical Skills and Simulation Center (RCSSC) for clinical skills instruction and patient simulation.

Health Mentors Program: This program is an innovative longitudinal approach to teaching clinical medicine in multidisciplinary groups, pairing a patient living with chronic disease and an integrated group of students representing Sidney Kimmel Medical College and the Colleges of Pharmacy, Nursing and Health Professions.

Anatomy: Students are instructed in anatomy by professors in the Department of Pathology, Anatomy & Cell Biology at Sidney Kimmel Medical College. Students will be completing the laboratory portion of the course in a newly-designed, 32,200 square-foot, multi-room laboratory. Six dissection rooms are each equipped with high-definition monitors, and at each dissection table are computers loaded with anatomical education and reference software.

Jefferson University – East Falls Campus

Physician Assistant Program
Hayward Hall 224
4201 Henry Avenue
Philadelphia, PA 19144
Phone: 215-951-2908
Email: paprogram@philau.edu

PROGRAM HIGHLIGHTS

Accreditation: Continuing

Degree Offered: Master (MSPAS)

Start Date: July annually

Program Length: 25 months

Class Capacity: 52 students

Tuition: $90,020

CASPA Participant: Yes

Supplemental Application: No

Yellow Ribbon: No

Admissions: Rolling

Application Deadline: November 1

PREREQUISITE COURSEWORK

Biology with lab (8 credits), Chemistry with lab (8 credits), Anatomy with lab (4 credits), Physiology with lab (4 credits), Microbiology with lab (4 credits), Statistics or Mathematics (3 credits), Psychology (3 credits), College Writing (3 credits), Medical Terminology (1 credit). Prerequisites must be completed with a grade "C" or better and within the last 10 years. AP credits are accepted provided they are listed on your college transcript.

GPA Requirement: Overall GPA 3.25; Science GPA 3.25

Healthcare Experience: 200 hours

PA Shadowing: Preferred, not required

Required Standardized Testing: None

Letters of Recommendation: Three required; preferably one academic, one patient care and one additional academic or patient care

Seat Deposit: $2,000

THOMAS JEFFERSON UNIVERSITY EAST FALLS CAMPUS (FORMERLY PHILADELPHIA UNIVERSITY)

MISSION:

The mission of the Jefferson Physician Assistant Program is to provide students with the foundation of knowledge, technical skills and critical thinking necessary to competently perform the functions of the physician assistant profession in an ethical, empathetic manner working with a licensed practicing physician. A secondary focus is to prepare students to provide comprehensive medical services to diverse under-served patient populations in inner-city and rural locations.

CLASS OF 2020

Overall GPA: 3.70

Science GPA: 3.60

PANCE SCORES

5-year First Time Pass: 96%

Most Recent First Time Pass: 97%

CURRICULUM STRUCTURE

Didactic: 12 months

Clinical: 13 months

Rotations: 8 mandatory, 2 elective (each 5 weeks)

UNIQUE PROGRAM FEATURES

Program: Philadelphia University merged with Thomas Jefferson University on July 1, 2017. The Philadelphia University PA Program is now one program offered at two campuses. This program is now referred to as the Jefferson University PA Program East Falls Campus & Jefferson University PA Program New Jersey Campus. The same curriculum is delivered on both East Falls and the New Jersey campuses.

Admissions Preference: Graduates from Jefferson and Stockton University are granted preferential admissions.

325

University of Pittsburgh

Physician Assistant Studies
3010 William Pitt Way
Pittsburgh, PA 15238
Phone: 412-624-6743
Email: mlacovey@pitt.edu

PROGRAM HIGHLIGHTS

Accreditation: Continuing

Degree Offered: Master (MS)

Start Date: January annually

Program Length: 24 months

Class Capacity: 48 students

Tuition: $88,638 (in-state); $105,375 (out-of-state)

CASPA Participant: Yes

Supplemental Application: No

Yellow Ribbon: No

Admissions: Rolling

Application Deadline: November 1

PREREQUISITE COURSEWORK

Anatomy with lab and Physiology (2 semesters), Biology with lab (2 semesters), Chemistry with lab (2 semesters), English Composition/Writing (2 semesters), Microbiology with lab (1 semester), Organic Chemistry with lab (1 semester), Intro Psychology (1 semester), Upper level Psychology (1 semester), Statistics (1 semester), Medical Terminology (1 semester or 1 credit). Prerequisite coursework must be completed by August 31st of the year of application. AP credits are accepted provided they are listed on your college transcript.

GPA Requirement: Overall GPA 3.0; Prerequisite Science GPA 3.0

Healthcare Experience: 500 hours

PA Shadowing: Preferred, not required

Required Standardized Testing: None

Letters of Recommendation: Three required; one from a professor, one from a supervisor of healthcare experience, and one character reference describing your commitment to leadership and service

Seat Deposit: $1,000

UNIVERSITY OF PITTSBURGH

MISSION:

The mission of the Physician Assistant (PA) Studies Program is to advance the PA profession and improve the health of our communities and the nation by: Developing and graduating a workforce of diverse and inclusive certified PAs with the required clinical knowledge, affective behaviors, and psychomotor skills to practice individualized health care in inter-professional teams; Promoting a lifelong desire for continued learning, scholarly activity, service to the community and advocacy within the PA profession; Contributing and coordinating research about the PA profession and the science, delivery, and administration of health care; and serving all communities of our school, city, and the world.

CLASS OF 2020

Male: 23%

Female: 77%

Overall GPA: 3.61

Science GPA: 3.60

GRE Verbal: 62nd percentile

GRE Quantitative: 55th percentile

GRE Analytical: 68th percentile

Average Healthcare Experience: 2,532 hours

Average Shadowing Experience: 60 hours

Average Age: 24

PANCE SCORES

5-year First Time Pass: 94%

Most Recent First Time Pass: 95%

CURRICULUM STRUCTURE

Didactic: 12 months

Clinical: 12 months

Rotations: 7 mandatory, 2 elective (each 5 weeks)

UNIQUE PROGRAM FEATURES

Affiliations: The Pitt PA program has a unique relationship with UPMC, one of the most renowned academic medical centers in the US. UPMC, an integrated health care delivery system focused on recruiting and retaining superb physicians and researchers, has developed internationally renowned centers in transplantation, cancer, neurosurgery, psychiatry, rehabilitation, geriatrics and women's health, among others.

PA Student Society: The program has a very active student society that is active in professional events and community service.

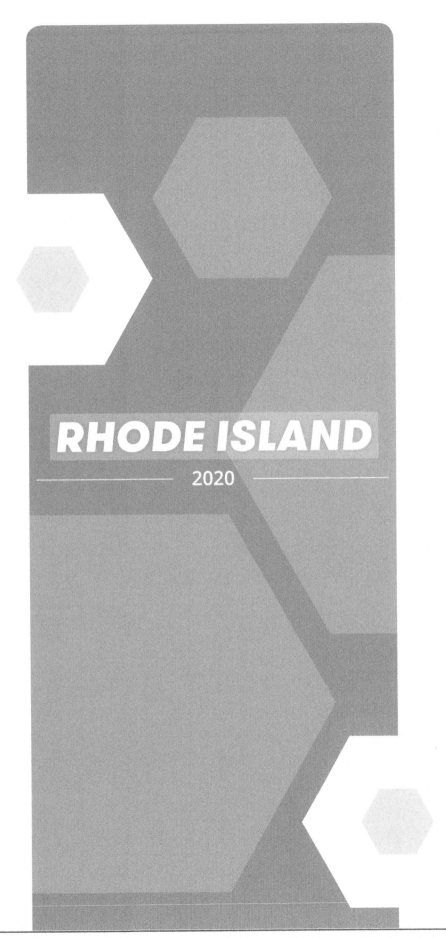

RHODE ISLAND

2020

Bryant University

1150 Douglas Pike
Smithfield, RI 02917
Phone: 401-232-6556
Email: pa_program@bryant.edu

PROGRAM HIGHLIGHTS

Accreditation: Continuing

Degree Offered: Master (MSPAS)

Start Date: January annually

Program Length: 27 months

Class Capacity: 45 students

Tuition: $100,724

CASPA Participant: Yes

Supplemental Application:
Yes ($50 fee)

Yellow Ribbon: No

Admissions: Rolling

Application Deadline: October 1

PREREQUISITE COURSEWORK

Biology with lab (8 credits),
Chemistry with lab (8 credits),
Human Anatomy and Physiology
(8 credits), Microbiology (3 credits),
Biochemistry or Organic Chemistry
with lab (3-4 credits), Psychology
(3 credits), Statistics (3 credits).
Prerequisites must be completed
with a grade of "C" or better and
by September 1st of the year of
application. AP credits are not
accepted.

GPA Requirement: Overall GPA 3.0;
Prerequisite GPA 3.0

Healthcare Experience: 2,000 hours

PA Shadowing: Not required

Required Standardized Testing: GRE

Letters of Recommendation: Three
required; no one specific

Seat Deposit: $800

BRYANT UNIVERSITY

MISSION:

To improve universal access to health care by graduating highly competent and confident Physician Assistants prepared to provide exceptional quality, patient-centered ethical health care in a collaborative environment.

NO CLASS STATISTICS REPORTED

PANCE SCORES

5-year First Time Pass: 97% (based on three years of data)

Most Recent First Time Pass: 95%

CURRICULUM STRUCTURE

Didactic: 15 months

Clinical: 12 months

Rotations: 11 mandatory, 1 elective (each 5 weeks)

UNIQUE PROGRAM FEATURES

Didactics: The human anatomy course takes place at Brown University's medical education building.

Facilities: The program has all new, high-tech classrooms and laboratories, including a high-fidelity simulation lab and a physical exam lab.

Johnson & Wales University

8 Abbott Park Place
Providence, RI 02903
Phone: 401-598-2381
Email: kspolidoro@jwu.edu

PROGRAM HIGHLIGHTS

Accreditation: Probation

Degree Offered: Master (MSPAS)

Start Date: June annually

Program Length: 24 months

Class Capacity: 36 students

Tuition: $94,392

CASPA Participant: Yes

Supplemental Application: No

Yellow Ribbon: Yes

Admissions: Rolling

Application Deadline: March 1

PREREQUISITE COURSEWORK

Anatomy and Physiology with lab (8 credits), Biology with lab (8 credits), Chemistry (Organic and Biochemistry preferred) with lab (8 credits), Math (3 credits), English (6 credits), Psychology or Sociology or Behavioral Science (6 credits). A&P must be completed within 7 years of matriculation. Prerequisites must be completed with a grade "C" or better. AP credits are not accepted.

GPA Requirement: Overall GPA 3.0; Science GPA 3.0

Healthcare Experience: 250 hours

PA Shadowing: Required (no specific number of hours)

Required Standardized Testing: GRE

Letters of Recommendation: Three required; no one specific

Seat Deposit: $1,000

JOHNSON & WALES UNIVERSITY

MISSION:

The mission of the Physician Assistant Studies program at JWU is to educate students to become collaborative practitioners with the respect, empathy and trust inherent to patient-centered, humanistic health care.

CLASS OF 2021

Male: 14%

Female: 86%

Overall GPA: 3.68

Science GPA: 3.62

GRE Verbal: 59th percentile

GRE Quantitative: 46th percentile

GRE Analytical: 67th percentile

Average Healthcare Experience: 2,880 hours

PANCE SCORES

5-year First Time Pass: 97% (based on four years of data)

Most Recent First Time Pass: 94%

CURRICULUM STRUCTURE

Didactic: 12 months

Clinical: 12 months

Rotations: 7 mandatory, 2 elective (each 5 weeks)

UNIQUE PROGRAM FEATURES

Admissions Preference: Articulation agreements are in place with local colleges and universities (Providence College, University of Rhode Island), with the goal of recruiting students local to the area who desire to practice in Rhode Island upon completion of their training.

Facilities: JWU offers an innovative, state-of-the-art facility specifically for the PA program, equipped with lecture halls with global teleconferencing capabilities, "active learning" classrooms, cadaver-based anatomy lab with access to e-study guides at each dissection station, and a clinical practice center similar to a hospital emergency room.

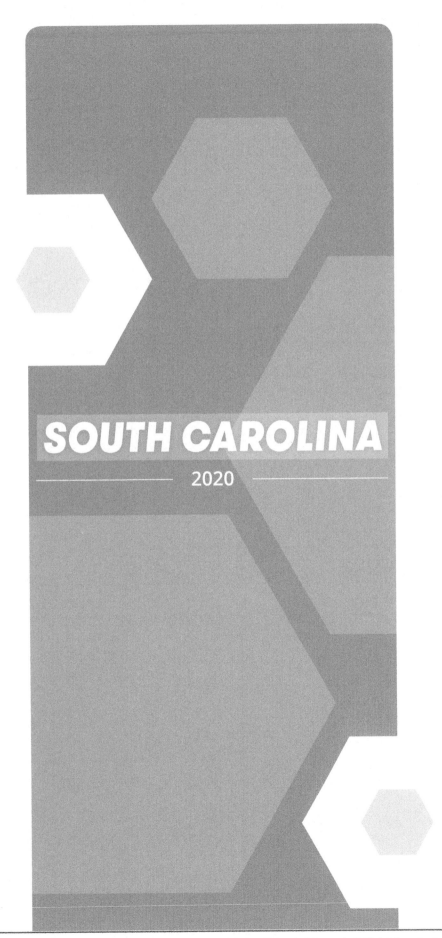

SOUTH CAROLINA

2020

Charleston Southern University

9200 University Blvd
Charleston, SC 29406
Phone: 843-863-7427
Email: paprogram@csuniv.edu

PROGRAM HIGHLIGHTS

Accreditation: Provisional

Degree Offered: Master (MMS)

Start Date: January annually

Program Length: 24 months

Class Capacity: 25 students

Tuition: $93,000

CASPA Participant: Yes

Supplemental Application: No

Yellow Ribbon: Yes

Admissions: Rolling

Application Deadline: September 1

PREREQUISITE COURSEWORK

Human Anatomy and Physiology with lab (8 credits), Microbiology with lab (4 credits), Organic Chemistry or Biochemistry with lab (4 credits), Upper level Biology, Chemistry or Physics (6 credits), Statistics (3 credits), Medical Terminology (1 credit). Prerequisites must be completed with a grade "C" or better and within the last 7 years. Applicants may apply with two remaining prerequisites provided they complete each with a grade "B" or better and before September 1st. AP credits are not accepted.

GPA Requirement: Overall GPA 3.0; Science GPA 3.0

Healthcare Experience: 1,000 hours

PA Shadowing: Preferred, not required

Required Standardized Testing: GRE

Letters of Recommendation: Three required; two must be from a healthcare setting and one of these must include a medical provider (PA, NP, MD, DO)

Seat Deposit: $1,000

CHARLESTON SOUTHERN UNIVERSITY

MISSION:

The mission of the Charleston Southern University Master of Medical Science in physician assistant studies program is to educate compassionate and highly motivated individuals in a Christian environment who excel in providing patient-centered care, practicing as an interprofessional team, serving as leaders in their communities and advancing the PA profession.

CLASS OF 2020

Male: 23%

Female: 77%

Minority: 16%

Overall GPA: 3.50

Science GPA: 3.40

PANCE SCORES

5-year First Time Pass: N/A

Most Recent First Time Pass: N/A (have not graduated a class yet)

CURRICULUM STRUCTURE

Didactic: 12 months

Clinical: 12 months

Rotations: 7 mandatory, 2 elective (each 5 weeks)

Graduate Research Project: Required for graduation

UNIQUE PROGRAM FEATURES

Facilities: A state of the art Health Science Building has recently been built to house the PA Program. It includes a cadaver lab, a simulation lab, a dry skills lab, debriefing rooms, exam rooms, lecture space and a computer lab for the program.

Curriculum: The program recognizes that not all students learn in the same way and has thus developed a curriculum structure to include lecture, small group, problem-based learning, high-fidelity simulation and practical hands-on training.

333

Francis Marion University

PO Box 100547
Florence, SC 29502
Phone: 843-661-1659
Email: eshefton@fmarion.edu

PROGRAM HIGHLIGHTS

Accreditation: Probation

Degree Offered: Master (MSPAS)

Start Date: August annually

Program Length: 27 months

Class Capacity: 32 students

Tuition: $68,348 (in-state);
$136,696 (out-of-state)

CASPA Participant: Yes

Supplemental Application: Yes ($41 fee)

Yellow Ribbon: No

Admissions: Non-rolling

Application Deadline: January 15

PREREQUISITE COURSEWORK

Anatomy and Physiology with lab (8 credits),
General Biology with lab (4 credits), Microbiology
with lab (4 credits), General Chemistry with lab
(8 credits), Organic Chemistry with lab (4 credits),
Statistics or Biostatistics (3 credits), Psychology
(6 credits), Medical Terminology (1 credit).
Prerequisites must be completed within the last
10 years.

GPA Requirement: Overall GPA 3.0; Prerequisite
GPA 3.0

Healthcare Experience: 250 hours

PA Shadowing: Preferred, not required

Required Standardized Testing: GRE (minimum
combined score 290 required, with 140 on each
of the verbal and quantitative sections)

Letters of Recommendation: Three required;
preferably from former professors or
professional associates/supervisors who can
attest to your academic potential

Seat Deposit: $500

FRANCIS MARION UNIVERSITY

MISSION:

The Francis Marion University Physician Assistant
Program seeks to educate excellent primary care
physician assistants to become compassionate,
ethical, and clinically skillful graduates who are
ready to provide health care services with personal
and professional integrity.

NO CLASS STATISTICS REPORTED

PANCE SCORES

5-year First Time Pass: 78% (based on one year of
data)

Most Recent First Time Pass: 78%

CURRICULUM STRUCTURE

Didactic: 15 months

Clinical: 12 months

Rotations: 7 mandatory, 1 elective, 1 primary care
elective (each 4 weeks)

UNIQUE PROGRAM FEATURES

Facilities: The PA program is housed in
a new building that has state of the art
equipment that gives a great opportunity
for learning. It is equipped with the latest
teaching technology in medical education
including a simulation center, an OSCE
suite, physical exam and anatomy labs, large
classrooms, and space for students to study
and gather.

Medical University of South Carolina

College of Health Professions
151-A Rutledge Avenue, MSC 960
Charleston, SC 29425
Phone: 843-792-3326
Email: chpstusv@musc.edu

PROGRAM HIGHLIGHTS

Accreditation: Continuing

Degree Offered: Master (MSPAS)

Start Date: May annually

Program Length: 27 months

Class Capacity: 60 students

Tuition: $57,918 (in-state);
$95,837 (out-of-state)

CASPA Participant: Yes

Supplemental Application: Yes ($80 fee)

Yellow Ribbon: No

Admissions: Non-rolling

Application Deadline: September 1

PREREQUISITE COURSEWORK

Statistics or Biostatistics (3 credits), General Chemistry I and II with lab (8 credits), Organic or Biochemistry (3 credits), Biology with lab (4 credits), Human Anatomy with lab (4 credits), Human Physiology with lab (4 credits), Microbiology with lab (4 credits), Medical Terminology (1 credit), Developmental Psychology or Human Growth and Development (3 credits). Prerequisites must be completed with a grade "C" or better and within the last 10 years. AP credits are not accepted.

GPA Requirement: Overall GPA 3.0; Prerequisite GPA 3.0

Healthcare Experience: Required (no specific number of hours)

PA Shadowing: Preferred, not required

Required Standardized Testing: GRE, CASPer

Letters of Recommendation: Three required; at least one should be from a health care provider, preferably a PA or physician

Seat Deposit: $1,000

MEDICAL UNIVERSITY OF SOUTH CAROLINA

MISSION:

To graduate highly competent physician assistants who are compassionate, culturally aware and attuned to the primary healthcare needs of the people of South Carolina and beyond.

CLASS OF 2021

Male: 24%

Female: 76%

Minority: 20%

Overall GPA: 3.64

Prerequisite GPA: 3.62

GRE Total: 55th percentile

Average Age: 25.4

PANCE SCORES

5-year First Time Pass: 97%

Most Recent First Time Pass: 98%

CURRICULUM STRUCTURE

Didactic: 15 months

Clinical: 12 months

Rotations: 8 mandatory, 1 elective (each 5 weeks)

Graduate Project: Required for graduation

UNIQUE PROGRAM FEATURES

Admissions Preference: Approximately 50% of each class is made up of South Carolina residents.

Community Service: MUSC PA students are involved in various projects in the local community as well as international mission trips.

North Greenville University

405 Lancaster Avenue
Greer, SC 29650
Phone: 864-663-0266
Email: paadmissions@ngu.edu

PROGRAM HIGHLIGHTS

Accreditation: Provisional

Degree Offered: Master (MMS)

Start Date: January annually

Program Length: 24 months

Class Capacity: 30 students

Tuition: $106,848

CASPA Participant: Yes

Supplemental Application: No

Yellow Ribbon: No

Admissions: Rolling

Application Deadline: August 1

PREREQUISITE COURSEWORK

Anatomy and Physiology I and II with lab (8 credits), General Biology with lab (4 credits), Other Biology course (3 credits), Microbiology (3 credits), General Chemistry with lab (4 credits), Other Chemistry course (3 credits), Psychology (3 credits), Statistics (3 credits). Prerequisites must be completed with a grade "B" or better and ideally within the last 5-7 years. Up to two prerequisites may be in progress at the time of application.

GPA Requirement: Overall GPA 3.0; Prerequisite GPA 3.0

Healthcare Experience: Preferred, not required

PA Shadowing: Preferred, not required

Required Standardized Testing: GRE (optional if you already have a Master's degree or higher)

Letters of Recommendation: Three required; each from a professional source

Seat Deposit: $1,500

NORTH GREENVILLE UNIVERSITY

MISSION:

To develop well-informed and compassionate PAs who provide patient centered and service oriented medical care in diverse environments.

NO CLASS STATISTICS REPORTED

PANCE SCORES

5-year First Time Pass: 100% (based on one year of data)

Most Recent First Time Pass: 100%

CURRICULUM STRUCTURE

Didactic: 12 months

Clinical: 12 months

Rotations: 7 mandatory, 1 elective (each 4 weeks except Family Medicine, which is 12 weeks)

UNIQUE PROGRAM FEATURES

Goals: Program goals are aimed at employment in South Carolina in the primary care sector and with underserved populations.

Applicant Selection: The NGU PA program values fair admissions practices, evaluating applicants using the following objective criteria: Transcripts (Overall Academic Strength and Science Aptitude); GRE; Letters of 'Professional' Recommendation; Paid Health Care Experience; Provider Shadowing and Volunteerism. Each of these items will be given a weighted point value (based on preset objective criteria) and the combined score will be used to rank candidates for interview (pre-screen matrix). The higher your score, the better your odds of being interviewed. Additionally, all North Greenville University graduates and military veterans who meet the PA Program admission requirements will be invited for an interview.

International Rotation: Students have the opportunity to complete an international elective rotation in Nicaragua, Dominican Republic, or India.

Presbyterian College

503 South Broad Street
Clinton, SC 29325
Phone: 864-938-3746
Email: jhtyson@presby.edu

PROGRAM HIGHLIGHTS

Accreditation: Provisional

Degree Offered: Master (MPAS)

Start Date: October annually

Program Length: 24 months

Class Capacity: 32 students

Tuition: $94,000 (including fees)

CASPA Participant: Yes

Supplemental Application: No

Yellow Ribbon: Not specified

Admissions: Rolling

Application Deadline: April 1

PREREQUISITE COURSEWORK

Anatomy and Physiology I and II with lab (8 credits), Organic Chemistry with lab (4 credits), Psychology (3 credits), Microbiology with lab (3 credits), Genetics (3 credits) all completed within the last 7 years; General Chemistry I and II with lab (8 credits), Biology I and II with lab (8 credits) both completed within the last 10 years; English (6 credits), Statistics or Algebra or Calculus or Finite Math or other equivalent math (6 credits), Humanities or Social Science (6 credits), Medical Terminology no time limit on these. Prerequisites must be completed with a grade "B" or better, with the exception of Organic Chemistry, which must be completed with a "C" or better. Prerequisites must be completed by July 31st prior to matriculation. AP credits may be accepted.

GPA Requirement: Overall GPA 3.2; Science GPA 3.2

Healthcare Experience: 250 hours

PA Shadowing: 50 hours (counts towards healthcare experience)

Required Standardized Testing: GRE

Letters of Recommendation: Three required; one from a certified PA or physician, one from a professor holding a doctoral degree OR a second from a certified PA or physician, and one of your choice who has knowledge of your work ethic, academic record, volunteer work or other activities and can comment on your ability to succeed in the PA program

Seat Deposit: $1,500

PRESBYTERIAN COLLEGE

MISSION:

The compelling purpose of Presbyterian College Physician Assistant Studies Program, as part of a church-related college, is to develop within the framework of Christian faith the medical, mental, moral, physical, and spiritual capacities of each student in preparation for a lifetime of service to our patients and those in need in our society.

NO CLASS STATISTICS REPORTED

PANCE SCORES

5-year First Time Pass: N/A

Most Recent First Time Pass: N/A (have no graduated a class yet)

CURRICULUM STRUCTURE

Didactic: 12 months

Clinical: 12 months

Rotations: 7 mandatory, 1 elective (each 5 weeks)

UNIQUE PROGRAM FEATURES

Early Clinical Exposure: There are targeted opportunities to shadow clinicians during the first year to provide students with early experiences in the healthcare field. This will also help strengthen didactic learning.

Student Bios: Available on the program website to learn more about current students enrolled in the program.

Physician Assistant Studies Program

School of Medicine
University of South Carolina
Columbia, SC 29208
Phone: 803-216-3950
Email: paprogram@uscmed.sc.edu

PROGRAM HIGHLIGHTS

Accreditation: Probation

Degree Offered: Master (MSPAS)

Start Date: January annually

Program Length: 27 months

Class Capacity: 30 students

Tuition: $52,815 (in-state); $91,896 (out-of-state)

CASPA Participant: Yes

Supplemental Application: Yes ($50 fee)

Yellow Ribbon: No

Admissions: Rolling

Application Deadline: September 1

PREREQUISITE COURSEWORK

Human Anatomy and Physiology I and II with lab (8 credits), Genetics (3 credits), General Chemistry I and II with lab (8 credits), Organic Chemistry with lab (4 credits), Biochemistry (3 credits), Microbiology (3 credits), Introductory Psychology or higher (3 credits), Statistics (3 credits), Medical Terminology (1 credit). At most two prerequisites may be pending at the time of application. Prerequisites must be completed within the last 7 years.

GPA Requirement: Overall GPA 3.0; Science GPA 3.0

Healthcare Experience: 500 hours

PA Shadowing: 50 hours (recommended, counts towards healthcare experience)

Required Standardized Testing: GRE

Letters of Recommendation: Three required; no one specific

Seat Deposit: $1,000

UNIVERSITY OF SOUTH CAROLINA SCHOOL OF MEDICINE

MISSION:

The USC School of Medicine–Columbia Masters in Science in Physician Assistant Studies Program strives to produce highly competent, compassionate physician assistants who are committed to lifelong learning and advancing the PA profession. The program is dedicated to producing physician assistants who deliver high-quality, patient-centered care, excel as members of an interprofessional health care team, while making significant contributions to the health care needs of South Carolina and the nation.

CLASS OF 2019

Overall GPA: 3.71

Science GPA: 3.63

GRE Total: 306

Average Healthcare Experience: 1,445 hours

PANCE SCORES

5-year First Time Pass: 95% (based on one year of data)

Most Recent First Time Pass: 95%

CURRICULUM STRUCTURE

Didactic: 15 months

Clinical: 12 months

Rotations: 8 mandatory, 2 elective (each 4-8 weeks)

Capstone Project: Required for graduation

UNIQUE PROGRAM FEATURES

Admissions Preference: Applicants who have served their communities or their countries through volunteer activities, military service, or employment opportunities greatly enhance the cultural perspective of the class. The PA Program is committed to attracting students from geographically underserved regions such as Area Health Education Centers (AHEC) in South Carolina, as well as students from different racial, ethnic, and socioeconomic backgrounds. Preference is given to South Carolina residents, USC alumni, and US veterans.

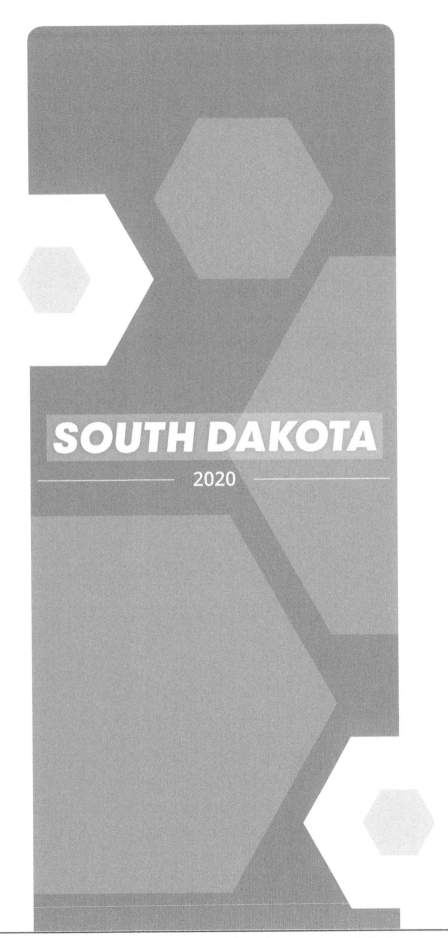

SOUTH DAKOTA

2020

The University of South Dakota

Physician Assistant Studies
414 East Clark Street, Julian Hall 120
Vermillion, SD 57069
Phone: 605-658-5926
Email: pa@usd.edu

PROGRAM HIGHLIGHTS

Accreditation: Continuing

Degree Offered: Master (MS)

Start Date: July annually

Program Length: 24 months

Class Capacity: 25 students

Tuition: $33,909 (in-state); $84,487 (out-of-state)

CASPA Participant: Yes

Supplemental Application: Yes ($35 fee)

Yellow Ribbon: No

Admissions: Not reported

Application Deadline: September 1

PREREQUISITE COURSEWORK

Biology (8 credits), Chemistry with lab (8 credits), Anatomy and Physiology with lab (8 credits), Microbiology with lab (4 credits), Biochemistry (3 credits), General Psychology (3 credits), Abnormal Psychology (3 credits), Statistics (2 credits). Prerequisites should be completed within the last 10 years and by June 1st of the year of planned matriculation. Prerequisites must be completed with a grade "C" or better.

GPA Requirement: Overall GPA 3.0; Prerequisite GPA 3.0

Healthcare Experience: 500 hours

PA Shadowing: Preferred, not required

Required Standardized Testing: Not required

Letters of Recommendation: Three required; preferably from college professors and PAs, MDs or other healthcare professionals with whom you have worked

Seat Deposit: $200

UNIVERSITY OF SOUTH DAKOTA

MISSION:

The Physician Assistant Studies Program at the University of South Dakota provides a comprehensive primary care education that prepares graduates to deliver high-quality healthcare to meet the needs of patients in South Dakota and the surrounding region.

CLASS OF 2020

Overall GPA: 3.80

Science GPA: 3.77

Average Healthcare Experience: 2.7 years

Average Age: 25

PANCE SCORES

5-year First Time Pass: 95%

Most Recent First Time Pass: 96%

CURRICULUM STRUCTURE

Didactic: 12 months

Clinical: 12 months

Rotations: 8 mandatory, 2 elective (each 6 weeks)

Master's Project: Required for graduation

UNIQUE PROGRAM FEATURES

Admissions Preference: The admissions committee gives preference to applicants with an overall and prerequisite GPA of 3.2 or greater, desire for practice in primary care or medically underserved area, direct patient contact of 1,000 hours or greater, and those with strong ties to South Dakota (resident, one or both parents are residents, graduated from high school in South Dakota, graduated from an accredited South Dakota University or College). However, the program also accepts non-resident students and encourages them to apply.

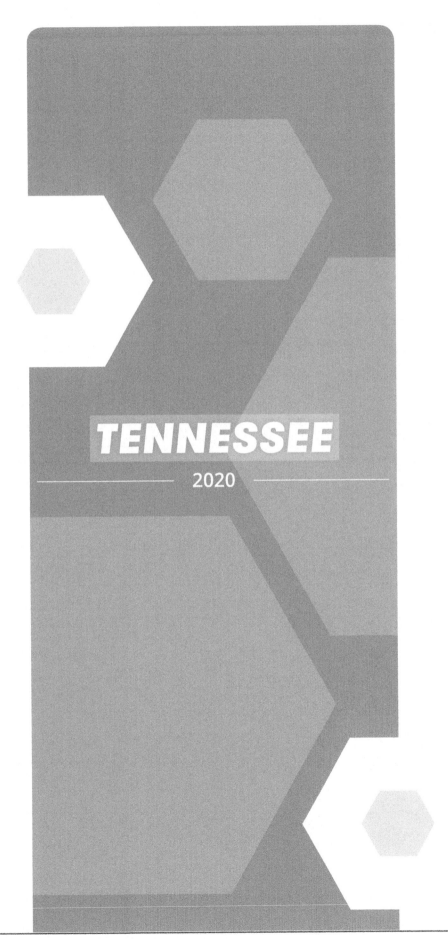

TENNESSEE
2020

Bethel University, Paris Campus

302B Tyson Avenue
Paris, TN 38242
Phone: 731-407-7650
Email: paprogram@bethelu.edu

PROGRAM HIGHLIGHTS

Accreditation: Continuing
Degree Offered: Master (MSPAS)
Start Date: January annually
Program Length: 27 months
Class Capacity: 50 students
Tuition: $87,500

CASPA Participant: Yes
Supplemental Application: Yes ($75 fee)
Yellow Ribbon: No
Admissions: Rolling
Application Deadline: September 1

PREREQUISITE COURSEWORK

General Biology I and II, General Chemistry I and II, Human Anatomy and Physiology I and II, Microbiology or Bacteriology, Psychology, Human Genetics. No prerequisites older than 5 years will be accepted, unless you have been employed full time in the health care field since completion of those prerequisites. Prerequisites must be completed with a grade "C" or better and by September 1st prior to the year of matriculation. Recommended courses: Biochemistry, Organic Chemistry, Cell Biology, Pharmacology, Immunology, Intro Statistics, Critical Thinking.

GPA Requirement: No minimum

Healthcare Experience: Preferred, not required

PA Shadowing: 40 hours

Required Standardized Testing: GRE

Letters of Recommendation: Three required; two from a PA, MD, DO, or NP and one from a university professor or advisor

Seat Deposit: $1,000

BETHEL UNIVERSITY

MISSION:

The Physician Assistant Program's mission is to create opportunities for the members of the learning community interested in healthcare to ultimately graduate as exceptional and compassionate healthcare professionals who practice medicine within an ethical framework grounded in Christian principles.

CLASS OF 2021

Overall GPA: 3.40

Science GPA: 3.30

GRE Total: 304

GRE Analytical: 3.8

Average Healthcare Experience: >1,900 hours

Average Shadowing Experience: 250 hours

Average Age: 25

PANCE SCORES

5-year First Time Pass: 95%

Most Recent First Time Pass: 90%

CURRICULUM STRUCTURE

Didactic: 12 months

Clinical: 15 months

Rotations: 8 mandatory, 3 elective (each 5 weeks)

UNIQUE PROGRAM FEATURES

Business of Medicine: This course is taken during clinical year and educates students on group practice models, management, human resources, insurance products, CPT and ICD coding, third party reimbursement as well as the potential impact of health care reform.

Community Service: The students participate in several volunteer commitments throughout the year including volunteering at a free clinic, toy drives, and 5k runs.

Christian Brothers University

650 East Parkway South
Memphis, TN 38104
Phone: 901-321-3388
Email: pas@cbu.edu

PROGRAM HIGHLIGHTS

Accreditation: Provisional

Degree Offered: Master (MSPAS)

Start Date: January annually

Program Length: 29 months

Class Capacity: 32 students

Tuition: $93,120

CASPA Participant: Yes

Supplemental Application: No

Yellow Ribbon: Yes

Admissions: Rolling

Application Deadline: October 1

PREREQUISITE COURSEWORK

General Biology I and II with lab, Anatomy and Physiology I and II with lab, General Chemistry I and II with lab, Organic Chemistry I and II, Microbiology with lab, Psychology, Statistics, Medical Terminology. Prerequisites must be completed with a grade "C" or better. If a course has been repeated, the repeat grade will be used in GPA calculations. AP credits are accepted if they were accepted at the undergraduate level.

GPA Requirement: Overall GPA 3.0; Prerequisite GPA 3.0

Healthcare Experience: Preferred, not required

PA Shadowing: Not required

Required Standardized Testing: CASPer

Letters of Recommendation: Two required; should be from health care professionals

Seat Deposit: $750

CHRISTIAN BROTHERS UNIVERSITY

MISSION:

To educate and prepare diverse and exemplary individuals to become caring, competent, ethical, and professional physician assistants who can practice clinically in a wide variety of settings and positively affect their patients, the community, and the health care system through evidence-based and preventive medicine, leadership, life-long learning, utilization of information technology, the provision of health care to the medically underserved, interdisciplinary team care, patient advocacy, and the delivery of primary health care for all patients.

CLASS OF 2021

Male: 38%

Female: 62%

Minority: 28%

Overall GPA: 3.48

Prerequisite GPA: 3.36

Average Healthcare Experience: 2,825 hours

Average Age: 24

PANCE SCORES

5-year First Time Pass: N/A

Most Recent First Time Pass: N/A (have not graduated a class yet)

CURRICULUM STRUCTURE

Didactic: 15 months

Clinical: 14 months

Rotations: 8 mandatory, 1 elective (each 6 weeks)

UNIQUE PROGRAM FEATURES

Admissions Preference: Preference is given to residents of the metro Memphis area and those living in the Mid-South, CBU students and alumni, and applicants with service in the armed forces.

Lincoln Memorial

6965 Cumberland Gap Parkway
Harrogate, TN 37752
Phone: 423-869-6669
Email: paadmissions@lmunet.edu

PROGRAM HIGHLIGHTS

Accreditation: Continuing

Degree Offered: Master (MMS)

Start Date: May annually

Program Length: 27 months

Class Capacity: 96 students

Tuition: $90,125

CASPA Participant: Yes

Supplemental Application:
Yes ($50 fee)

Yellow Ribbon: No

Admissions: Rolling

Application Deadline: November 1

PREREQUISITE COURSEWORK

General Biology I and II with lab (8-10 credits), General Chemistry I and II with lab (8-10 credits), Organic Chemistry I with lab and Organic Chemistry II with lab or Biochemistry (8-10 credits), Human Anatomy with lab (3-4 credits), Human Physiology (3-4 credits), Microbiology with lab (3-4 credits), General Psychology (3 credits), Psychology Elective (3 credits), English (6 credits), Mathematics (3 credits), Statistics (2-3 credits), Medical Terminology (2 credits). Prerequisites must be completed with a grade "C" or better. Prerequisites may be in progress at the time of application. Recommended courses: Biochemistry, Biostatistics, Advanced Psychology, Cell Biology, Embryology, Epidemiology, Histology, Immunology, Parasitology, Pathogenic Bacteriology, Abnormal Psychology, Human Sexuality, Physics, Technical Writing, Advanced Chemistry and Quantitative Analysis.

GPA Requirement: Overall GPA 2.8; Science GPA 2.8

Healthcare Experience: 150 hours

PA Shadowing: 40 hours (20 of these hours must be in a primary care setting)

Required Standardized Testing: GRE

Letters of Recommendation: Three required; one must be from a PA, one from a PA, MD, dentist, podiatrist, or optometrist, and one from an academic advisor, science/math professor, or current/recent employer

Seat Deposit: $500

LINCOLN MEMORIAL UNIVERSITY

MISSION:

To educate future Physician Assistants to provide quality healthcare with an emphasis in primary care to the medically underserved of Appalachia and beyond.

CLASS OF 2020

Overall GPA: 3.49

Science GPA: 3.38

GRE Verbal: 152

GRE Quantitative: 150

GRE Analytical: 3.9

PANCE SCORES

5-year First Time Pass: 94%

Most Recent First Time Pass: 92%

CURRICULUM STRUCTURE

Didactic: 14 months

Clinical: 13 months

Rotations: 8 mandatory, 1 elective, 1 selective (each 4-8 weeks)

Capstone Project: Required for graduation

UNIQUE PROGRAM FEATURES

Facilities: The school has a clinical exam center and simulation lab where students are able to experience a variety of simulated medical scenarios, using trained simulated patients, simulated devices and an actual medical and surgical facility that could be found in a clinic or hospital "real world" setting.

Mission Trips: Each year PA students and faculty organize and participate in mission trips to places like Peru, Honduras, Nicaragua and Guatemala, as well as participate in other leadership endeavors.

347

Lipscomb University

One University Park Drive
Nashville, TN 37204
Phone: 615-966-7247
Email: paschool@lipscomb.edu

PROGRAM HIGHLIGHTS

Accreditation: Provisional

Degree Offered: Master (MPAS)

Start Date: September annually

Program Length: 27 months

Class Capacity: 50 students

Tuition: $110,015 (including fees)

CASPA Participant: Yes

Supplemental Application: No

Yellow Ribbon: No

Admissions: Rolling

Application Deadline: December 1

PREREQUISITE COURSEWORK

Biology (8 credits to include any of the following: Cell Biology with lab, Microbiology with lab, Immunology, Virology, Molecular Basis of Human Disease, Molecular Biology with lab or Genetics), Human Anatomy and Physiology I and II with lab (8 credits), Chemistry (8 credits to include any of the following: General Chemistry I and II with lab, Organic Chemistry I and II or Chemistry for Health Sciences with lab), Psychology (3 credits), Statistics (3 credits). Prerequisites must be completed with a grade "C" or better and within the last 7 years for science prerequisites. AP credits may be accepted for the Statistics and Psychology requirements.

GPA Requirement: Overall GPA 3.0; Prerequisite GPA 3.0

Healthcare Experience: Required (no specific number of hours)

PA Shadowing: Required (no specific number of hours)

Required Standardized Testing: Not required

Letters of Recommendation: Three required; highly recommended that one be from a PA

Seat Deposit: $1,500

LIPSCOMB UNIVERSITY

MISSION:

The Lipscomb University School of Physician Assistant Studies is focused on educating students to become physician assistants who will provide service to their community as an integral part of the healthcare team. Our mission is built on a framework of Christian ethics rooted in faith and is committed to producing knowledgeable and compassionate healthcare providers of the highest quality. Our graduates will be servant leaders in medicine that work to improve patients' health across the lifespan.

CLASS OF 2021

Overall GPA: 3.70

Science GPA: 3.61

Average Healthcare Experience: 831 hours

Average Shadowing Experience: 90 hours

PANCE SCORES

5-year First Time Pass: N/A

Most Recent First Time Pass: N/A (have not graduated a class yet)

CURRICULUM STRUCTURE

Didactic: 15 months

Clinical: 12 months

Rotations: 7 mandatory, 1 elective (each 6 weeks)

UNIQUE PROGRAM FEATURES

Religious Focus: Lipscomb University is committed to uniting Christian faith and practice with academic excellence. They believe that you are called to serve in the healthcare industry, and they engage in local partnerships with Vanderbilt, Meharry, Heritage, HCA and Sarah Cannon to best prepare you for a number of hands-on careers to match your professional calling.

MILLIGAN COLLEGE

MISSION:

To prepare physician assistants as servant leaders who provide clinical expertise while making positive contributions to the profession, the communities they practice in, and society as a whole.

CLASS OF 2021

Overall GPA: 3.68

Science GPA: 3.66

GRE Total: 305

PANCE SCORES

5-year First Time Pass: N/A

Most Recent First Time Pass: N/A (have not graduated a class yet)

CURRICULUM STRUCTURE

Didactic: 15 months

Clinical: 13 months

Rotations: 7 mandatory, 1 elective (each 6 weeks)

UNIQUE PROGRAM FEATURES

Religious Focus: The program offers a course titled Christ and Calling in Healthcare, which entails an examination of how contemporary Western cultures shape how Christians understand their faith, and an exploration of how Christians in healthcare are affected by this and respond to these challenges as a healthcare employee on a daily basis and by taking part in medical missions and service to others.

Facilities: The Ballad Health Physician Assistant Center, housed in Milligan's B. D. Phillips Building, has an open floor plan with 13 patient exam tables, eight of which are equipped with medical equipment including ophthalmoscopes, otoscopes, blood pressure cuffs, thermometers, wall desks, and privacy curtains that separate each area. The Center is used to train students in a wide array of clinical competencies, including communication, history taking, physical examination, counseling, and patient safety. Clinical skills training, such as practice with urinary catheter trainers, IV injection manikin arms, casting, and suturing, also take place in the MSHA PA Center.

South College

Physician Assistant Studies
400 Goody's Lane
Knoxville, TN 37922
Phone: 865-251-1800
Email:
pa_program@southcollegetn.edu

PROGRAM HIGHLIGHTS

Accreditation: Continuing

Degree Offered: Master (MHS)

Start Date: October annually

Program Length: 27 months

Class Capacity: 85 students

Tuition: $101,250

CASPA Participant: Yes

Supplemental Application: Yes ($95 fee)

Yellow Ribbon: Yes

Admissions: Not reported

Application Deadline: March 1

PREREQUISITE COURSEWORK

Anatomy and Physiology I and II with lab (8 credits), General Chemistry I and II with lab (8 credits), Biology I and II with lab (8 credits), English (6 credits), Statistics or other Advanced Math (6 credits), Humanities or Social Science (6 credits). AP credits are accepted provided they are listed on your college transcript. Recommended courses: Genetics, Microbiology, Immunology, Organic Chemistry, Biochemistry, other advanced Bio/Chem courses.

GPA Requirement: Overall GPA 2.75; Science GPA 2.75; Prerequisite GPA 2.75

Healthcare Experience: Preferred, not required

PA Shadowing: Preferred, not required

Required Standardized Testing: GRE

Letters of Recommendation: Three required; one must be from a physician, PA or NP

Seat Deposit: $1,500

SOUTH COLLEGE - KNOXVILLE

MISSION:

The mission of the South College Masters of Health Science in Physician Assistant Studies program is to educate highly qualified physician assistants, preparing them to become competent, compassionate, and comprehensive healthcare providers for clinical practice in rural and urban areas, focusing on underserved communities.

CLASS OF 2019

Overall GPA: 3.51

GRE Verbal: 155

GRE Quantitative: 154

GRE Analytical: 4.0

Average Healthcare Experience: 1,501 hours

PANCE SCORES

5-year First Time Pass: 97%

Most Recent First Time Pass: 96%

CURRICULUM STRUCTURE

Didactic: 15 months

Clinical: 12 months

Rotations: 7 mandatory, 1 elective (each 6 weeks)

Capstone Research Project: Required for graduation

UNIQUE PROGRAM FEATURES

VET-UP: This program is specifically designed for medics and corpsmen candidates as a bridging program to enter the Physician Assistant Program at South College. Candidates must have 4 years military service as a medic or corpsmen and be in the process of completing a BS degree with a focus on health sciences.

South College

616 Marriott Drive
Nashville, TN 37214
Phone: 629-802-3000
Email: panashville@south.edu

PROGRAM HIGHLIGHTS

Accreditation: Provisional

Degree Offered: Master (MHS)

Start Date: October annually

Program Length: 27 months

Class Capacity: 30 students

Tuition: $101,250

CASPA Participant: Yes

Supplemental Application: Yes ($95 fee)

Yellow Ribbon: Yes

Admissions: Not reported

Application Deadline: March 1

PREREQUISITE COURSEWORK

Anatomy and Physiology I and II with lab (8 credits), General Chemistry I and II with lab (8 credits), Biology I and II with lab (8 credits), English (6 credits), Statistics or other Advanced Math (6 credits), Humanities or Social Science (6 credits). AP credits are accepted provided they are listed on your college transcript. Recommended courses: Genetics, Microbiology, Immunology, Organic Chemistry, Biochemistry, other advanced Bio/Chem courses.

GPA Requirement: Overall GPA 2.75; Science GPA 2.75; Prerequisite GPA 2.75

Healthcare Experience: Preferred, not required

PA Shadowing: Not required

Required Standardized Testing: GRE

Letters of Recommendation: Three required; one must be from a physician, PA or NP

Seat Deposit: $1,500

SOUTH COLLEGE - NASHVILLE

MISSION:

The mission of the South College, Nashville Campus, Masters of Health Science in Physician Assistant Studies program is to educate highly qualified physician assistants, preparing them to become competent, compassionate, and comprehensive healthcare providers for clinical practice in rural and urban areas, who will mature into leaders within the medical community.

CLASS OF 2021

Overall GPA: 3.43

Science GPA: 3.38

Average Healthcare Experience: 5,313 hours

PANCE SCORES

5-year First Time Pass: N/A

Most Recent First Time Pass: N/A (have not graduated a class yet)

CURRICULUM STRUCTURE

Didactic: 15 months

Clinical: 12 months

Rotations: 7 mandatory, 1 elective (each 6 weeks)

Capstone Research Project: Required for graduation

UNIQUE PROGRAM FEATURES

VET-UP: This program is specifically designed for medics and corpsmen candidates as a bridging program to enter the Physician Assistant Program at South College. Candidates must have 4 years military service as a medic or corpsmen and be in the process of completing a BS degree with a focus on health sciences.

Trevecca Nazarene University

333 Murfreesboro Road
Nashville, TN 37210
Phone: 615-248-1225
Email: Admissions_PA@trevecca.edu

PROGRAM HIGHLIGHTS

Accreditation: Continuing

Degree Offered: Master (MSM)

Start Date: May annually

Program Length: 27 months

Class Capacity: 50 students

Tuition: $92,300

CASPA Participant: Yes

Supplemental Application: No

Yellow Ribbon: No

Admissions: Not reported (though early application is recommended)

Application Deadline: October 1

PREREQUISITE COURSEWORK

Human Anatomy and Physiology with lab (8 credits), General Chemistry I and II with lab (8 credits), Microbiology with lab (3-4 credits), General Psychology (3 credits), Developmental Psychology (3 credits), Medical Terminology (1 credit or certificate). Prerequisites must be completed within 7 years of matriculation. No more than two prerequisites should be pending for the spring semester prior to matriculation. Recommended courses: Immunology, Pathophysiology, Genetics, Molecular or Cell Biology, Biochemistry, Organic Chemistry.

GPA Requirement: Overall GPA 3.25; Science GPA 3.25

Healthcare Experience: 250 hours

PA Shadowing: 10 hours

Required Standardized Testing: GRE (minimum score of 300)

Letters of Recommendation: Three required; one must be from a PA

Seat Deposit: $500

TREVECCA NAZARENE UNIVERSITY

MISSION:

To prepare professionally competent physician assistants who will use their skills to serve their communities in compassionate ministry.

CLASS OF 2021

Overall GPA: 3.70

Science GPA 3.76

GRE Total: 307

PANCE SCORES

5-year First Time Pass: 99%

Most Recent First Time Pass: 98%

CURRICULUM STRUCTURE

Didactic: 15 months

Clinical: 12 months

Rotations: 7 mandatory, 1 elective (each 6 weeks)

UNIQUE PROGRAM FEATURES

Medical Mission Trips: Students can participate in rotations and trips to Zambia, Swaziland, and Haiti.

Community Service: Trevecca's PA students participate in learning experiences with The Clinic at Mercury Courts and Room In The Inn, which serve Nashville's medically underserved and homeless population.

University of Tennessee Health Science Center

Master of Medical Science Physician Assistant Program
66 North Pauline St. #116
Memphis, TN 38163
Phone: 901-448-8000
Email: paprograminfo@uthsc.edu

PROGRAM HIGHLIGHTS

Accreditation: Continuing

Degree Offered: Master (MMS-PA)

Start Date: January annually

Program Length: 24 months

Class Capacity: 30 students

Tuition: $49,154 (in-state); $81,518 (out-of-state)

CASPA Participant: Yes

Supplemental Application: No

Yellow Ribbon: Yes

Admissions: Rolling

Application Deadline: August 1

PREREQUISITE COURSEWORK

Anatomy and Physiology with lab (8 credits), Biology with lab (8 credits), Microbiology (3 credits), Chemistry with lab (8 credits), Medical Terminology (1 credit), General Psychology or Sociology or Anthropology (3 credits), Math (3 credits). Prerequisites must be completed with a grade "C" or better and by the time of application submission. For any course that has been repeated, the grades will be averaged to calculate a final grade. Recommended courses: Cell Biology, Molecular Biology, Genetics.

GPA Requirement: Overall GPA 3.0; Science GPA 3.0

Healthcare Experience: 500 hours (can include shadowing hours)

PA Shadowing: Preferred, not required

Required Standardized Testing: GRE (combined score of 300 is considered competitive)

Letters of Recommendation: Three required; preferably from a professor, an MD and a PA

Seat Deposit: $1,000

UNIVERSITY OF TENNESSEE HEALTH SCIENCE CENTER (MEMPHIS)

MISSION:

The mission of the University of Tennessee Health Science Center's Physician Assistant program is to prepare a diverse group of highly skilled Physician Assistant practitioners who are dedicated to improving access and providing high quality primary and/or specialty health care as part of interprofessional teams and who are committed to lifelong learning and to increasing the knowledge base of the profession.

NO CLASS STATISTICS REPORTED

PANCE SCORES

5-year First Time Pass: 97% (based on four years of data)

Most Recent First Time Pass: 100%

CURRICULUM STRUCTURE

Didactic: 12 months

Clinical: 12 months

Rotations: 9 mandatory, 2 elective (each 4 weeks)

Capstone Project: Required for graduation

UNIQUE PROGRAM FEATURES

Academic Medical Center: This is the only program in TN that boasts being part of an academic medical center and providing students with access to the resources therein.

Applicants: The program factors in Tennessee residence when reviewing applications, and historically about half of the students in each class are from Tennessee.

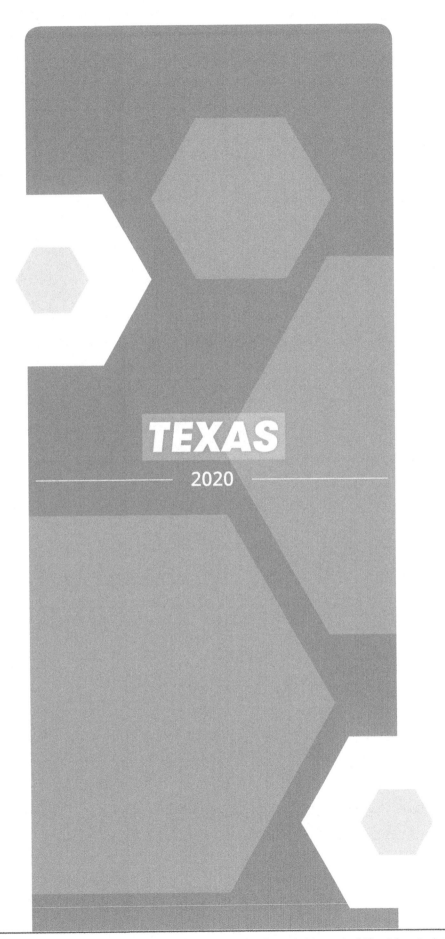

TEXAS

2020

Baylor College of Medicine

1 Baylor Plaza
Physician Assistant Program, M108
Houston, TX 77030
Phone: 713-798-3663
Email: paprogram@bcm.edu

PROGRAM HIGHLIGHTS

Accreditation: Continuing

Degree Offered: Master (MSPA)

Start Date: June annually

Program Length: 30 months

Class Capacity: 40 students

Tuition: $66,730

CASPA Participant: Yes

Supplemental Application: No (but $50 fee)

Yellow Ribbon: No

Admissions: Non-rolling

Application Deadline: September 1

PREREQUISITE COURSEWORK

Anatomy with lab (4 credits), Physiology with lab (4 credits), Microbiology with lab (4 credits), Genetics (3 credits), General Chemistry I and II with lab (8 credits), Organic Chemistry with lab (4 credits), Statistics (3 credits), General Psychology (3 credits), Humanities Elective (3 credits), English Composition (3 credits). Science prerequisites must be completed within the last 7 years and non-science within the last 10 years. All prerequisites must be completed by May of the year of matriculation and with a grade "C" or better. AP credits are not accepted. Recommended courses: Medical Terminology.

GPA Requirement: Overall GPA 3.2; Science GPA 3.2

Healthcare Experience: Preferred, not required

PA Shadowing: Preferred, not required

Required Standardized Testing: GRE (minimum 153 verbal, 144 quantitative, and 3.5 analytical)

Letters of Recommendation: Three required; no one specific

Seat Deposit: $300

BAYLOR COLLEGE OF MEDICINE

MISSION:

To educate physician assistants who will provide excellent healthcare to individuals and communities in a broad range of settings. The core values embraced by the program's faculty include honesty, integrity, self-motivation, flexibility, lifelong learning, reflective practice, teamwork, and primary concern for the patient's welfare.

CLASS OF 2021

Male: 12%

Female: 88%

Minority: 37%

Overall GPA: 3.70

GRE Verbal: 78th percentile

GRE Quantitative: 74th percentile

GRE Analytical: 54th percentile

Average Age: 24

PANCE SCORES

5-year First Time Pass: 97%

Most Recent First Time Pass: 97%

CURRICULUM STRUCTURE

Didactic: 13 months

Clinical: 17 months

Rotations:
11 mandatory
(each 4-8 weeks)

Master's Research Paper: Required for graduation

UNIQUE PROGRAM FEATURES

Texas Medical Center: As the largest medical center in the world it offers world class facilities for the training of fellows, residents, medical, psychology, pharmacy, nursing, and social work students and others in the allied health disciplines.

Interdisciplinary Education: Team-based instruction occurs within the didactic and clinical phases of the curriculum with experiences involving various mixes of medical, nurse anesthesia, physician assistant, pharmacy, social work, and nursing students to ensure a rich experience in the area of role socialization.

Curriculum: Working with standardized patients in Baylor's Simulation Program for Clinical Performance Improvement, PA students practice and receive feedback on their history taking, examination, and counseling skills.

Enrichment Pathways: Students have the option to pursue specialized interests through enrichment tracks offered in collaboration with the School of Medicine. Pathways open to PA students include medical ethics and global health. PA students may also opt to earn a Diploma in Tropical Medicine through the Baylor College of Medicine National School of Tropical Medicine.

Community Involvement: An important element of the PA program curriculum is the service learning requirement, which provides students with early exposures to underserved members of the Houston community and the social and medical issues that beset linguistically isolated individuals.

Hardin-Simmons University

2434 Hickory St.
Abilene, TX 79698
Phone: 325-670-1702
Email: PAdept@hsutx.edu

PROGRAM HIGHLIGHTS

Accreditation: Provisional

Degree Offered: Master (MPAS)

Start Date: August annually

Program Length: 27 months

Class Capacity: 30 students

Tuition: $77,682 (including fees)

CASPA Participant: Yes

Supplemental Application: No

Yellow Ribbon: No

Admissions: Rolling

Application Deadline: December 1

PREREQUISITE COURSEWORK

Anatomy (4 credits), Physiology (4 credits), Biology (8 credits), Chemistry (4 credits), Organic Chemistry (4 credits), English (3 credits), Microbiology (4 credits), Statistics (3 credits), Psychology (3 credits), Sociology or additional Psychology (3 credits). You may have courses planned or in progress at the time of application. AP credits are accepted provided they are listed on your college transcript.

GPA Requirement: Overall GPA 3.0; Science GPA 3.0

Healthcare Experience: Preferred, not required

PA Shadowing: Preferred, not required

Required Standardized Testing: GRE, CASPer (recommended)

Letters of Recommendation: Three required; no one specific

Seat Deposit: $500

HARDIN-SIMMONS UNIVERSITY (ABILENE)

MISSION:

The mission of the Hardin-Simmons University PA Program is to develop and prepare compassionate, professional PA providers who are committed to life-long leadership, learning, and community service. Graduates will work as part of the healthcare team to deliver exceptional healthcare to rural West Texas and under-served communities worldwide.

CLASS OF 2020

Minority: 30%

Overall GPA: 3.66

Science GPA: 3.63

GRE Verbal: 153.47

GRE Quantitative: 151.87

GRE Analytical: 3.98

Average Healthcare Experience: 2,439 hours

PANCE SCORES

5-year First Time Pass: N/A

Most Recent First Time Pass: N/A (have not graduated a class yet)

CURRICULUM STRUCTURE

Didactic: 14 months

Clinical: 13 months

Rotations: 8 mandatory, 2 elective (each 5 weeks)

Capstone Project: Required for graduation

UNIQUE PROGRAM FEATURES

Community Service: The PA Program curriculum requires 50 hours of community service. Students may volunteer in many different ways, including an annual medical mission trip. In spring 2018, the PA Dept., collaborating with Buckner International, went to Peru where they treated 714 people in 5 days. The trip wrapped up with a visit to Machu Picchu.

Interservice PA Program

3599 Winfield Scott
IPAP, Building #2841, Suite 2512
Fort Sam Houston, TX 78234
Phone: 210-221-8004
Email: maria.r.charles.civ@mail.mil

PROGRAM HIGHLIGHTS

Accreditation: Continuing

Degree Offered: Master (MSPA)

Start Date: August annually

Program Length: 29 months

Class Capacity: 200 students

Tuition: $0

CASPA Participant: No

Supplemental Application: No

Yellow Ribbon: No

Admissions: Not reported

Application Deadline: None

PREREQUISITE COURSEWORK

A minimum of 60 semester hours with emphasis in science coursework. SAT, Basic Life Support, and the Service Unique Applicant Package must also be completed.

GPA Requirement: Overall GPA 2.50; Science GPA 3.0

Healthcare Experience: Preferred, not required

PA Shadowing: Not required

Required Standardized Testing: None

Letters of Recommendation: Three required; from a PA, their commanding officer, and another from their immediate supervisor

Seat Deposit: None

INTERSERVICE

MISSION:

To provide the uniformed services with highly competent, compassionate physician assistants who model integrity, strive for leadership excellence, and are committed to lifelong learning.

NO CLASS STATISTICS REPORTED

PANCE SCORES

5-year First Time Pass: 96%

Most Recent First Time Pass: 86%

CURRICULUM STRUCTURE

Didactic: 16 months

Clinical: 13 months

Rotations: 11 mandatory, 1 elective (variable duration)

Master's Thesis: Required for graduation

UNIQUE PROGRAM FEATURES

Applicants: This program is only for Service members of the Army, Navy, Air Force, Coast Guard, Army Reserves, and Army National Guard. Marine Corps applicants are also encouraged to apply. There is no direct civilian pathway for students to directly enter with program without joining one of the above military services.

Rotations: Students are assigned to a single core site where they complete the majority of their rotations.

TTUHSC Physician Assistant Program

3600 N. Garfield
Midland, TX 79705
Phone: 432-620-1120
Email: health.professions@ttuhsc.edu

PROGRAM HIGHLIGHTS

Accreditation: Continuing

Degree Offered: Master (MPAS)

Start Date: May annually

Program Length: 27 months

Class Capacity: 60 students

Tuition: $32,125 (in-state); $84,875 (out-of-state)

CASPA Participant: Yes

Supplemental Application: Yes ($75 fee)

Yellow Ribbon: No

Admissions: Rolling

Application Deadline: October 1

PREREQUISITE COURSEWORK

Genetics (3 credits), Microbiology (4 credits), Anatomy and Physiology (8 credits), Organic Chemistry or Biochemistry (4 credits), Psychology (3 credits), Statistics (3 credits). No more than 9 credits of prerequisite courses may be in progress at the time of application. Prerequisite courses completed within the last 7 years are preferred. AP credits are not accepted.

GPA Requirement: Overall GPA 3.0; Science GPA 3.0

Healthcare Experience: Preferred, not required

PA Shadowing: Preferred, not required

Required Standardized Testing: GRE

Letters of Recommendation: Three required; no one specific

Seat Deposit: $125

TEXAS TECH UNIVERSITY HEALTH SCIENCES CENTER

MISSION:

The mission of the Texas Tech University Health Sciences Center School of Health Professions Physician Assistant Program is to provide comprehensive medical education to physician assistant students. Through an environment of academic excellence and the promotion of life-long learning and professionalism, graduates will be prepared to practice patient-centered primary care, increasing access to healthcare for communities of West Texas and beyond.

CLASS OF 2021

Minority: 5%

Overall GPA: 3.56

Science GPA: 3.46

GRE Verbal: 53rd percentile

GRE Quantitative: 37th percentile

GRE Analytical: 52nd percentile

Average Age: 26.1

PANCE SCORES

5-year First Time Pass: 96%

Most Recent First Time Pass: 91%

CURRICULUM STRUCTURE

Didactic: 15 months

Clinical: 12 months

Rotations: 7 mandatory, 1 selective (each 6 weeks)

Master's Project: Required for graduation

UNIQUE PROGRAM FEATURES

Applications: Priority in application review and invitation for interview will be given to those applicants who have verified CASPA, the supplemental application complete, and official GRE scores reported by August 1.

Rotations: Applicants are assigned to a single region where they complete the majority of their clinical rotations. No region is limited to one city however. Example regions include El Paso, Lubbock, Amarillo, Abilene, and Odessa/Midland.

Admissions Preference: In accordance with the mission and goals of the PA Program, special consideration may be given to the following applicants: Residents from the 108 counties in the service area of TTUHSC; veterans; residents from underserved populations; or residents from economically or environmentally disadvantaged backgrounds.

PA Admissions
3500 Camp Bowie Boulevard
Fort Worth, TX 76107
Phone: 817-735-2003
Email: padmissions@unthsc.edu

PROGRAM HIGHLIGHTS

Accreditation: Continuing

Degree Offered: Master (MPAS)

Start Date: August annually

Program Length: 30 months

Class Capacity: 75 students

Tuition: $21,360 (in-state, including fees); 79,320 (out-of-state, including fees)

CASPA Participant: Yes

Supplemental Application: No (but $40 fee)

Yellow Ribbon: No

Admissions: Rolling

Application Deadline: October 1

PREREQUISITE COURSEWORK

Psychology (3 credits), Statistics (3 credits), Anatomy with lab (4 credits), Physiology with lab (4 credits), Organic Chemistry with lab (4 credits), Microbiology with lab (4 credits), Genetics (3 credits). Prerequisites must be completed with a grade "C" or better and prior to December 31st of the application year. AP credits are accepted provided they are listed on your college transcript.

GPA Requirement: Overall GPA 3.0

Healthcare Experience: Preferred, not required

PA Shadowing: Preferred, not required

Required Standardized Testing: GRE

Letters of Recommendation: Two required; highly recommended that one be from a PA with whom you have worked or shadowed

Seat Deposit: None

UNIVERSITY OF NORTH TEXAS HEALTH SCIENCES CENTER - FORT WORTH

MISSION:

The mission of the Program is to create solutions for a healthier community by preparing graduates with knowledge and skills needed for physician assistant practice, emphasizing primary care medicine and meeting the healthcare needs of underserved populations.

CLASS OF 2021

Overall GPA: 3.76

Science GPA: 3.70

GRE Total: 65th percentile

PANCE SCORES

5-year First Time Pass: 100%

Most Recent First Time Pass: 99%

CURRICULUM STRUCTURE

Didactic: 18 months

Clinical: 12 months

Rotations: 8 mandatory, 4 elective (each 4 weeks)

Master's Project: Required for graduation

UNIQUE PROGRAM FEATURES

Early Application: The program highly recommends applying early due to its rolling admissions. To be considered for the first interview day of the cycle, an applicant should have his/her application and all supporting materials submitted no later than the end of July.

Early Clinical Exposure: Students complete supervised clinical experiences throughout the didactic portion of the curriculum to begin to integrate classroom knowledge with clinical learning.

Rotations: Every student completes a rotation dedicated to working with an underserved population.

Dual Degree: The program offers a dual PA/MPH degree option.

361

Department of Physician Assistant
Studies
7703 Floyd Curl Drive, MSC 6249
San Antonio, TX 78229
Phone: 210-567-4240
Email: pastudies@uthscsa.edu

PROGRAM HIGHLIGHTS

Accreditation: Continuing

Degree Offered: Master (MPAS)

Start Date: June annually

Program Length: 30 months

Class Capacity: 45 students

Tuition: $36,683 (in-state);
$84,212 (out-of-state)

CASPA Participant: Yes

Supplemental Application: Yes ($60 fee)

Yellow Ribbon: No

Admissions: Non-rolling

Application Deadline: October 1

PREREQUISITE COURSEWORK

Human Anatomy and Physiology I
and II with lab (8 credits), General
Chemistry I and II with lab (8
credits), Organic Chemistry with
lab (4 credits), Microbiology with
lab (4 credits), Genetics (3 credits),
Psychology (3 credits), Statistics (3
credits). All prerequisites must be
completed within the last 10 years,
with a grade "C" or better, and by
the application deadline. AP credits
are accepted provided they are
listed on your college transcript.

GPA Requirement: Overall GPA 3.0;
Science GPA 3.0

Healthcare Experience: Preferred,
not required

PA Shadowing: Preferred, not
required

Required Standardized Testing: GRE

Letters of Recommendation: Two
required; no one specific

Seat Deposit: Not specified

UNIVERSITY OF TEXAS - HEALTH SCIENCES CENTER AT SAN ANTONIO

MISSION:

The Mission of the Department of Physician Assistant Studies at the University of Texas Health Science Center, San Antonio is to prepare outstanding physician assistants to recognize and treat acute and chronic illness and promote health. The Department of Physician Assistant Studies makes lives better by improving the health care, health outcomes and the wellbeing of patients and their families through education, practice, service and research.

CLASS OF 2021

Male: 27%

Female: 73%

Minority: 62%

Overall GPA: 3.54

Science GPA: 3.47

Average Healthcare
Experience: 4,574 hours

Average Shadowing
Experience: 233 hours

Average Age: 24

PANCE SCORES

5-year First Time Pass: 99%

Most Recent First Time Pass:
98%

CURRICULUM STRUCTURE

Didactic: 14 months

Clinical: 16 months

Rotations: 10 mandatory,
5 elective (each 4 weeks)

Research Project: Required for
graduation

UNIQUE PROGRAM FEATURES

Interprofessional Education: There are a number of interprofessional educational opportunities available throughout the Physician Assistant Studies curriculum within the School of Health Professions. Additionally, the TeamSTEPPS course of instruction is a required component of the PA studies curriculum and is embedded within PHAS 6004, Preventative Medicine and Public Health.

University of Texas - Medical Branch at Galveston

301 University Boulevard
Galveston, TX 77555-1145
Phone: 409-772-3048
Email: pasadmis@utmb.edu

PROGRAM HIGHLIGHTS

Accreditation: Continuing

Degree Offered: Master (MPAS)

Start Date: July annually

Program Length: 26 months

Class Capacity: 90 students

Tuition: $39,689 (in-state, including fees); $86,443 (out-of-state, including fees)

CASPA Participant: Yes

Supplemental Application: Yes ($35 fee)

Yellow Ribbon: No

Admissions: Rolling

Application Deadline: September 1

PREREQUISITE COURSEWORK

Biological Sciences with lab (8 credits), Microbiology or Bacteriology with lab (3-4 credits), Immunology or Virology (3 credits), Genetics (3 credits), Human Anatomy with lab (4 credits), Human Physiology with lab (4 credits), Chemistry with lab (8 credits), Organic Chemistry or Biochemistry with lab (3-4 credits), Behavioral Sciences (6 credits), Statistics (3 credits), Medical Terminology (2-3 credits). Prerequisites must be completed with a grade "C" or better.

GPA Requirement: Overall GPA 3.0; Science GPA 3.0

Healthcare Experience: Preferred, not required

PA Shadowing: Preferred, not required

Required Standardized Testing: GRE

Letters of Recommendation: Three required; recommended that letters be from professors, college advisors, clinicians or employers

Seat Deposit: $1,000

UNIVERSITY OF TEXAS MEDICAL BRANCH AT GALVESTON

MISSION:

To develop and graduate academically and clinically exceptional physician assistants.

CLASS OF 2021

Male: 18%

Female: 82%

Minority: 46%

Overall GPA: 3.66

Science GPA: 3.58

GRE Verbal: 153

GRE Quantitative: 152

Average Age: 25

PANCE SCORES

5-year First Time Pass: 98%

Most Recent First Time Pass: 94%

CURRICULUM STRUCTURE

Didactic: 12 months

Clinical: 14 months

Rotations: 11 mandatory, 1 elective (each 4 weeks)

UNIQUE PROGRAM FEATURES

Admissions Preference: Preference is given to Texas residents, however, all applicants are considered.

The University of Texas Rio Grande Valley

The Graduate College
Marialice Shary Shivers Bldg. 1.158
1201 West University Drive
Edinburg, TX 78539
Phone: 956-665-2298
Email: pad@utrgv.edu

PROGRAM HIGHLIGHTS

Accreditation: Continuing

Degree Offered: Master (MPAS)

Start Date: August annually

Program Length: 28 months

Class Capacity: 100 students

Tuition: $19,930 (in-state); $48,890 (out-of-state)

CASPA Participant: Yes

Supplemental Application: Yes ($50 fee)

Yellow Ribbon: No

Admissions: Rolling

Application Deadline: September 1

PREREQUISITE COURSEWORK

General Biology I and II (6 credits), Genetics (3 credits), Microbiology (3 credits), Anatomy and Physiology I and II (6 credits), General Chemistry I and II (6 credits), Organic Chemistry or Biochemistry (3 credits), Statistics (3 credits), Intro Psychology or Abnormal Psychology (3 credits). All prerequisites must be completed by the application deadline. At least 15 credits must be completed within the last 5 years. Recommended courses: Spanish, Medical Terminology.

GPA Requirement: Overall GPA 3.0

Healthcare Experience: Preferred, not required

PA Shadowing: Preferred, not required

Required Standardized Testing: GRE

Letters of Recommendation: Three required; preferably one from a professor, one from a healthcare provider you have shadowed or worked with, and one from an employer/supervisor

Seat Deposit: None

UNIVERSITY OF TEXAS - RIO GRANDE VALLEY

MISSION:

The mission of the Department of Physician Assistant (DPA) at The University of Texas Rio Grande Valley is to provide an innovative advanced medical education to physician assistant students who will transform health care delivery to the multicultural population of South Texas. The DPA promotes the importance of lifelong learning and self-evaluation in its students.

CLASS OF 2021

Male: 28%

Female: 72%

Minority: 81%

Overall GPA: 3.57

Science GPA: 3.52

Average Age: 25.1

PANCE SCORES

5-year First Time Pass: 93%

Most Recent First Time Pass: 91%

CURRICULUM STRUCTURE

Didactic: 12 months

Clinical: 16 months

Rotations: 8 mandatory, 1 elective (each 4 weeks)

Capstone Project: Required for graduation

UNIQUE PROGRAM FEATURES

Diversity: The University of Texas Rio Grande Valley is the second largest Hispanic serving institution in the US with over 24,000 enrolled. UTRGV is a veteran friendly campus and the veteran's department on campus works well with the PA department in assisting those veteran students in the PA program.

Spanish Language: Fluency or experience with the Spanish language is desirable given the location of the program and is taken into consideration at the time of application.

UT Southwestern

5323 Harry Hines Boulevard
Dallas, TX 75390-9090
Phone: 214-648-1701
Email:
PA.SSHP@UTSouthwestern.edu

PROGRAM HIGHLIGHTS

Accreditation: Continuing

Degree Offered: Master (MPAS)

Start Date: May annually

Program Length: 30 months

Class Capacity: 60 students

Tuition: $41,149 (in-state, including fees); $87,629 (out-of-state, including fees)

CASPA Participant: Yes

Supplemental Application: No

Yellow Ribbon: No

Admissions: Non-rolling

Application Deadline: September 1

PREREQUISITE COURSEWORK

Human Anatomy with lab (4 credits), Human Physiology with lab (4 credits), Genetics (3 credits), Psychology (3 credits), General Chemistry with lab (8 credits), Organic Chemistry with lab (4 credits), Microbiology with lab (4 credits), Statistics (3 credits). Prerequisites must be completed in the last 10 years and must be complete at the time of application. Prerequisites must be completed with a grade "C" or better. Recommended courses: Biochemistry, Cellular Biology, Human Sexuality, Immunology, Medical Terminology, Pharmacology, Spanish.

GPA Requirement: Overall GPA 3.0; Science GPA 3.0

Healthcare Experience: Preferred, not required

PA Shadowing: Preferred, not required

Required Standardized Testing: GRE

Letters of Recommendation: Three required; no one specific

Seat Deposit: None

UT SOUTHWESTERN - SCHOOL OF HEALTH PROFESSIONS

MISSION:

The mission of the Physician Assistant Studies Program is to: excel in the art and science of physician assistant education and promote inter-professional primary health care delivery to a diverse and dynamic population; to encourage leadership, service, and excellence among our faculty, staff, students, and graduates; and to foster a commitment to evidence-based practice, quality improvement, and patient safety.

CLASS OF 2019

Male: 26%

Female: 74%

Overall GPA: 3.66

Science GPA: 3.77

GRE Total: 307

Average Age: 24

PANCE SCORES

5-year First Time Pass: 100%

Most Recent First Time Pass: 100%

CURRICULUM STRUCTURE

Didactic: 15 months

Clinical: 15 months

Rotations: 9 mandatory, 1 elective (each 4-8 weeks)

Research Project: Required for graduation

UNIQUE PROGRAM FEATURES

Admissions Preference: At least 90% of each class is comprised of Texas residents based on current state laws.

Clinical Experiences: Students will experience clinical training at two new state-of-the-art on campus teaching hospitals and have opportunities for international clinical experiences.

365

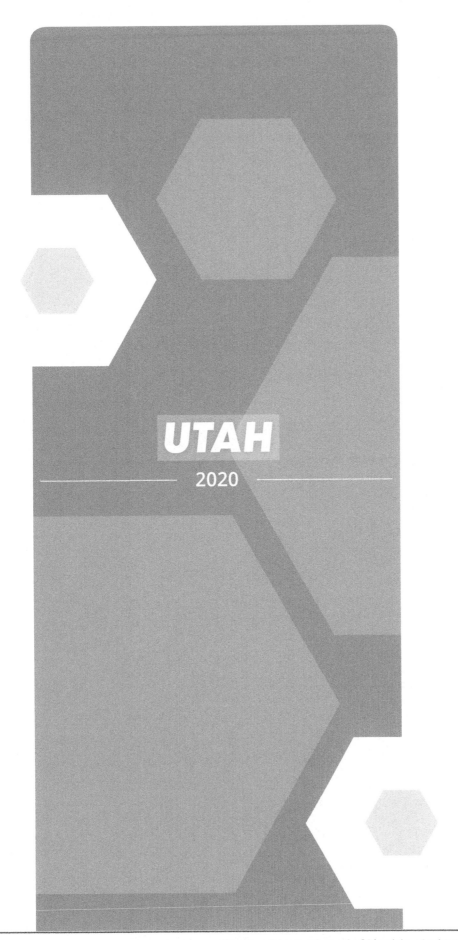

UTAH

2020

Rocky Mountain University of Health Professions

122 East 1700 South, Building 3
Provo, UT 84606
Phone: 801-375-5125
Email: admissions@rmuohp.edu

PROGRAM HIGHLIGHTS

Accreditation: Continuing
Degree Offered: Master (MPAS)
Start Date: May annually
Program Length: 28 months
Class Capacity: 50 students
Tuition: $113,658

CASPA Participant: Yes
Supplemental Application: No
Yellow Ribbon: No
Admissions: Non-rolling
Application Deadline: October 1

PREREQUISITE COURSEWORK

Human Anatomy with lab (3-4 credits), Human Physiology with lab (3-4 credits), General Biology with lab (4 credits), Microbiology with lab (4 credits), General Chemistry with lab (8-10 credits), Statistics (2-3 credits), College Algebra or higher (3 credits), Psychology (3 credits), Medical Terminology (1-3 credits). Anatomy, Physiology, Microbiology and Medical Terminology must be completed within the last 10 years. Prerequisites must be completed with a grade "C" or better. Up to 9 credits of prerequisite coursework may be in progress or planned at the time of application. AP credits are accepted for the Math requirement. Recommended courses: Genetics or Cellular Biology, Organic Chemistry or Biochemistry, Technical Writing.

GPA Requirement: Overall GPA 3.2; Science GPA 3.0

Healthcare Experience: 250 hours

PA Shadowing: Preferred, not required

Required Standardized Testing: GRE (combined score of 298 and 3.5 analytical is required), CASPer

Letters of Recommendation: Three required; strongly recommended that one be from a PA or physician

Seat Deposit: $1,000

ROCKY MOUNTAIN UNIVERSITY OF HEALTH PROFESSIONS

MISSION:

The mission of the RMUoHP PA Program is to educate students to become competent physician assistants who value and provide comprehensive, evidence-based, patient-centered care and are committed to lifelong-learning, professional excellence, and collaborative practice

NO CLASS STATISTICS REPORTED

PANCE SCORES

5-year First Time Pass: 97% (based on three years of data)

Most Recent First Time Pass: 100%

CURRICULUM STRUCTURE

Didactic: 16 months

Clinical: 12 months

Rotations:
7 mandatory,
1 elective (each
5 weeks)

UNIQUE PROGRAM FEATURES

Community Service: In accordance with their mission and goals, the RMUoHP PA program aims to admit students who have a history of community service within their circle of influence, evidenced through their CASPA application, in the hope that students will continue to serve in the communities in which they practice.

Curriculum: During the didactic phase of the program, students are challenged weekly with simulated patient encounters. This allows students to learn how to treat and care for patients in the didactic phase and prepare for their clinical experiences.

Extracurricular: Each year during the summer semester break, students have the opportunity to travel to Africa with faculty and university administration to provide humanitarian work and gain exposure to third-world clinical experiences. Students will spend time both in the clinics and hospitals as well as the local village.

369

University of Utah

375 Chipeta Way
Suite A
Salt Lake City, UT 84108
Phone: 801-581-7766
Email: admissions@upap.utah.edu

PROGRAM HIGHLIGHTS

Accreditation: Continuing

Degree Offered: Master (MPAS)

Start Date: May annually

Program Length: 27 months

Class Capacity: 64 students

Tuition: $75,108 (in-state, including fees); $111,640 (out-of-state, including fees)

CASPA Participant: Yes

Supplemental Application: No

Yellow Ribbon: Yes

Admissions: Non-rolling

Application Deadline: August 1

PREREQUISITE COURSEWORK

Human Anatomy with lab (4 credits), Human Physiology (4 credits), Biology (4 credits), Chemistry (8 credits). Prerequisites must be completed with a grade "C" or better and by the time of application. Anatomy and Physiology must be completed within the last 7 years. AP credits are not accepted. Recommended courses: Writing, Statistics, Microbiology, Genetics.

GPA Requirement: Overall GPA 3.0 (those with a 2.70 will be considered if they have a very strong application)

Healthcare Experience: 2,000 hours

PA Shadowing: Preferred, not required

Required Standardized Testing: CASPer

Letters of Recommendation: Three required; no one specific

Seat Deposit: $1,000

UNIVERSITY OF UTAH

MISSION:

To improve the quality of health and access to care, with a commitment to the medically underserved, by educating students to become highly proficient, socially conscious, and accountable physician assistants (PAs) in the primary care model.

CLASS OF 2021

Male: 58%

Female: 42%

Minority: 33%

Overall GPA: 3.52

Science GPA: 3.51

Average Healthcare Experience: 9,462 hours

Average Age: 29

PANCE SCORES

5-year First Time Pass: 95%

Most Recent First Time Pass: 93%

CURRICULUM STRUCTURE

Didactic: 15 months

Clinical: 12 months

Rotations: 7 mandatory, 2 elective (duration not specified); at least one is in a rural location

Master's Project: Required for graduation

UNIQUE PROGRAM FEATURES

Rotations: Students can choose to do an elective rotation in Thailand, Nepal or Guatemala.

Community Engagement: Community Engagement at UPAP is a structured learning experience that combines community service with preparation and reflection. Students can complete opportunities at Head Start Migrant Farm Worker Program, the Student-Run Free Clinic at Maliheh, Doctor's Free Clinic and the Salt Lake Community Action Program.

Extracurricular: PASSED (Physician Assistant Students Supporting Equity & Diversity) is an accredited group that is dedicated to promoting cultural and community awareness, civic involvement, social justice and the reduction of disparity in healthcare as we strive to refine our practice of medicine, professionalism and the skills necessary to become culturally competent, patient centered health care providers.

Affiliate Campus: The program has received accreditation for a distant campus in St. George, Utah, in the health sciences facilities on the campus of Dixie State University. Requirements for candidates interested in the St. George Campus will be the same as those for the Salt Lake City campus.

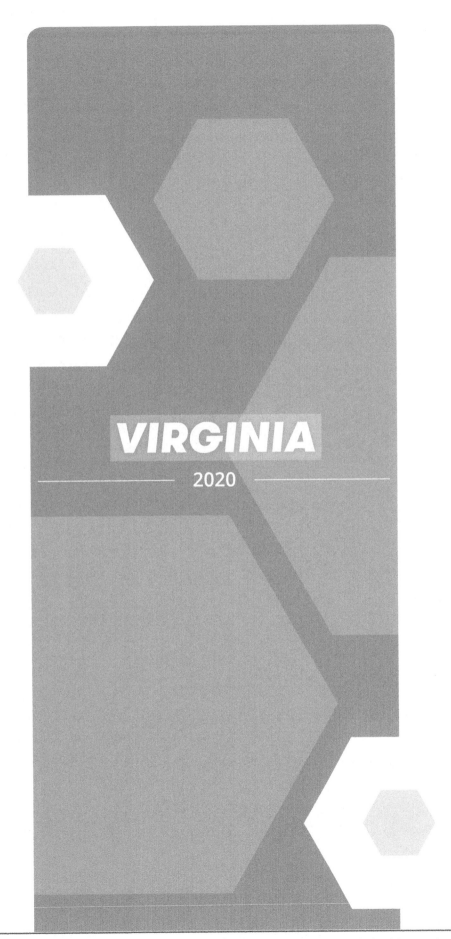

VIRGINIA
2020

Eastern Virginia Medical School

700 West Olney Road
Suite 1155
Norfolk, VA 23501
Phone: 757-446-7158
Email: paprogram@evms.edu

PROGRAM HIGHLIGHTS

Accreditation: Continuing

Degree Offered: Master (MPA)

Start Date: January annually

Program Length: 28 months

Class Capacity: 80 students

Tuition: $84,448 (in-state); $103,334 (out-of-state)

CASPA Participant: Yes

Supplemental Application: Yes (no fee)

Yellow Ribbon: No

Admissions: Non-rolling

Application Deadline: March 1

PREREQUISITE COURSEWORK

Anatomy and Physiology I and II (6 credits), General Chemistry (3 credits), Organic Chemistry or Biochemistry (3 credits), Microbiology or Cell Biology (3 credits), Introductory Psychology (3 credits), additional Psychology (3 credits), Math or Statistics or Physics (3 credits). Prerequisites must be completed with a grade "B-" or better and by the application deadline. Anatomy, Physiology, Organic Chemistry or Biochemistry, Microbiology or Cell Biology and additional Psychology must be completed within 10 years of the application deadline.

GPA Requirement: Overall GPA 3.0

Healthcare Experience: Preferred, not required (though most accepted students have >2,000 hours)

PA Shadowing: Not required

Required Standardized Testing: CASPer

Letters of Recommendation: Three required; no one specific

Seat Deposit: $500

EASTERN VIRGINIA MEDICAL SCHOOL

MISSION:

The mission of the EVMS Physician Assistant Program is to prepare students to provide healthcare in a broad range of medical settings by training them in the medical arts and sciences in an inclusive, multicultural environment dedicated to the delivery of patient-centered care, while fostering a strong commitment to clinical and community partnerships.

CLASS OF 2020

Male: 24%

Female: 76%

Minority: 25%

Overall GPA: 3.39

Prerequisite GPA: 3.87

Average Healthcare Experience: 3,338 hours

Average Age: 27.2

PANCE SCORES

5-year First Time Pass: 96%

Most Recent First Time Pass: 91%

CURRICULUM STRUCTURE

Didactic: 16 months

Clinical: 12 months

Rotations: 7 mandatory, 2 elective (each 5 weeks)

Service Learning Practicum: Required for graduation

UNIQUE PROGRAM FEATURES

Clinical Skills Curriculum: EVMS houses the Sentara Center for Simulation and Immersive Learning, which uses standardized patients in a controlled environment to teach clinical history taking and physical exam skills.

Fellowship: The Fellowship in Pediatric Urgent Care is a collaboration between Eastern Virginia Medical School and Children's Specialty Group (CSG) – one of the largest pediatric specialty medicine practices in Virginia. Fellows receive a generous monthly stipend as a CSG employee.

Early Assurance: The Early Assurance Program (EAP) exists to offer outstanding and qualified undergraduate students with firm interests in a career as a PA and in attending EVMS the opportunity to gain early assurance of acceptance into the PA program at EVMS before beginning their final year of college. Students at Randolph-Macon College, William & Mary, Norfolk State University, Virginia Wesleyan University and Christopher Newport University are eligible.

Emory & Henry College

565 Radio Hill Road
Marion, VA 24354
Phone: 276-944-6493
Email: ldowell@ehc.edu

PROGRAM HIGHLIGHTS

Accreditation: Provisional

Degree Offered: Master (MPAS)

Start Date: May annually

Program Length: 27 months

Class Capacity: 34 students

Tuition: $83,608

CASPA Participant: Yes

Supplemental Application: No (but $30 fee)

Yellow Ribbon: No

Admissions: Rolling

Application Deadline: March 1

PREREQUISITE COURSEWORK

Human Anatomy and Physiology I and II with lab (8 credits), Biology with lab (8 credits), Chemistry with lab (4 credits), Organic Chemistry or Biochemistry with lab (4 credits), Genetics (3 credits), Statistics (3 credits), Medical Terminology (2 credits). Up to three prerequisites may be pending completion at the time of application. Prerequisites must be completed with a grade "C" or better. AP courses are not accepted. Recommended courses: English Composition, Intro Psychology, Abnormal Psychology, Developmental Psychology, Sociology and/or Cultural Anthropology, Physics.

GPA Requirement: Overall GPA 3.0; Science GPA 2.7; Prerequisite GPA 3.0

Healthcare Experience: 300 hours (plus 100 community service/volunteer hours)

PA Shadowing: 20 hours

Required Standardized Testing: GRE

Letters of Recommendation: Three required; one from a PA with whom you have shadowed for 20 or more hours, one from a professor familiar with your academic work, and one from a work supervisor (either volunteer or paid work)

Seat Deposit: $500

EMORY & HENRY COLLEGE

MISSION:

To provide a collaborative, interprofessional culture that prepares highly-competent healthcare professionals who exhibit exemplary professionalism; provide culturally sensitive, mindful, patient/client-centered healthcare services; and actively contribute to the advancement of their professions and communities through leadership, scholarship, and service.

CLASS OF 2021

Male: 24%

Female: 76%

Minority: 10.34%

Overall GPA: 3.42

Science GPA: 3.34

Prerequisite GPA: 3.46

GRE Verbal: 53rd percentile

GRE Quantitative: 33rd percentile

GRE Written: 52nd percentile

Average Healthcare Experience: 3,741 hours

Average Shadowing Experience: 135 hours

Average Age: 26.1

PANCE SCORES

5-year First Time Pass: 83% (based on one year of data)

Most Recent First Time Pass: 83%

CURRICULUM STRUCTURE

Didactic: 13 months

Clinical: 14 months

Rotations: 10 mandatory, 1 elective (each 4-8 weeks)

Practice Based Learning Project: Required for graduation

UNIQUE PROGRAM FEATURES

Admissions Preference: Admissions preference is given to individuals in the following categories: Emory & Henry college alumni; individuals who have served their country via service in the Armed Forces, Public Health Service, AmeriCorps or with the Peace Corps; long-term (>10 year) residents of Southwest Virginia; students from environmentally and economically disadvantaged backgrounds; and minority applicants.

Facilities: The PA Lab is used to teach students how to conduct physical examinations and patient assessments. The lab includes twenty exam bays, set up to simulate an outpatient examination room, including wall mounted cameras for student observation. Additionally, the PA lab houses many advanced skills task trainers including ophthalmoscopic and otoscopic trainers, auscultation trainers, airway trainers, breast and pelvic exam trainers, IV and IO access trainers, and injection trainers.

Early Clinical Exposure: Students will begin on-site clinical experiences in the first week of the program at the Mel Leaman Free Clinic, a clinic that provides healthcare to the area's uninsured, low-income individuals.

James Madison University

Physician Assistant Program
235 Martin Luther King, Jr. Way,
MSC 4315
Harrisonburg, VA 22807
Phone: 540-568-2395
Email: paprogram@jmu.edu

PROGRAM HIGHLIGHTS

Accreditation: Continuing

Degree Offered: Master (MPAS)

Start Date: August annually

Program Length: 28 months

Class Capacity: 32 students

Tuition: $68,495 (in-state);
$88,168 (out-of-state)

CASPA Participant: Yes

Supplemental Application: Yes ($60 fee)

Yellow Ribbon: No

Admissions: Rolling

Application Deadline: August 1

PREREQUISITE COURSEWORK

Human or Mammalian Physiology (1 semester), Human or Mammalian Anatomy with lab (1 semester), Biochemistry (1 semester), Genetics (1 semester), Microbiology (1 semester), Medical Terminology (1 semester). Anatomy and Physiology must be completed with a grade "B" or better. All other prerequisites can be completed with a grade "C" or better. Prerequisites (except Medical Terminology) must be completed within 7 years of matriculation. Prerequisites do not need to be completed by the time of application.

GPA Requirement: No minimum (overall GPA 3.0 preferred)

Healthcare Experience: 1,000 hours

PA Shadowing: Preferred, not required

Required Standardized Testing: GRE

Letters of Recommendation: Three required; preferably from prior supervisors/employers, university professors, and/or medical professionals (clinicians) who have observed you working or volunteering in a patient care environment

Seat Deposit: $500

JAMES MADISON UNIVERSITY

MISSION:

The mission of the James Madison University Physician Assistant Program is to provide educational opportunities for students to develop the knowledge, skills, and attitudes necessary to function as primary care physician assistants, serving the medical needs of the Commonwealth of Virginia and society in general including rural and medically underserved areas.

CLASS OF 2021

Male: 28%

Female: 72%

Overall GPA: 3.53

Science GPA: 3.51

GRE Verbal: 66th percentile

GRE Quantitative: 49th percentile

GRE Written: 70th percentile

Average Healthcare Experience: 4,299 hours

Average Age: 25.1

PANCE SCORES

5-year First Time Pass: 99%

Most Recent First Time Pass: 96%

CURRICULUM STRUCTURE

Didactic: 16 months

Clinical: 12 months

Rotations: 9 mandatory, 1 elective (each 4 weeks)

Capstone Project: Required for graduation

UNIQUE PROGRAM FEATURES

Promotores de Salud: The PDS program trains Hispanic men and women to be health resource persons who are able to provide friends, family, and co-workers with culturally appropriate health information. JMU PA assistant students serve as the primary instructors of the 40-hour training. PA students get the benefit of practicing presentation skills while also getting to experience working with Spanish interpreters.

International Rotations: Students have the opportunity to do an international rotation in Trujillo, Peru.

White Coats On Call: Each winter, the JMU PA Program participates in this annual grassroots lobbying effort. Students from many of the Virginia PA programs come together during the General Assembly in Richmond to inform their senators and delegates about the challenges facing the practice of medicine in the commonwealth of Virginia.

Admissions Preference: Preference is given to military veterans. Any United States veteran who completes the admissions process is guaranteed an on-campus interview.

Student-Engaged Medical Clinic: Through a federal grant funded collaboration with a local free clinic, students get early clinical exposure during didactic year by seeing patients, taking histories and performing physical exams under the direct supervision of a preceptor.

Murphy Deming College of Health Sciences MSPA Program

100 Baldwin Boulevard
Fishersville, VA 22939
Phone: 540-887-4110
Email:
MDCHSadmit@marybaldwin.edu

PROGRAM HIGHLIGHTS

Accreditation: Probation

Degree Offered: Master (MSPA)

Start Date: January annually

Program Length: 27 months

Class Capacity: 30 students

Tuition: $87,360

CASPA Participant: Yes

Supplemental Application: No (but $45 fee)

Yellow Ribbon: Yes

Admissions: Rolling

Application Deadline: October 1

PREREQUISITE COURSEWORK

Biology with lab (3-4 credits), Human or Vertebrate Anatomy with lab (3-4 credits), Human or Vertebrate Physiology with lab (3-4 credits), Microbiology with lab (3-4 credits), Chemistry with lab (3-4 credits), Organic Chemistry or Biochemistry (3-4 credits), Psychology (6 credits, 1 must be an upper level course), Statistics (3 credits), Medical Terminology (1-2 credits). All courses must be completed prior to September 1st other than Medical Terminology. Prerequisites must be completed with a grade "C" or better. Anatomy, Physiology, Chemistry and Medical Terminology must be completed within 10 years of application.

GPA Requirement: Overall GPA 3.0

Healthcare Experience: Preferred, not required

PA Shadowing: Preferred, not required

Required Standardized Testing: GRE

Letters of Recommendation: Three required; no one specific

Seat Deposit: $2,000

MARY BALDWIN UNIVERSITY

MISSION:

The mission of the MSPA Program at Mary Baldwin University is to academically and clinically prepare students for PA practice as compassionate, effective, qualified clinicians able to serve in a variety of medical specialty areas and settings in collaboration with licensed physicians. This is accomplished in an environment promoting diversity along with respect for self and others. The MSPA Program is committed to leadership, interprofessional education, and collaborative practice. The Program's mission is realized in a dynamic and holistic learning environment dedicated to critical reasoning, engaged learning and scholarship, and innovative teaching with a strong commitment to service, especially for those in underserved or disadvantaged areas. Veritably, the Program holds that the primary goal of medical training is service to humanity.

NO CLASS STATISTICS REPORTED

PANCE SCORES

5-year First Time Pass: 100% (based on two years of data)

Most Recent First Time Pass: 100%

CURRICULUM STRUCTURE

Didactic: 15 months

Clinical: 12 months

Rotations: 7 mandatory, 1 elective (each 6 weeks)

UNIQUE PROGRAM FEATURES

Facilities: The new Health Sciences Building is a three-story facility that is the flagship building in Fishersville, Virginia. Completed in June 2014, this facility includes four large classrooms, six seminar rooms, nine clinical laboratories including three simulation suites, two research spaces, faculty/staff offices and numerous collaborative learning spaces.

Students: Although Mary Baldwin was traditionally an all-girls school, it has accepted both male and female students into its graduate programs for approximately 30 years. They are also a military friendly institution.

Articulation Agreements: Murphy Deming College of Health Sciences PA program has articulation agreements with the following institutions and gives preference to applicants who meet the criteria of those agreements: Mary Baldwin University, Bridgewater College, Ferrum College, Virginia Military Institute, Columbia College, Eastern Mennonite University.

Radford University

101 Elm Avenue SE
Roanoke, VA 24013
Phone: 540-985-4016
Email: rhadley1@radford.edu

PROGRAM HIGHLIGHTS

Accreditation: Continuing

Degree Offered: Master (MSPA)

Start Date: August annually

Program Length: 27 months

Class Capacity: 42 students

Tuition: $80,295

CASPA Participant: Yes

Supplemental Application: No

Yellow Ribbon: No

Admissions: Rolling

Application Deadline: November 1

PREREQUISITE COURSEWORK

Anatomy and Physiology I and II with lab (8 credits), General Chemistry I and II with lab (8 credits), Biochemistry or Cell Biology (3 credits), Microbiology with lab (4 credits), Genetics or Immunology (3 credits), Statistics (3 credits), Medical Terminology (1 credit), Psychology (6 credits, 1 course must be upper level). At least 12 credits of this coursework must be completed in the last 3 years. Prerequisites must be completed with a grade "C" or better. AP credits are accepted.

GPA Requirement: Overall GPA 3.0

Healthcare Experience: 500 hours

PA Shadowing: Not required

Required Standardized Testing: GRE

Letters of Recommendation: Three required; preferably one each from an academic advisor/professor, a clinical supervisor or employer, and a healthcare professional with whom you have worked

Seat Deposit: $500

RADFORD UNIVERSITY

MISSION:

The mission of the Radford University Carilion Physician Assistant Program is to graduate ethical, competent, and compassionate PAs who are well versed in the art and science of medicine and are prepared to effectively function as members and leaders of the interprofessional healthcare team.

NO CLASS STATISTICS REPORTED

PANCE SCORES

5-year First Time Pass: 97%

Most Recent First Time Pass: 95%

CURRICULUM STRUCTURE

Didactic: 15 months

Clinical: 12 months

Rotations: 8 mandatory, 2 elective (duration not specified)

Capstone Project: Required for graduation

UNIQUE PROGRAM FEATURES

Recent Merger: The Radford University PA program began in 1997 as the Jefferson College of Health Sciences PA program until the merger of Jefferson College of Health Sciences with Radford University in July of 2019. The program is now within the Waldron College of Health and Human Services. The prior Jefferson College of Health Sciences campus is now known as "Radford University, Carilion", and continues to be located near downtown Roanoke, in the same facilities as previously. The PA program curriculum, faculty, location, and clinical rotations remain unchanged from previous years.

377

Shenandoah University

1460 University Drive
Winchester, VA 22601
Phone: 540-542-6208
Email: pa@su.edu

PROGRAM HIGHLIGHTS

Accreditation: Continuing

Degree Offered: Master (MSPAS)

Start Date: July annually

Program Length: 30 months

Class Capacity: 60 students

Tuition: $97,965 (including fees)

CASPA Participant: Yes

Supplemental Application: No

Yellow Ribbon: Yes

Admissions: Rolling

Application Deadline: October 1

PREREQUISITE COURSEWORK

Human Anatomy and Physiology with lab (8 credits), General or Introductory Chemistry with lab (4 credits), Biochemistry or Organic Chemistry with lab (3-4 credits), Microbiology with lab (4 credits), Abnormal Psychology (3 credits), Developmental Psychology (3 credits), Math (3 credits), Medical Terminology (1-3 credits). Prerequisites should be completed within the last 10 years and Anatomy and Physiology should preferably be completed within the last 5 years and at the same institution. Prerequisites must be completed with a grade "C" or better.

GPA Requirement: Overall GPA 3.0; Science GPA 3.0; Prerequisite GPA 3.0

Healthcare Experience: Preferred, not required

PA Shadowing: Preferred, not required

Required Standardized Testing: GRE

Letters of Recommendation: Three required; no one specific

Seat Deposit: $500

SHENANDOAH UNIVERSITY

MISSION:

The mission of the Shenandoah University Division of Physician Assistant Studies is to provide a comprehensive educational program in a collaborative and supportive environment to develop highly skilled, well-educated, compassionate primary-care oriented physician assistants who are capable of providing high quality, patient-centered health care in a variety of settings.

CLASS OF 2021

Overall GPA: 3.55

Science GPA: 3.50

Prerequisite GPA: 3.70

GRE Verbal: 56th percentile

GRE Quantitative: 43rd percentile

GRE Analytical: 59th percentile

Average Healthcare Experience: 3,810 hours

Average Shadowing Experience: 192 hours

Average Age: 25

PANCE SCORES

5-year First Time Pass: 98%

Most Recent First Time Pass: 100%

CURRICULUM STRUCTURE

Didactic: 16 months

Clinical: 14 months

Rotations: 7 mandatory (primary care emphasis), 1 elective, 1 community preceptorship (each 4-8 weeks)

UNIQUE PROGRAM FEATURES

Admissions Preference: Preference will be given to candidates who can demonstrate a commitment to practice in primary care in rural or urban medically underserved areas. Candidates requesting this preference must do so in the form of a letter that is uploaded with their CASPA application. Applicants should include their rationale for the request along with documentation supporting the commitment to primary care practice in underserved communities.

Didactic: Each student is required to take at least one 3 credit professional elective course that is interdisciplinary in nature.

Medical Mission Trip: Students have the opportunity to explore the world and experience health care in other countries through medical mission trips to countries such as Nicaragua.

Rotations: Students can complete their clinical rotations abroad at locations like Clinica Madre de Cristo in Trujillo, Peru.

Performing Arts Medicine: PA students have the opportunity to earn a certificate in Performing Arts Medicine through the Division of athletic training.

Dual-Degree Option: The Physician Assistant Studies & Master Of Public Health Dual Degree Program offers students an opportunity to earn a Master Of Public Health Degree (MPH) in conjunction with training in the Physician Assistant (PA) Studies program.

South University

2151 Old Brick Road
Glen Allen, VA 23060
Phone: 804-727-6894
Email:
richmondpaprogram@southuniversity.edu

PROGRAM HIGHLIGHTS

Accreditation: Provisional

Degree Offered: Master (MSPA)

Start Date: January annually

Program Length: 27 months

Class Capacity: 36 students

Tuition: $84,600

CASPA Participant: Yes

Supplemental Application: No

Yellow Ribbon: No

Admissions: Non-rolling

Application Deadline: August 1

PREREQUISITE COURSEWORK

Human Anatomy with lab (1 course), Human Physiology with lab (1 course), General Biology (2 courses), General Chemistry with labs (2 courses), Biochemistry or Organic Chemistry with lab (1 course), Microbiology with lab (1 course). Prerequisites must be completed with a grade "C" or better and be completed prior to application submission. AP credits are accepted.

GPA Requirement: Overall GPA 3.0; Science GPA 3.0

Healthcare Experience: Preferred, not required

PA Shadowing: Preferred, not required

Required Standardized Testing: GRE

Letters of Recommendation: Three required; at least one must be from a PA, MD, DO or NP

Seat Deposit: $1,000

SOUTH UNIVERSITY, RICHMOND

MISSION:

The South University Physician Assistant (MS) exists to educate a diverse student population as providers of high-quality, cost-efficient health care who will make a positive impact while practicing the art and science of medicine with physician collaboration.

CLASS OF 2021

Male: 19%

Female: 81%

Minority: 39%

Overall GPA: 3.39

PANCE Scores

5-year First Time Pass: 100% (based on one year of data)

Most Recent First Time Pass: 100%

CURRICULUM STRUCTURE

Didactic: 15 months

Clinical: 12 months

Rotations: 7 mandatory, 1 elective (each 5 weeks)

UNIQUE PROGRAM FEATURES

Admissions Preference: Preference is given to applicants with: GRE scores at or above the 50th percentile, overall GPA at or above 3.3 and science GPA at or above 3.15.

University of Lynchburg

1501 Lakeside Drive
Department of PA Medicine
Lynchburg, VA 24501
Phone: 434-544-8876
Email: pa@lynchburg.edu

PROGRAM HIGHLIGHTS

Accreditation: Continuing
Degree Offered: Master (MPAM)
Start Date: June annually
Program Length: 27 months
Class Capacity: 40 students
Tuition: $86,660

CASPA Participant: Yes
Supplemental Application: Yes ($50 fee)
Yellow Ribbon: No
Admissions: Rolling
Application Deadline: January 15

PREREQUISITE COURSEWORK

Biology with lab (8 credits), General
Chemistry or Introductory Chemistry
with lab (4 credits), Organic Chemistry
or Biochemistry with lab (4 credits),
Human Anatomy with lab (4 credits),
Human Physiology with lab (4 credits),
Microbiology with lab (3-4 credits),
Genetics (3 credits), Psychology (3
credits), Statistics (3 credits), Social
Sciences (3 credits). Prerequisites
must be completed with a grade "C" or
better. AP credits are accepted.

GPA Requirement: Overall GPA 3.0;
Science GPA 3.0; Prerequisite GPA 3.0

Healthcare Experience: 500 hours

PA Shadowing: 8 hours

Required Standardized Testing: GRE or
MCAT

Letters of Recommendation: Three
required; one from a physician, PA, or
NP

Seat Deposit: $1,000

UNIVERSITY OF LYNCHBURG

MISSION:

The mission of the University of Lynchburg School of PA
Medicine is to educate PAs to become compassionate health
care providers with an emphasis on teamwork, communication,
human diversity and patient-centered care. The dynamic
interdisciplinary advanced curriculum will facilitate the highest
standard of patient care while also creating leaders within
medicine, local and global communities, and accelerating the
advancement of the profession.

CLASS OF 2021

Male: 37.5%

Female: 62.5%

Overall GPA: 3.52

GRE Verbal: 152

GRE Quantitative: 153

GRE Written: 4.0

Average Age: 25

Healthcare Experience: 2,090
hours

PANCE SCORES

5-year First Time Pass: 99%
(based on three years of
data)

Most Recent First Time Pass:
96%

CURRICULUM STRUCTURE

Didactic: 12 months

Clinical: 15 months (including
summative)

Rotations: 7 mandatory,
4 elective (each 2-8 weeks)

Master's Research: Required
for graduation

UNIQUE PROGRAM FEATURES

Facilities: The program
boasts an anatomy lab
featuring flat screen
monitors and 21 cadaver
stations as well as
custom-designed PA
program space in the
Graduate Health Science
Building, which features
advanced equipment and
technology.

Doctoral Option: The
program has developed
a doctoral option (DMSc)
where students who
complete the MPAM
program can engage in an
additional 9-12 months
of instruction to include
a clinical fellowship and
coursework in leadership,
healthcare management,
organizational behavior,
disaster medicine, and
global health.

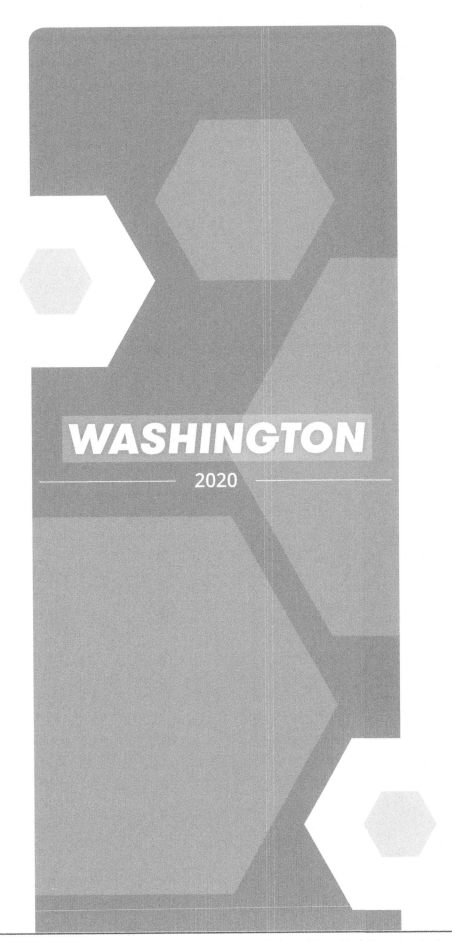

WASHINGTON
2020

Heritage University

3240 Fort Road
Toppenish, WA 98948
Phone: 509-865-0707
Email: PA_HU@heritage.edu

PROGRAM HIGHLIGHTS

Accreditation: Probation

Degree Offered: Master (MSPA)

Start Date: May annually

Program Length: 24 months

Class Capacity: 32 students

Tuition: $80,750

CASPA Participant: Yes

Supplemental Application: Yes ($25 fee)

Yellow Ribbon: Yes

Admissions: Early application highly encouraged

Application Deadline: November 1

PREREQUISITE COURSEWORK

Human Anatomy and Physiology I and II (6 credits), Microbiology with lab (3 credits), Human Sciences (6 credits), Math (3 credits). A&P must be completed within the last 5 years. Prerequisites must be completed with a grade "B" or better. All should be completed by January 15th prior to the May start date. Recommended courses: Organic Chemistry, General or Cell Biology, General or Inorganic Chemistry, Biochemistry, Molecular Biology, Genetics.

GPA Requirement: Overall GPA 3.0; Science GPA 3.0

Healthcare Experience: 1,000 hours (500 hours must be within the last 5 years)

PA Shadowing: Preferred, not required

Required Standardized Testing: None

Letters of Recommendation: Three required; preferably one from a PA, one from a physician, and one from a supervisor

Seat Deposit: $500

HERITAGE UNIVERSITY

MISSION:

The mission of the program is to increase access to healthcare, particularly in small, rural, and underserved areas, by educating future Physician Assistants who will provide high quality medical care in a compassionate and competent manner.

CLASS OF 2019

Male: 51%

Female: 49%

Minority: 39%

Overall GPA: 3.33

Science GPA: 3.31

Faculty to Student Ratio: 1:8

Average Healthcare Experience: 4,818 hours

Average Age: 29

PANCE SCORES

5-year First Time Pass: 82% (based on three years of data)

Most Recent First Time Pass: 89%

CURRICULUM STRUCTURE

Didactic: 12 months

Clinical: 12 months

Rotations: 7 mandatory (variable duration)

Master's Research Project: Required for graduation

UNIQUE PROGRAM FEATURES

Didactic: The program offers Spanish for Medical Professionals during the spring didactic semester.

Rural and Underserved Focus: Most rotations take place in rural or underserved communities, primarily in Washington, Idaho, Montana and Alaska. Most of these learning centers are based in small towns that have smaller hospitals with active emergency departments, a few key specialists, and a good family medicine or internal medicine base.

Continuity Clinic: The clinical phase is integrated so that students spend 2-3 days each week in a family medicine environment and the other days in specialty settings.

383

University of Washington

4311 11th Avenue NE
Ste. 200
Seattle, WA 98105
Phone: 206-616-4001
Email: medex@uw.edu

PROGRAM HIGHLIGHTS

Accreditation: Continuing

Degree Offered: Master (MCHS)

Start Date: July annually

Program Length: 27 months

Class Capacity: 140 students (divided among 4 campuses)

Tuition: $81,612

CASPA Participant: Yes

Supplemental Application: Yes (no fee)

Yellow Ribbon: No

Admissions: Non-rolling

Application Deadline: September 1

PREREQUISITE COURSEWORK

Human Anatomy and Physiology I and II (6 credits), General Biology (3 credits), Microbiology (3 credits), Chemistry (3 credits), Statistics (3 credits), English (6 credits). Prerequisites must be completed by the application deadline and with a grade "B-" or better. It is strongly recommended that prerequisites be completed within the last 5-7 years. AP credits will only be accepted for English requirements. Recommended courses: Biochemistry, Genetics, Social Sciences.

GPA Requirement: Overall GPA 3.0 (for the Last 60 Credits)

Healthcare Experience: 2,000 hours

PA Shadowing: Preferred, not required

Required Standardized Testing: GRE (unless applicant has a prior master's degree)

Letters of Recommendation: Three required; preferably one from a PA/NP and one from a physician

Seat Deposit: $500

UNIVERSITY OF WASHINGTON

MISSION:

MEDEX Northwest, the University of Washington School of Medicine's Physician Assistant Program, is committed to educating experienced health personnel from diverse backgrounds to practice medicine with physician supervision. The program provides a broad, competency-based curriculum that focuses on primary care with an emphasis on underserved populations. MEDEX encourages life-long learning to meet ever-changing health care needs. As a pioneer in PA education, MEDEX continues to be innovative in identifying, creating, and filling new niches for PAs as a strategy for expanding health care access.

CLASS OF 2020

Male: 45%

Female: 55%

Minority: 32%

Average Age: 30

PANCE SCORES

5-year First Time Pass: 91%

Most Recent First Time Pass: Varies by campus from 77-98%

CURRICULUM STRUCTURE

Didactic: 15 months

Clinical: 12 months

Rotations: 6 mandatory, 1 elective (each 4 weeks, except primary care which is 4 months)

Capstone Project: Required for graduation

UNIQUE PROGRAM FEATURES

Campuses: MEDEX Northwest currently operates four classroom sites as a strategy to better serve potential students throughout the five-state northwest service region. Sites that offer a master's degree are Seattle, WA, Spokane, WA, Tacoma, WA and Anchorage, AK. Beginning in 2020, a new campus will be added in Kona, HI.

Rural and Underserved Focus: The program trains students in primary care in rural and underserved areas. Students complete a four-month family medicine rotation and travel to different sites to work with a variety of populations. The core MEDEX mission of primary care and access for rural and medically underserved populations is a recurring theme across the curriculum.

Admissions Preference: MEDEX is committed to training physician assistants who will serve where they are most needed. Preference is given to applicants from the WWAMI service region (Washington, Wyoming, Alaska, Montana, Idaho) and Nevada, and from other rural or medically underserved areas. MEDEX looks for prior work experience in an area that is medically underserved and gives preference to applicants who seem likely to continue such work. Preference is also given to applicants with military experience.

Competitive Applicants: The MEDEX website lists a number of factors and stats of competitive applicants so you can see how you match up.

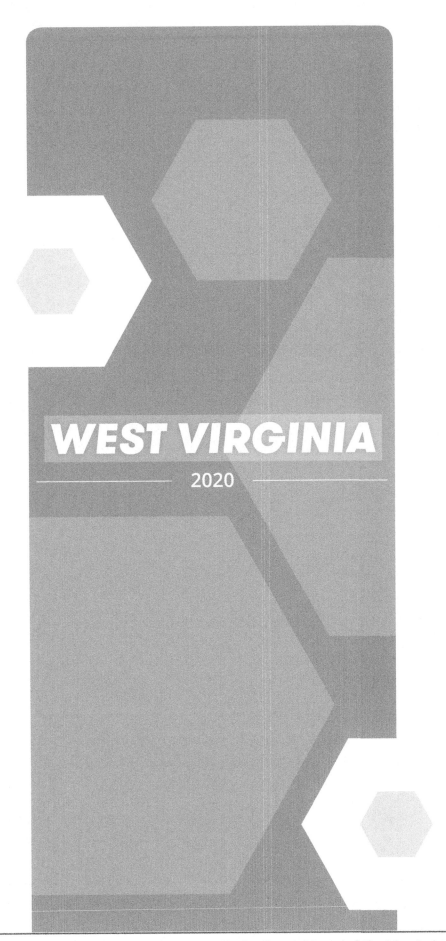

WEST VIRGINIA
2020

Alderson-Broaddus University

101 College Hill Drive
PO Box 2036
Philippi, WV 26416
Phone: 304-457-6315
Email: pa@ab.edu

PROGRAM HIGHLIGHTS

Accreditation: Continuing
Degree Offered: Master (MSPAS)
Start Date: May annually
Program Length: 27 months
Class Capacity: 36 students
Tuition: $96,950

CASPA Participant: Yes
Supplemental Application: Yes (no fee)
Yellow Ribbon: No
Admissions: Rolling
Application Deadline: March 1

PREREQUISITE COURSEWORK

Human Anatomy and Physiology with lab (8 credits), Microbiology with lab (4 credits), Chemistry with lab (4 credits), Statistics (3 credits), Organic Chemistry or Biochemistry with lab (4 credits), Upper Level Science Courses (8 credits). Prerequisites may be in progress at the time of application and should be completed within the last 7 years. AP credits generally do not fulfill prerequisite requirements.

GPA Requirement: Overall GPA 3.0; Science GPA 3.0; Prerequisite GPA 3.0 (the most competitive applicants should possess overall and science GPAs of 3.2)

Healthcare Experience: Preferred, not required

PA Shadowing: 40 hours

Required Standardized Testing: GRE

Letters of Recommendation: Three required; no one specific

Seat Deposit: $500

ALDERSON-BROADDUS UNIVERSITY

MISSION:

The mission of the Alderson-Broaddus College Physician Assistant Studies Program is to academically and clinically prepare physician assistants who deliver high-quality, patient-centered, primary and specialty care, with physician supervision, to diverse populations.

CLASS OF 2021

Male: 36%
Female: 64%
Minority: 16%
Overall GPA: 3.60
Science GPA: 3.54
Prerequisite GPA: 3.61
GRE Verbal: 151.3
GRE Quantitative: 152.5
GRE Analytical: 3.93
Average Age: 23.5

PANCE SCORES

5-year First Time Pass: 94%
Most Recent First Time Pass: 96%

CURRICULUM STRUCTURE

Didactic: 15 months
Clinical: 12 months
Rotations: 8 mandatory, 1 elective (each 4-8 weeks)
Capstone Project: Required for graduation

UNIQUE PROGRAM FEATURES

Facilities: The program recently renovated many of its classrooms and labs to state of the art facilities to improve the student experience.

Tradition: The program was the first to offer a PA Bachelor's degree in 1968 and has since graduated over 1700 PAs, one third of which practice in West Virginia. The program has graduates in all 48 contiguous United States.

387

PROGRAM HIGHLIGHTS

Accreditation: Continuing

Degree Offered: Master (MPAS)

Start Date: January annually

Program Length: 28 months

Class Capacity: 30 students

Tuition: $86,593 (including fees)

CASPA Participant: Yes

Supplemental Application: Yes ($50 fee)

Yellow Ribbon: No

Admissions: Rolling

Application Deadline: August 1

PREREQUISITE COURSEWORK

Human Anatomy and Physiology with lab (8 credits), General Biology with lab (4 credits), Microbiology with lab (4 credits), Chemistry with lab (8 credits), Organic Chemistry I and II with lab (8 credits), Statistics (1 semester), College Algebra or higher (1 semester), Psychology (1 semester). Prerequisites may be in progress at the time of application and must be completed with a grade "C" or better. Recommended courses: Biochemistry, Medical Terminology.

GPA Requirement: Overall GPA 3.0

Healthcare Experience: Preferred, not required

PA Shadowing: Not required

Required Standardized Testing: GRE

Letters of Recommendation: Three required; one should be from a PA or physician

Seat Deposit: $1,000

UNIVERSITY OF CHARLESTON

MISSION:

The mission of the University of Charleston Physician Assistant Program is to prepare competent physician assistants who value and provide comprehensive, patient-centered, culturally sensitive primary care, and are committed to lifelong-learning, professional growth, community health, and caring for underserved populations.

CLASS OF 2020

Male: 20%

Female: 80%

Overall GPA: 3.60

Science GPA: 3.50

GRE Verbal: 151

GRE Quantitative: 152

GRE Analytical: 4.0

Average Healthcare Experience: 2,017 hours

Average Volunteer Experience: 943 hours

Average Shadowing Experience: 284 hours

Average Age: 24

PANCE SCORES

5-year First Time Pass: 97%

Most Recent First Time Pass: 86%

CURRICULUM STRUCTURE

Didactic: 16 months

Clinical: 12 months

Rotations: 7 mandatory, 1 elective (each 5 weeks)

UNIQUE PROGRAM FEATURES

Pass/Fail Grading: The program utilizes a pass/fail grading system to facilitate a culture where students strive to elevate their classmates to provide the best care possible for patients, rather than work to outperform one another.

Active and Collaborative Learning: The program strongly values utilizing innovative educational methods using a variety of approaches beyond standard lecture, including case-based, problem-based, and team-based instruction. Students are challenged to develop clinical reasoning skills, think critically, enhance interpersonal and communication skills, apply evidence-based resources, and problem-solve as clinicians and as members of an interdisciplinary healthcare team. This is accomplished through simulated clinical experiences with standardized patients and state of the art simulation mannequins.

Synthesized Medicine Curriculum: Instead of courses addressing content separately in clinical medicine, diagnostic skills, and pharmacotherapeutics, the UC PA program has been designed to integrate all of these components together into specialty-based modules (e.g. Cardiovascular, Pulmonology, Pediatrics) to enhance learning and retention.

Reflective Practice Portfolio Project: Towards the end of the didactic component, students are challenged to reflect deeply on their knowledge and skill base in order to identify their strengths and weaknesses. They are then responsible for developing specific plans to address their weaknesses. This project helps prepare students to become well-rounded clinicians who have cultivated a consistent pattern of self-reflective practice.

West Liberty University

208 University Drive
College Union Box 173
West Liberty, WV 26074
Phone: 304-336-5098
Email: paprogram@westliberty.edu

PROGRAM HIGHLIGHTS

Accreditation: Continuing

Degree Offered: Master (MSPAS)

Start Date: July annually

Program Length: 24 months

Class Capacity: 19 students

Tuition: $55,440 (in-state); $82,960 (out-of-state)

CASPA Participant: Yes

Supplemental Application: Yes ($25 fee)

Yellow Ribbon: No

Admissions: Rolling

Application Deadline: October 1

PREREQUISITE COURSEWORK

General Chemistry with lab (8 credits) or Inorganic Chemistry + Organic Chemistry + Biochemistry with labs (minimum of 8 credits for all three), Microbiology with lab (4 credits), Human Anatomy and Physiology with lab (8 credits), Psychology (1 course), Humanities or Social Science (3 credits), English or Writing (6 credits), Mathematics (3 credits). No more than two prerequisites may be in progress at the time of application and all must have been completed in the US. AP credits are not accepted. Recommended courses: Genetics.

GPA Requirement: Overall GPA 3.0; Science GPA 3.0

Healthcare Experience: Preferred, but not required

PA Shadowing: Preferred, not required

Required Standardized Testing: GRE, CASPer

Letters of Recommendation: Three required; at least one from an employer or a professor

Seat Deposit: $500

WEST LIBERTY UNIVERSITY

MISSION:

West Liberty University's Physician Assistant Studies Program is committed to providing high-quality education to physician assistant candidates, who as an integral part of the health-care team, will provide empathetic and competent care to the patients they serve, including those in underserved areas.

NO CLASS STATISTICS REPORTED

PANCE SCORES

5-year First Time Pass: 94%

Most Recent First Time Pass: 86%

CURRICULUM STRUCTURE

Didactic: 12 months

Clinical: 12 months

Rotations: 7 mandatory, 2 elective (each 5 weeks)

Literature Review: Required for graduation

UNIQUE PROGRAM FEATURES

State Institution: This institution is state funded, meaning that they have a preference for residents of West Virginia and for prior graduates of West Liberty University, though neither of these is a requirement for admission into the program.

Early Admissions: For applicants who would like to be considered for an invitation to participate in an early interview session, their CASPA application must be verified along with the supplemental application and $25 fee submitted by August 1st of the year of application.

Small Class Size: The program accepts a maximum of 19 students per year. This ensures a close-knit class and individualized attention from faculty. Additionally, you can read about each student and their past experiences on the program website.

Interview Process: Candidates will be issued two screening exams during the interview process: English Composition and Medical Terminology. Applicants must be proficient in writing and reading comprehension to be accepted into the program. The Medical Terminology evaluation will not be used to determine acceptance into the program but rather to see where the applicant stands at the time of matriculation.

West Virginia University

West Virginia University

PO Box 9225
Morgantown, WV 26506-9225
Phone: 304-293-5466
Email: jjmomen@hsc.wvu.edu

PROGRAM HIGHLIGHTS

Accreditation: Provisional

Degree Offered: Master (MHS)

Start Date: January annually

Program Length: 28 months

Class Capacity: 25 students

Tuition: $124,254 (in-state); $167,873 (out-of-state)

CASPA Participant: Yes

Supplemental Application: No

Yellow Ribbon: No

Admissions: Rolling

Application Deadline: July 31

PREREQUISITE COURSEWORK

Biology with lab (4 credits), General Chemistry with lab (8 credits), Organic or Biochemistry with lab (4 credits), Human Anatomy with lab (4 credits), Human Physiology (3 credits), Microbiology (3 credits), Psychology (3 credits), Statistics (3 credits), Medical Terminology (1 credit). Prerequisites must be completed with a grade "C" or better and within 10 years prior to matriculation. AP credits are not accepted. No more than two prerequisites may be outstanding at the time of interview.

GPA Requirement: Overall GPA 3.0; Prerequisite GPA 3.0

Healthcare Experience: 80 hours (shadowing may count towards the requirement)

PA Shadowing: Preferred, not required

Required Standardized Testing: GRE

Letters of Recommendation: Three required; one from a college or university professor, one from a supervisor of the clinical experience including evidence of how the student contributed to the delivery of care, and a third from either of the two preceding categories

Seat Deposit: $1,000

WEST VIRGINIA UNIVERSITY

MISSION:

The Division of Physician Assistant Studies is committed to improving health and quality of life for individuals within and beyond the state of West Virginia. The Division is dedicated to providing physician assistants to address health care needs by offering a high quality education program that strives for excellence in education and clinical practice. The Division, through a commitment to evidence-based practice, contributes to scholarship in the field. The program provides a model for addressing health disparity through an understanding of health and health policy, as well as awareness of demographic risk factors for health and quality of life as applied both locally and globally.

NO CLASS STATISTICS REPORTED

PANCE SCORES

5-year First Time Pass: N/A

Most Recent First Time Pass: N/A (have not graduated a class yet)

CURRICULUM STRUCTURE

Didactic: 15 months

Clinical: 12 months

Rotations: 7 mandatory, 2 elective, 1 rural (each 4-8 weeks)

UNIQUE PROGRAM FEATURES

Admissions: All residents of West Virginia and West Virginia University graduates meeting the minimum WVU physician assistant program admissions requirements will be offered an on-campus interview.

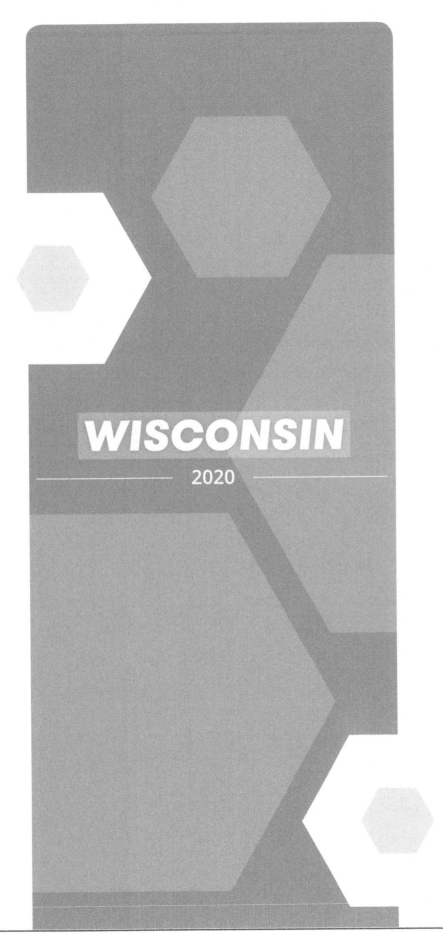

WISCONSIN
2020

Carroll University

100 N. East Avenue
Waukesha, WI 53186
Phone: 262-524-7361
Email: painfo@carrollu.edu

PROGRAM HIGHLIGHTS

Accreditation: Continuing

Degree Offered: Master (MSPAS)

Start Date: June annually

Program Length: 24 months

Class Capacity: 20 students

Tuition: $80,634

CASPA Participant: Yes

Supplemental Application: No (but $50 supplemental fee)

Yellow Ribbon: No

Admissions: Non-rolling

Application Deadline: October 1

PREREQUISITE COURSEWORK

Anatomy (1 semester), Physiology (1 semester), Microbiology (1 semester), other Biological Sciences (2 semesters), Chemistry (4 semesters), Psychology (2 semesters), Statistics (1 semester). Anatomy and Physiology must be completed within 5 years of matriculation. AP courses are accepted for General Psychology, General Biology I, General Chemistry I and Statistics. Prerequisites must be completed with a grade "C" or better. No more than two prerequisites may be pending at the time of application. Recommended courses: Pathophysiology, Medical Terminology, Epidemiology, Pharmacology, Foreign Language.

GPA Requirement: Overall GPA 3.0; Science GPA 3.0

Healthcare Experience: 500 hours

PA Shadowing: Preferred, not required

Required Standardized Testing: GRE

Letters of Recommendation: Three required; preferably from a college instructor, a supervisor from a work or volunteer clinical experience, and a health care professional such as a PA, NP, MD or DO

Seat Deposit: $500

CARROLL UNIVERSITY

MISSION:

The Mission of the Master of Science in Physician Assistant Studies Program is to educate physician assistants to provide comprehensive quality health care to all, respectful of patient/ client values, committed to ethical principles and grounded in evidence-based practice and clinical reasoning. Graduates will contribute to the profession and communities and be prepared to practice medicine in a variety of primary care settings under the supervision of physicians. Graduates will also be prepared to provide service to medically underserved communities and diverse patient populations.

CLASS OF 2021

Male: 30%

Female: 70%

Overall GPA: 3.79

Science GPA: 3.77

GRE Verbal:
58th percentile

GRE Quantitative:
57th percentile

Average Healthcare Experience: 1,244 hours

PANCE SCORES

5-year First Time Pass: 98%

Most Recent First Time Pass: 95%

CURRICULUM STRUCTURE

Didactic: 12 months

Clinical: 12 months

Rotations: 7 mandatory, 1 elective (each 4-8 weeks)

Capstone Project: Required for graduation

UNIQUE PROGRAM FEATURES

Early Clinical Exposure: Exposure in the first year through supervised clinical practicums (Foundations of Cultural Competence and Health Disparities Courses) provides students with hands-on patient/ client experience that allows students to integrate classroom learning with practical and clinical applications while providing service to the community. This helps students to develop clinical skills, and emphasizes wellness and prevention across the lifespan.

Admissions Preference: Carroll graduates receive additional points towards admission during the admissions process. Approximately 10-25% of accepted students per year are prior Carroll graduates.

Facilities & Technology: The Michael and Mary Jaharis Science Laboratories offer new portable technology, anatomical models and computer-aided dissections through the Anatomage dissection table. The program also has a cadaver dissection lab.

Rotations: International rotations are available for the elective rotation.

393

Concordia University

12800 N. Lake Shore Drive
Mequon, WI 53097
Phone: 262-243-4437
Email: erica.galligan@cuw.edu

PROGRAM HIGHLIGHTS

Accreditation: Continuing

Degree Offered: Master (MSPAS)

Start Date: May annually

Program Length: 26 months

Class Capacity: 30 students

Tuition: $83,630

CASPA Participant: Yes

Supplemental Application: Yes ($10 fee)

Yellow Ribbon: No

Admissions: Rolling

Application Deadline: September 1

PREREQUISITE COURSEWORK

General Chemistry with lab (2 semesters), Organic Chemistry with lab (1 semester), Biochemistry (1 semester), Microbiology with lab (1 semester), Human Anatomy and Physiology with lab (2 semesters), Biology with lab (2 semesters), Genetics (1 semester), Psychology (1 semester), Statistics (1 semester), College Algebra or higher (1 semester), Medical Terminology (1 semester). Prerequisites must be completed at the time of application (aside from one non-science prerequisite) and with a grade "C" or better. A&P and Medical Terminology are recommended to be completed within 5 years of application. Recommended courses: Nutrition, Pharmacology, Immunology, additional Psychology courses.

GPA Requirement: Overall GPA 3.2 Prerequisite GPA 3.2

Healthcare Experience: 500 hours

PA Shadowing: 24 hours

Required Standardized Testing: CASPer

Letters of Recommendation: Three required; one from a PA you have shadowed, one from an employer/supervisor of your healthcare experience, and one other professional/academic/character letter

Seat Deposit: $500

CONCORDIA UNIVERSITY

MISSION:

Our mission in the PA program is to educate students who are committed to caring for patients in mind, body and spirit with an emphasis on continual lifelong learning.

NO CLASS STATISTICS REPORTED

PANCE SCORES

5-year First Time Pass: 96%

Most Recent First Time Pass: 100%

CURRICULUM STRUCTURE

Didactic: 15 months

Clinical: 11 months

Rotations: 9 mandatory, 2 elective (each 4 weeks)

UNIQUE PROGRAM FEATURES

Focus: This program has a focus on primary care, preventive medicine, and health literacy and students will work with a variety of primary care and medically underserved populations. The program is also faith-based and committed to engaging mind and spirit for service to Christ in the church and the world.

Facilities: The program boasts a newly renovated cadaver lab and a simulation lab for student learning.

Rotations: International rotations are available.

Marquette University

1700 Building
P.O. Box 1881
Milwaukee, WI 53233
Phone: 414-288-5688
Email: Pastudies@marquette.edu

PROGRAM HIGHLIGHTS

Accreditation: Continuing

Degree Offered: Master (MPAS)

Start Date: August annually

Program Length: 33 months

Class Capacity: 55 students

Tuition: $43,350 per year

CASPA Participant: Yes

Supplemental Application: Yes ($65 fee)

Yellow Ribbon: No

Admissions: Non-rolling

Application Deadline: September 1

PREREQUISITE COURSEWORK

Biology (2 semesters), General Chemistry with lab (1-2 semesters), Biochemistry (1 semester), Psychology or other Social Science (1 semester), Statistics (1 semester), Medical Terminology (1 semester). AP credit is accepted for Psychology and Statistics. Highly recommended that courses be completed in the last 5 years and taken at a 4-year institution. Prerequisites must be completed with a grade "C" or better.

GPA Requirement: Overall GPA 3.0

Healthcare Experience: 200 hours

PA Shadowing: Not required

Required Standardized Testing: GRE

Letters of Recommendation: Three required; one from someone who knows you academically, one from someone who knows your work ethic, and one from someone who knows you personally

Seat Deposit: $1,500

MARQUETTE UNIVERSITY

MISSION:

Our mission is to develop physician assistants in the Jesuit tradition who realize their full potential as excellent clinicians and national leaders. We pursue this for ad majorem Dei gloriam, the greater glory of God, and the benefit of the human community.

NO CLASS STATISTICS REPORTED

PANCE SCORES

5-year First Time Pass: 100%

Most Recent First Time Pass: 100%

CURRICULUM STRUCTURE

Didactic: 21 months

Clinical: 12 months

Rotations: 11 mandatory, 6 elective (each 2-6 weeks)

Capstone Project: Required for graduation

UNIQUE PROGRAM FEATURES

Admissions Preference: Approximately 50% of each class is chosen from Marquette undergraduate students and 50% is chosen from external candidates.

Rotations: An international internal medicine rotation is available in Belize and a rural medicine rotation in Alaska.

University of Wisconsin

1725 State Street
Health Science Center 4033
La Crosse, WI 54601
Phone: 608-785-8470
Email: paprogram@uwlax.edu

PROGRAM HIGHLIGHTS

Accreditation: Continuing

Degree Offered: Master (MSPAS)

Start Date: May annually

Program Length: 24 months

Class Capacity: 25 students

Tuition: $35,657 (in-state);
$87,345 (out-of-state)

CASPA Participant: Yes

Supplemental Application: Yes ($50 fee)

Yellow Ribbon: No

Admissions: Non-rolling

Application Deadline: August 1

PREREQUISITE COURSEWORK

Human Anatomy and Physiology I and II (2 semesters), Microbiology (1 semester), additional Health Related Upper Division Biological Science (at least 11 total biology credits with 2 lab courses), General Chemistry (1 semester), Organic Chemistry (1 semester), Biochemistry (1 semester and at least 11 total chemistry credits with 2 lab courses), Precalculus or Calculus (1 semester), Statistics (1 semester), Psychology (1 semester). Prerequisites may be in progress/planned at the time of application.

GPA Requirement: Overall GPA 3.0; Science GPA 3.0

Healthcare Experience: Preferred, not required

PA Shadowing: Not required

Required Standardized Testing: GRE

Letters of Recommendation: Three required; no one specific

Seat Deposit: $1,000

UNIVERSITY OF WISCONSIN - LA CROSSE

MISSION:

The mission of our program is to educate highly competent and compassionate physician assistants who excel in meeting the healthcare needs of the regions served by the partner institutions.

CLASS OF 2021

Overall GPA: 3.89

Science GPA: 3.86

GRE Verbal: 157

GRE Quantitative: 158

Average Healthcare Experience: 1,940 hours

Average Age: 22.3

PANCE SCORES

5-year First Time Pass: 100%

Most Recent First Time Pass: 100%

CURRICULUM STRUCTURE

Didactic: 12 months

Clinical: 12 months

Rotations: 7 mandatory, 2 selective, 2 elective (each 4 weeks)

Capstone Project: Required for graduation

UNIQUE PROGRAM FEATURES

Clinical Affiliation: The program is affiliated with the Mayo Clinic Health System, Gundersen Health System and Marshfield Clinic Health System, where students complete many of their clinical rotations.

Facilities: The Health Science Center serves as the PA Program home with space for didactic lectures, exam rooms, and a study lounge. It is home to the Medical Dosimetry Program, Occupational Therapy Program, Physical Therapy Program, and Radiation Therapy Program.

Admissions Preference: Keeping in line with the program mission, the program aims to accept applicants who plan to work in the Wisconsin and Minnesota areas.

PROGRAM HIGHLIGHTS

Accreditation: Continuing

Degree Offered: Master (MPAS)

Start Date: May annually

Program Length: 24 months

Class Capacity: 58 students

Tuition: $35,445 (in-state); $72,094 (out-of-state); $49,868 (Minnesota residents)

CASPA Participant: Yes

Supplemental Application: Yes (no fee – included in CASPA)

Yellow Ribbon: Yes

Admissions: Non-rolling

Application Deadline: August 1

PREREQUISITE COURSEWORK

Mammalian Biology with lab, Microbiology with lab, Biochemistry, Human Anatomy, Human Physiology, Statistics (1 semester), Psychology (1 semester). Physiology must be taken within 3 years of matriculation. Up to two prerequisite courses may be outstanding at the time of application.

GPA Requirement: Overall GPA 3.2; Science GPA 3.2

Healthcare Experience: 1,000 hours

PA Shadowing: Not required

Required Standardized Testing: None

Letters of Recommendation: Three required; at least one should be from someone with whom you have worked in a healthcare setting

Seat Deposit: None

UNIVERSITY OF WISCONSIN - MADISON

MISSION:

The mission of the University of Wisconsin-Madison Physician Assistant Program is to educate professionals committed to the delivery of comprehensive health care in a culturally and ethnically sensitive manner, with an emphasis on primary health care for populations and regions in need.

NO CLASS STATISTICS REPORTED

PANCE SCORES

5-year First Time Pass: 98%

Most Recent First Time Pass: 96%

CURRICULUM STRUCTURE

Didactic: 12 months

Clinical: 12 months

Rotations: 4 mandatory (each 8 weeks), elective (either one 8-week or two 4-week electives)

Capstone Project: Required for graduation

UNIQUE PROGRAM FEATURES

Acceptance: For applicants who meet the 3.20 minimum GPA requirement, the following considerations are made: trends in grades, recent coursework, prerequisite coursework, difficulty of coursework, course load, quality of school, graduate work and academic record statement.

Rotations: Students have the opportunity to take part in international rotations. All students are also required to complete one rotation at a rural site or with an underserved population.

Distance Education Option: The program offers a 3-year distance education option with 2 years of part time didactic work and 1 year of full time clinical work in the student's home community. It is generally reserved for students who have a desire to practice in their home rural or underserved community.

wisPACT: There is a northern Wisconsin community track option where students attend live lectures and discussions via video conferencing at UW-Marathon County as well. It is generally reserved for those who want to practice in northern Wisconsin.

Dual Degree: Students can complete a dual degree MPH/PA program, where the 1st year consists of MPH coursework and the 2nd and 3rd years comprise the PA program.

Student Testimonials: These are available on the website for applicants to get an insider perspective on the program.

Appendix I: List of Programs Requiring the GRE

Anne Arundel Community College

Arcadia University

Augusta University

Baldwin Wallace University

Barry University

Baylor College of Medicine

Bethel University

Boston University School of Medicine PA Program

Bryant University

Butler University

Campbell University

Carroll University

Case Western Reserve University

Central Michigan University

Chapman University

Charleston Southern University

Chatham University

Clarkson University

College of Saint Scholastica

CUNY York College

Des Moines University

DeSales University

Dominican University

Duke University Medical Center

East Carolina University

Eastern Michigan University

Elon University

Emory & Henry College

Emory University

Florida Gulf Coast University

Florida International University Herbert Wertheim College of Medicine

Florida State University

Francis Marion University

Franciscan Missionaries of Our Lady University

George Washington University

Grand Valley State University

Hardin-Simmons University (Abilene)

Harding University

High Point University

Idaho State University

Indiana State University

Indiana University School of Health and Rehabilitation Sciences

James Madison University

Johnson & Wales University

Keiser University

Kettering College

Lake Erie College

Lenoir-Rhyne University

Lincoln Memorial University

Lock Haven University

Long Island University

Louisiana State University - New Orleans

Louisiana State University Health Sciences Center Shreveport

Lynchburg College

Marietta College

Marist College

Marquette University

Mary Baldwin University (Murphy Deming College of Health Sciences)

Marywood University

Medical University of South Carolina

Mercer University

Mercyhurst University

Methodist University

MGH Institute of Health Professions

Midwestern University (Downers Grove)

Midwestern University (Glendale)

Milligan College

Misericordia University

Mississippi College

Missouri State University

Monmouth University

Mount St. Joseph University

North Greenville University

Northeastern State University - OK

Northern Arizona University

Northwestern University

Nova Southeastern University, Fort Lauderdale

Nova Southeastern University, Fort Myers

Nova Southeastern University, Jacksonville

Nova Southeastern University, Orlando

Ohio Dominican University

Ohio University

Oregon Health & Science University

Penn State University

Radford University

Rocky Mountain College

Rocky Mountain University of Health Professions

Rosalind Franklin Univ of Medicine
Rush University
Saint Catherine University
Salus University
Seton Hall University
Shenandoah University
South College
South University in Savannah
South University, Richmond
Southern Illinois University
St. Ambrose University
Stanford University
Stephens College
SUNY Upstate Medical Center
Temple University Lewis Katz School of Medicine
Texas Tech University Health Sciences Center
Touro University Nevada
Trevecca Nazarene University
University of Saint Francis (Fort Wayne) University
University of Alabama at Birmingham
University of Arkansas
University of Colorado
University of Detroit Mercy
University of Dubuque
University of Evansville
University of Florida
University of Iowa
University of Kentucky
University of Missouri - Kansas City
University of Mount Union
University of Nebraska

University of New England
University of New Mexico
University of North Carolina - Chapel Hill
University of North Texas HS Center Ft Worth
University Of Oklahoma, Oklahoma City
University of Oklahoma, Tulsa
University of Pittsburgh
University of Saint Francis (Fort Wayne)
University of South Alabama
University of South Carolina
University of South Florida
University of Southern California (LA)
University of St. Francis
University of Tennessee Health Science Center (Memphis)
University of Texas - HS Center at San Antonio
University of Texas - Medical Branch at Galveston
University of Texas Rio Grande Valley
University of the Cumberlands
University of Toledo
University of Washington
University of Wisconsin - La Crosse
UT Southwestern - School of Health Professions
Wake Forest University (Bowman Gray)
Wayne State University
Weill Cornell Medicine Graduate School of Medical Sciences
Wingate University
Yale University School of Medicine
Yale University School of Medicine (Online)

Appendix II: List of Programs Not Requiring the GRE

Arizona School of Health Sciences

Augsburg College

Bay Path University

Bethel University

California Baptist University

Charles R. Drew University

College of Saint Mary

Concordia University

Cuyahoga Community College/Cleveland State University

D'youville College

Daemen College

Dominican University of California

Drexel University

Duquesne University

Eastern Virginia Medical School

Franklin College

Franklin Pierce University

Gannon University

Gardner Webb University

Heritage University

Hofstra University

Howard University

Interservice

Jefferson University East Falls Campus

King's College

Le Moyne College

Loma Linda University

Marshall B. Ketchum University

MCPHS University (Boston)

MCPHS University (Manchester/Worcester)

Mercy College

Miami-Dade College

New York Institute of Technology

Northeastern University

Oklahoma City University

Pace University-Lenox Hill Hospital, NYC

Pace University, Pleasantville

Pacific University

Pennsylvania College of Technology

Philadelphia College of Osteopathic Medicine

Quinnipiac University

Red Rocks Community College

Rochester Institute of Technology

Rutgers University

Sacred Heart University

Saint Francis University

Saint Louis University

Samuel Merritt University

Seton Hill University

Slippery Rock University

South University, Tampa

Southern California University of Health Sciences

Springfield College

St. John's University

Stony Brook University

Sullivan University

SUNY Downstate Medical Center

The CUNY School of Medicine

Thomas Jefferson University

Touro College (Bay Shore)

Touro College (Manhattan)

Touro University - California

Towson University CCBC - Essex

Union College

University of Bridgeport

University of California-Davis

University of Charleston

University of Dayton

University of Findlay

University of Incarnate Word

University of Manitoba

University of North Dakota

University of Saint Joseph

University of South Dakota

University of Tampa

University of the Pacific

University of Toledo

University of Toronto

University of Utah

University of Wisconsin - Madison

Wagner College

West Liberty University

Western Michigan University

Western University of Health Sciences

Westfield State University

Wichita State University

Appendix III: Schools Offering On-Campus Housing

AdventHealth University
Augusta University
Barry University
Central Michigan University
Chatham University
College of Saint Mary
College of Saint Scholastica
D'youville College
Daemen College
DeSales University
Dominican University
Drexel University
Eastern Michigan University
Florida Gulf Coast University
Francis Marion University
Gannon University
Grand Valley State University
Hardin-Simmons University (Abilene)
Harding University
Hofstra University
Howard University
Idaho State University
Indiana University School of Health and Rehabilitation Sciences
Interservice
Kettering College
King's College
Lenoir-Rhyne University
Lincoln Memorial University
Lock Haven University
Long Island University
Louisiana State University - New Orleans
Marietta College
Marquette University
Marywood University
MCPHS University (Manchester/Worcester)
Mercer University
Mercyhurst University
Methodist University
Midwestern University (Downers Grove)
Midwestern University (Glendale)
Milligan College
Missouri State University
Monmouth University
Mount St. Joseph University
New York Institute of Technology

Northeastern State University - OK
Northeastern University
Nova Southeastern University, Fort Lauderdale
Ohio Dominican University
Oklahoma City University
Pace University-Lenox Hill Hospital, NYC
Penn State University
Pennsylvania College of Technology
Rochester Institute of Technology
Rosalind Franklin Univ of Medicine
Rutgers University
Saint Catherine University
Saint Francis University
Slippery Rock University
Southern Illinois University
Springfield College
St. Ambrose University
Stanford University
Stony Brook University
Sullivan University
SUNY Downstate Medical Center
SUNY Upstate Medical Center
Thomas Jefferson University
Union College
University of Arkansas
University of Bridgeport
University of Charleston
University of Dayton
University of Dubuque
University of Evansville
University of Findlay
University of Florida
University of Missouri - Kansas City
University of Mount Union
University of Nebraska
University of North Carolina - Chapel Hill
University Of Oklahoma, Oklahoma City
University of Saint Joseph
University of South Dakota
University of South Florida
University of Southern California (LA)
University of Texas - Medical Branch at Galveston
University of Texas Rio Grande Valley
University of the Cumberlands
University of the Pacific
University of Utah

University of Wisconsin - Madison
UT Southwestern - School of Health Professions
Wagner College
Wayne State University
Weill Cornell Medicine Graduate School of
Medical Sciences

West Liberty University
Western University of Health Sciences
Wichita State University
Yale University School of Medicine

Appendix IV: Schools Without Overall GPA Minimum Requirements

Albany Medical College
Arcadia University
Bethel University (TN)
Boston University School of Medicine PA
Program
Charles R. Drew University
College of Saint Mary
Duke University Medical Center
Idaho State University
James Madison University
Kettering College
Marietta College
Methodist University

MGH Institute of Health Professions
Pacific University
Red Rocks Community College
Stanford University
St. John's University
Tufts University
University of Florida
University of Saint Francis (Fort Wayne)
Wake Forest University (Bowman Gray)
Weill Cornell Medicine Graduate School of
Medical Sciences
Wingate University
Yale University School of Medicine

Appendix V: CASPA GRE Codes by Program

Adventist University of Health Sciences	6985 Adventist U Hlth Sci CASPA
Albany Medical College	0403 Albany Medical Colg CASPA
Alderson Broaddus College	0522 Alderson Broaddus Coll CASPA
Anne Arundel Community College	0517 Anne Arundel CC MS Phys Asst CASPA
Arcadia University	1578 Arcadia U Phys Asst Prog CASPA
Baldwin Wallace University	0498 Baldwin Wallace U PA CASPA
Baylor College of Medicine	2149 Baylor College Medicine CASPA
Bethel University	0510 Bethel U MS Phys Asst CASPA
Boston University	0400 Boston U Schl Medicine CASPA
Bryant University	8825 Bryant U Phys Asst CASPA
Butler University	0477 Butler U Phys Asst CASPA
Campbell University	0406 Campbell U CUCPHS CASPA
Carroll University	0409 Carroll U CASPA
Case Western Reserve University	1703 Case Western Reserve U CASPA
Central Michigan University	0518 Central Michigan U CASPA
Chapman University	3681 Chapman U Phys Asst CASPA
Charleston Southern University	2179 Charleston Southern U CASPA
Chatham University	3879 Chatham U Phys Asst CASPA
Clarkson University	0285 Clarkson U CASPA
College of St. Scholastica	0552 Coll St Scholastica CASPA
Cornell University - Weill Cornell Medical School	0479 Weill Cornell Graduate School CASPA
CUNY York College	1984 York Coll CUNY CASPA
DeSales University	0540 DeSales U CASPA
Des Moines University	0447 Des Moines U Phys Asst CASPA
Dominican University	7340 Dominican U Phys Asst CASPA
Duke University	0422 Duke U Phys Asst CASPA
East Carolina University	0421 East Carolina U PA CASPA
Eastern Michigan University	3646 Eastern Mich U Phys Asst CASPA
Elon University	0398 Elon U Physician Asst CASPA
Emory & Henry College	7413 Emory & Henry Coll CASPA
Emory University	0459 Emory U Phys Asst CASPA
Florida Gulf Coast University	2066 Florida Gulf Coast U CASPA
Florida International University	0554 Florida Intl U CASPA
Florida State University	2122 Florida State U CASPA
Francis Marion University	0553 Francis Marion U CASPA
Gardner-Webb University	3648 Gardner Webb U Phys Asst CASPA
Harding University	0417 Harding U Phys Asst CASPA
Hardin-Simmons University	7453 Hardin Simmons U CASPA
High Point University	7291 High Point U Phys Asst CASPA
Indiana State University	7339 Indiana St U Phys Asst CASPA
Indiana University	3752 Indiana U Phys Asst Prog CASPA
Johnson & Wales University	0468 Johnson & Wales Phys Asst CASPA
Keiser University	0284 Keiser U CASPA
Kettering College	7341 Kettering Coll CASPA
Lenoir Rhyne University	7553 Lenoir Rhyne U Phys Asst CASPA
Lincoln Memorial University	0565 Lincoln Memorial U DCOM Phys Asst CASPA

Lock Haven University	8827 Lock Haven U Phys Asst CASPA
Louisiana State University HSC - New Orleans	0202 Louisiana St U New Orleans CASPA
Louisiana State University HSC - Shreveport	0423 LSU HSC PA Shreveport CASPA
Lynchburg College	3874 Lynchburg College Phys Asst CASPA
Marietta College	0937 Marietta Coll Phys Asst Program CASPA
Marist College	7412 Marist College CASPA
Marquette University	5872 Marquette U Phys Asst CASPA
Mary Baldwin University	3656 Mary Baldwin U Phys Asst CASPA
Mercer University	0441 Mercer U Phys Asst CASPA
Mercyhurst University	1614 Mercyhurst U Phys Asst CASPA
Methodist University	0399 Methodist U Phys Asst CASPA
MGH Institute of Health Professions	3865 MGH Inst Hlth Prof Phys Asst CASPA
Midwestern University - Glendale	0508 Midwestern U Phys Asst CASPA
Milligan College	7342 Milligan College CASPA
Mississippi College	0598 Mississippi College CASPA
Missouri State University	2189 Missouri State U CASPA
Monmouth University	3880 Monmouth U Phys Asst CASPA
Mount St. Joseph University	7328 Mt St Joseph U CASPA
North Greenville University	7362 North Greenville U CASPA
Northeastern University	7350 Northeastern U Phys Asst CASPA
Northeastern State University	7376 Northeastern State U CASPA Muskogee
Northern Arizona University	2118 Northern Arizona U CASPA
Northwestern University	4879 Northwestern U Phys Asst CASPA
Nova Southeastern University - Fort Lauderdale	0947 Nova Southeastern U Fort Lauderdale CASPA
Nova Southeastern University - Fort Myers	0951 Nova Southeastern U FT Myers CASPA
Nova Southeastern University - Jacksonville	0952 Nova Southeastern U Jacksonville CASPA
Nova Southeastern University - Orlando	0964 Nova Southeastern U Orlando CASPA
Ohio Dominican University	0436 Ohio Dominican U PA CASPA
Ohio University	0957 Ohio U Div Phys Asst CASPA
Oregon Health & Science University	4780 OHSU Phys Asst Prgm CASPA
Our Lady of the Lake College	7348 Our Lady Lake Coll CASPA
Penn State University	0900 Penn State Colg Medcn CASPA
Presbyterian College	2176 Presbyterian Coll CASPA
Radford University	4762 Radford U Phys Asst CASPA
Rocky Mountain College	7349 Rocky Mountain Coll CASPA
Rocky Mountain University	3660 Rocky Mountain U Phys Asst CASPA
Rosalind Franklin University	0276 Rosalind Franklin U Phys Asst CASPA
Rush University	0962 Rush U Phys Asst CASPA
Rutgers University	0544 Rutgers Sch Hlth Related Prof CASPA
Salus University	0432 Salus U Phys Asst CASPA
Shenandoah University	0414 Shenandoah U Phy Asst CASPA
Slippery Rock University	1583 Slippery Rock U CASPA
South College	1635 South Coll MS Hlth Sci CASPA
South University in Savannah - Georgia	0467 South U Savannah Phys Asst CASPA
South University - Richmond, VA	7147 South U Richmond VA CASPA
South University - Tampa	0454 South U Tampa Phys Asst CASPA
Southern Illinois University	0480 Southern Illinois U Phys Asst CASPA
St. Ambrose University	0420 St Ambrose PA CASPA
Saint Catherine University	0431 Saint Catherine U Phys Asst CASPA

Stephens College	1576 Stephens Coll Phys Asst Prog CASPA
Temple University	1746 Temple U Sch Medicine CASPA
Texas Tech University Health Sciences Center	3652 Texas Tech U Phys Asst CASPA
Touro University - Nevada	2174 Touro U CASPA
Trevecca Nazarene University	0532 Trevecca Nazarene U CASPA
Trine University	7343 Trine U CASPA
Tufts University	0438 Tufts U Pub Hlth Prog Phys Asst CASPA
Union College	3645 Union Coll Phys Asst CASPA
University of Alabama at Birmingham	0570 U Alabama Birmingham CASPA
University of Arkansas for Medical Sciences	0279 U Arkansas Med Sci CASPA
University of Bridgeport	7292 U Bridgeport Phys Asst CASPA
University of Charleston	8830 U Charleston Phys Asst CASPA
University of Colorado	3722 U Colorado Phys Asst CASPA
University of the Cumberlands	1608 U Cumberlands CASPA
University of Detroit Mercy	0509 U Detroit Mercy Phys Asst CASPA
University of Dubuque	1620 U Dubuque CASPA
University of Evansville	1765 U Evansville Phys Asst CASPA
University of Florida	0427 U Florida Phys Asst CASPA
University of Iowa	0466 U Iowa Phys Asst CASPA
University of Missouri - Kansas City	8831 U Missouri KC Phys Asst CASPA
University of Nebraska Medical Center	4917 U Nebraska Med Ctr Phys Asst CASPA
University of New England	0500 U New England Phys Asst CASPA
University of New Mexico	7347 U New Mexico Phys Asst CASPA
University of North Carolina	6945 U North Carolina Allied Hlth Sci CASPA
University of North Texas Health Science Center	6380 U North Texas HSC CASPA
University of Oklahoma - Oklahoma City	2180 U Oklahoma CASPA
University of the Pacific	7363 U of the Pacific CASPA
University of Pittsburgh	0452 U Pittsburgh Phys Asst CASPA
University of South Alabama	2169 U South Alabama CASPA
University of South Florida	8854 U South Florida Phys Asst CASPA
University of South Carolina	2178 U South Carolina CASPA
University of Southern California	1416 U Southern California Keck Sch Med CASPA
University of St. Francis - New Mexico	0523 U St Francis CASPA
University of St. Joseph	1417 U St Joseph CASPA
University of Tennessee Health Science Center	0201 U Tennessee Hlth Sci Ctr CASPA
University of Texas at San Antonio	7552 U Texas Hlth Sci Ctr San Antonio CASPA
University of Texas Medical Branch at Galveston	0437 U Texas Med Branch Phys CASPA
University of Toledo	1845 U Toledo CASPA
University of Washington MEDEX	0548 U Washington MEDEX NW CASPA
University of Wisconsin - La Crosse	0445 U Wisconsin La Crosse PA CASPA
Wake Forest University	5923 Wake Forest Sch Med Phys Asst CASPA
Wayne State University	3647 Wayne State U Phys Asst CASPA
Yale University	3983 Yale U Phys Asst Program CASPA

Appendix VI: Anatomy Format by Program

Cadaver Based Anatomy (Dissection, Prosection or Both)		Non-Cadaver Based Anatomy (3-D/Virtual Software, Models)
AdventHealth University	Quinnipiac University	Anne Arundel Community College
Albany Medical College	Radford University	Arcadia University (Pennsylvania)
Alderson-Broaddus University	Red Rocks Community College	Arizona School of Health Sciences
Arcadia University (Delaware)	Rochester Institute of Technology	Barry University
Augsburg University	Rocky Mountain College	Butler University
Augusta University	Rocky Mountain University of Health Professions	California Baptist University
Baldwin Wallace University	Rocky Vista University	California State University – Monterey Bay
Baylor College of Medicine	Rosalind Franklin University	Charleston Southern University
Bay Path University	Rush University	Chatham University
Bethel University (MN)	Saint Catherine University	Christian Brothers University
Bethel University (TN)	Saint Francis University	College of Saint Elizabeth
Boston University	Saint Louis University	CUNY York College
Bryant University	Salus University	Dominican University of California
Campbell University	Samford University	Dominican University of Illinois
Carroll University	Samuel Merritt University	East Carolina University
Case Western Reserve University	Seton Hall University	Franciscan Missionaries of Our Lady University
Chapman University	Seton Hill University	Francis Marion University
Charles R. Drew University	Shenandoah University	Franklin College
College of Saint Mary	Slippery Rock University	Gannon University (FL)
College of Saint Scholastica	Southern California University of Health Sciences	Gardner Webb University
Colorado Mesa University	Southern Illinois University	Harding University
Concordia University	South University (Georgia)	Heritage University
Cornell University	Springfield College	Indiana State University
CUNY School of Medicine	Stanford University	Keiser University
Daemen College	Stephens College	Lake Erie College
Desales University	Stony Brook University	Marshall B. Ketchum University
Des Moines University	St. Ambrose University	MCPHS University – Worcester
Drexel University	SUNY Downstate Medical Center	MCPHS University – Manchester
Duke University	SUNY Upstate Medical Center	Miami-Dade College
Duquesne University	Temple University	Monmouth University
D'Youville College	Texas Tech University Health Sciences Center	Mount St. Joseph University
Eastern Michigan University	Thomas Jefferson University (NJ)	North Greenville University
Eastern Virginia Medical School	Thomas Jefferson University – East Falls/Center City	Nova Southeastern University – Fort Myers
Elon University	Touro College (Manhattan)	Nova Southeastern University – Jacksonville
Emory & Henry College	Touro University (California)	
Emory University	Touro University (Nevada)	
Florida Gulf Coast University		
Florida International University		
Herbert Wertheim College of Medicine		
Florida State University		

Cadaver Based Anatomy (Dissection, Prosection or Both)		Non-Cadaver Based Anatomy (3-D/Virtual Software, Models)
Franklin Pierce University	Towson University CCBC – Essex	Nova Southeastern University – Orlando
Frostburg State University	Trevecca Nazarene University	Rutgers University
Gannon University (PA)	Trine University	Sacred Heart University
George Washington University	Tufts University	South College – Nashville
Grand Valley State University	Union College	South College – Knoxville
Hardin-Simmons University	University of Alabama at Birmingham	South University (Tampa)
High Point University	University of Arkansas	St. John's University
Hofstra University	University of Bridgeport	Sullivan University
Idaho State University	University of Colorado	Touro College (Bay Shore and Nassau University Medical Center)
Indiana University School of Health and Rehabilitation Sciences	University of Dayton	University of California-Davis
Interservice	University of Detroit – Mercy	University of Charleston
James Madison University	University of Dubuque	University of North Dakota
Johnson & Wales University	University of Evansville	University of Saint Joseph
King's College	University of Findlay	University of the Cumberlands
Le Moyne College	University of Florida College of Medicine	University of Washington (MEDEX)
Lenoir-Rhyne University	University of Iowa	Valparaiso University
Lincoln Memorial University	University of Kentucky	Westfield State University
Lipscomb University	University of Lynchburg	Wingate University
Lock Haven University	University of Missouri – Kansas City	Xavier University of Louisiana
Loma Linda University	University of Mount Union	
Long Island University	University of Nebraska	
Louisiana State University – New Orleans	University of Nevada Reno	
Louisiana State University – Shreveport	University of New England	
Marietta College	University of New Mexico	
Marist College	University of North Carolina	
Marquette University	University of North Texas Health Sciences Center – Fort Worth	
Mary Baldwin University	University of Oklahoma, Oklahoma City	
Marywood University	University of Oklahoma, Tulsa	
MCPHS University – Boston (in collaboration with Harvard)'	University of Pittsburgh	
Medical University of South Carolina	University of Saint Francis (Fort Wayne)	
Mercer University	University of South Alabama	
Mercy College	University of South Carolina	
Mercyhurst University	University of South Dakota	
Methodist University	University of South Florida	
MGH Institute of Health Professions	University of Southern California	

Cadaver Based Anatomy (Dissection, Prosection or Both)		Non-Cadaver Based Anatomy (3-D/Virtual Software, Models)
Midwestern University (Glendale) Midwestern University (Downers Grove) Milligan College Misericordia University Mississippi College Missouri State University Morehouse School of Medicine New York Institute of Technology Northeastern University Northern Arizona University Northwestern University Nova Southeastern University – Fort Lauderdale Ohio Dominican University Oklahoma City University Oregon Health & Science University Pace University – Lenox Hill Pace University – Pleasantville Pacific University Penn State University Pennsylvania College of Technology Pfeiffer University Philadelphia College of Osteopathic Medicine	University of St. Francis University of Tampa University of Tennessee University of Texas – Health Sciences Center at San Antonio University of Texas – Medical Branch at Galveston University of Texas – RGV University of Texas Southwestern University of the Pacific University of Toledo University of Utah University of Wisconsin – La Crosse University of Wisconsin – Madison Wagner College Wake Forest University Wayne State University Western Michigan University Western Univ of Health Sciences Wichita State University Yale School of Medicine Yale School of Medicine PA Online	

**Information unavailable for the following programs at the time of publication:
Central Michigan University
Clarkson University
Creighton University
Kettering College
Northwestern College
Ohio University
Presbyterian College
South University (Virginia)
University of La Verne
West Liberty University
West Virginia University